A BEAM OF INTENSE DARKNESS

Written by pioneering analyst and creative thinker, James Grotstein, *A Beam of Intense Darkness* offers a thorough overview and illuminating insight into the often-complex work of W. R. Bion.

This psychoanalytic classic sees Grotstein introduce over 30 key Bionian theories, comprehensively explaining them to the reader before offering his own insight and commentary. Grotstein first encountered Bion as his analysand and, later, as his friend. This book offers a level of insight only possible through such a close relationship, and offers a dialogue between Bion and Grotstein as they delve into the inner workings of the human psyche. Throughout, Grotstein offers his own original thoughts on topics such as projective *trans*identification, transcendent position and the truth drive.

With a new introduction from Nicola Abel-Hirsch, this book is an essential read for anyone interested in Bion's work and legacy.

James S. Grotstein, M.D. (1925–2015) was clinical professor of psychiatry at the David Geffen School of Medicine, UCLA, and training and supervising analyst at the New Center for Psychoanalysis and the Psychoanalytic Center of California, Los Angeles. He was on the editorial board of the *International Journal of Psychoanalysis* and past North American vice-president of the International Psychoanalytical Association. A world-renowned and prolific contributor to psychoanalytic literature, he is considered one of the foremost scholars and elucidators of the work of Wilfred Bion, who was also his analyst.

ROUTLEDGE MENTAL HEALTH CLASSIC EDITIONS

The *Routledge Mental Health Classic Edition* series celebrates Routledge's commitment to excellence within the field of mental health. These books are recognized as timeless classics covering a range of important issues and continue to be recommended as key reading for professionals and students in the area. With a new introduction that explores what has changed since the books were first published, and why these books are as relevant now as ever, the series presents key ideas to a new generation.

More Than Miracles:
The State of the Art of Solution-Focused
Brief Therapy (Classic Edition)
Steve de Shazer and Yvonne Dolan with Harry Korman,
Terry Trepper, Eric McCollum, and Insoo Kim Berg

Using Trauma-Focused Therapy Stories:
Interventions for Therapists, Children, and
Their Caregivers (Classic Edition)
By Pat Pernicano

Life and Loss:
A Guide to Help Grieving Children (Classic Edition)
Linda Goldman

Self-Supervision:
A Primer for Counselors and Human Service
Professionals (Classic Edition)
Patrick J. Morrissette

Before You See Your First Client:
55 Things Counselors, Therapists and Human Service
Workers Need to Know (Classic Edition)
Howard Rosenthal

African American Grief (Classic Edition)
Paul C. Rosenblatt and Beverly R. Wallace

Do Funerals Matter?
The Purposes and Practices of Death Rituals in
Global Perspective (Classic Edition)
William G. Hoy

Rhythms of Recovery:
Trauma, Nature, and the Body (Classic Edition)
Leslie E. Korn

Grief and Bereavement in Contemporary Society:
Bridging Research and Practice (Classic Edition)
Robert A. Neimeyer, Darcy L. Harris, Howard R. Winokuer,
and Gordon F. Thornton

Art Therapy, Trauma, and Neuroscience:
Theoretical and Practical Perspectives (Classic Edition)
Juliet L. King

Users and Abusers of Psychiatry:
A Critical Look at Psychiatric Practice (Classic Edition)
Lucy Johnstone

Psychotherapy: An Erotic Relationship:
Transference and Countertransference
Passions (Classic Edition)
David Mann

Collective Trauma, Collective Healing:
Promoting Community Resilience in the Aftermath
of Disaster (Classic Edition)
Jack Saul

Unlocking the Emotional Brain:
Eliminating Symptoms at Their Roots Using Memory
Reconsolidation (Classic Edition)
Bruce Ecker, Robin Ticic, and Laurel Hulley

The New Handbook of Counseling
Supervision (Classic Edition)
L. DiAnne Borders and Lori L. Brown

Therapy and the Postpartum Woman:
Notes on Healing Postpartum Depression for
Clinicians and the Women Who Seek their Help
Karen Kleiman

Beyond Empathy:
A Therapy of Contact-in-Relationship
Richard G. Erskine, Janet P. Moursund, and Rebecca L. Trautmann

Hidden Treasure:
A Map to the Child's Inner Self
Violet Oaklander

Married Women Who Love Women:
And More…
Carren Strock

Playing Sick? Untangling the Web of Munchausen Syndrome,
Munchausen by Proxy, Malingering, and Factitious Disorder
Marc D. Feldman

A Beam of Intense Darkness:
Wilfred Bion's Legacy to Psychoanalysis
James S. Grotstein

A BEAM OF INTENSE DARKNESS

Wilfred Bion's Legacy to Psychoanalysis

CLASSIC EDITION

James S. Grotstein

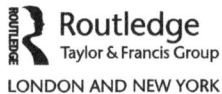
Routledge
Taylor & Francis Group

LONDON AND NEW YORK

Designed cover image: © Getty

Classic edition published 2024
by Routledge
4 Park Square, Milton Park, Abingdon, Oxon OX14 4RN

and by Routledge
605 Third Avenue, New York, NY 10158

Routledge is an imprint of the Taylor & Francis Group, an informa business

First edition published by Karnac 2007

British Library Cataloguing-in-Publication Data
A catalogue record for this book is available from the British Library

Library of Congress Cataloging-in-Publication Data
Names: Grotstein, James S., author.
Title: A beam of intense darkness : Wilfred Bion's legacy to psychoanalysis / James S. Grotstein.
Description: Abingdon, Oxon ; New York, NY : Routledge, 2024. |
Series: Routledge mental health classic editions | Originally published in 2007 in London by Karnac Books. | Includes bibliographical references and index. |
Identifiers: LCCN 2023027797 (print) | LCCN 2023027798 (ebook) |
ISBN 9781032391601 (hardback) | ISBN 9781032384764 (paperback) |
ISBN 9781003348665 (ebook)
Subjects: LCSH: Bion, Wilfred R. (Wilfred Ruprecht), 1897–1979. | Psychoanalysis.
Classification: LCC RC438.6.B54 G76 2024 (print) | LCC RC438.6.B54 (ebook) |
DDC 616.89/17—dc23/eng/20230817
LC record available at https://lccn.loc.gov/2023027797
LC ebook record available at https://lccn.loc.gov/2023027798

ISBN: 9781032391601 (hbk)
ISBN: 9781032384764 (pbk)
ISBN: 9781003348665 (ebk)

DOI: 10.4324/9781003348665

Typeset in Palatino
by codeMantra

To Wilfred Bion

My gratitude to you for allowing *Me* to become reunited with *me*—and for encouraging me to play with your ideas as well as my own.

CONTENTS

INTRODUCTION TO CLASSIC EDITION   xiii

ACKNOWLEDGEMENTS AND SOURCES OF INFORMATION   xvii

ABOUT THE AUTHOR   xxi

Prelude and prologue   1

1   An introduction   9

2   What kind of analyst was Bion?   27

3   What kind of person was Bion?   34

4   Bion's vision   36

5   Bion's legacy   44

6   Bion's metatheory   65

7   Bion on technique   82

8	Clinical vignette encompassing Bion's technical ideas	98
9	Bion, the mathematician, the mystic, the psychoanalyst	102
10	The "Language of Achievement"	109
11	Bion's discovery of O	114
12	The concept of the "transcendent position"	121
13	The quest for the truth, Part A: the "truth drive" as the hidden order of Bion's metatheory for psychoanalysis	135
14	The quest for the truth, Part B: curiosity about the truth as the "seventh servant"	139
15	Lies, "lies", and falsehoods	147
16	The container and the contained	151
17	"Projective transidentification": an extension of the concept of projective identification	168
18	Bion's work with groups	190
19	Bion's studies in psychosis	197
20	Transformations	213
21	Psychoanalytic functions and elements	235
22	Points, lines, and circles	239
23	The Grid	243
24	Fetal mental life and its caesura with postnatal mental life	256
25	What does it mean to dream? Bion's theory of dreaming	259

26   Dreaming, phantasying, and the "truth instinct"   290

27   "Become"   305

28   P-S ↔ D   308

29   L, H, and K and passion   311

30   Faith   315

31   Bion's discovery of zero ("no-thing")   319

Epilogue   327

W. R. BION BIBLIOGRAPHY   333

REFERENCES AND BIBLIOGRAPHY   341

INDEX   361

Ariadne's thread

The phrase "a beam of intense darkness" was conceived by Freud; he wrote it in a letter to Lou Andreas-Salome. Later, it was quoted by Bion to Grotstein.
As Grotstein recalls:

> Once, following an analytic session of mine, Bion, unusually for him, went to his bookshelf, pulled out a German edition of Freud's correspondence with Lou Andreas-Salome and translated it for me on the spot. I made instant notes about it moments afterwards: "When conducting an analysis, one must cast a beam of intense darkness so that something which has hitherto been obscured by the glare of the illumination can glitter all the more in the darkness." I have come to realize that this was the statement that was to become the Ariadne's thread that would run through Bion's later thinking ...
>
> (pp.1/2)

"A beam of intense darkness" may sound a strange, nonsensical kind of thing. However, it refers to the idea of switching off the light of what we know, plunging ourselves into darkness, and thereby allowing us to catch sight of what might ordinarily be obscured. Why "intense"? This is not about finding any old thing. It is about managing to see what may be right before our eyes, but unconsciously hidden because it is too immediate, overwhelming or challenging.

The importance of a "beam of intense darkness"—putting the glitter of what we think we know, our memories and desires, to one side—is central to Bion's later work. Indeed, in the quote above, Grotstein describes this as the "Ariadne's thread" running through Bion's later thinking. In Greek mythology, Ariadne, daughter of King Minos, helped her love Theseus escape from an impenetrable labyrinth by giving him a thread he could unravel as he walked into it. After slaying the half bull and half man Minotaur, Theseus could retrace his steps by following the thread.

Books about the work of Bion generally present his work chronologically. This publication's contents shows it to be different. It reflects Grotstein's journey in relation to Bion's work. In a sense, he plunges into the darkness, brushing aside what he already knows, his new understanding conjuring an Ariadne's thread: a guide for him and us to find our way through Bion's later work by.

Background

In 1968, aged 70, Bion accepted an invitation to move to California where he spent his last decade working and writing. In California, one of his patients was James Grotstein, who remained in analysis with Bion for six years, attending five times a week.

In 2018, the book *Of Things Invisible to Mortal Sight: Celebrating the Work of James S. Grotstein* (Ed. Annie Reiner) was published to celebrate Grotstein's work. Reading the papers that compose that publication, I was struck by the generous 'size' of both Grotstein's thinking and his life. A renowned psychoanalyst and psychoanalytic theorist himself, he was one of the first American analysts to import Klein to the States and to elucidate Bion's work. This was a big man and he is uniquely qualified to be a guide to Bion's work.

Grotstein's analysis with Bion

There has been considerable debate in the international psychoanalytical world about Bion's later work. Was he moving away from psychoanalysis, or more into the heart of it? What is fascinating about this book is that we get a picture of Bion's actual clinical work following his move to California.

This is Grotstein:

> Bion rarely conversed with me. He was the most disciplined analyst I have ever met. His respect for the analytic frame was always obvious. He would never repeat an interpretation, even if I told him that

I had not heard it. He would remind me that it could not be repeated: the time had passed. On one occasion he reminded me of Heraclitus' koan that one can never step into the same river twice. Virtually the entirety of his relationship with me during the analysis was interpretative. He interpreted frequently and often at length. Yet he was always "Kleinian"—but in his own way. I never read any of Bion's works while I was in analysis with him and was therefore surprised later when I read his concept of "abandoning memory and desire". He spoke and interpreted in an active and highly engaged manner; consequently, I don't know when he found the time to "abandon memory and desire". I recall, however, that like a scout, he doggedly tracked the sequence of my free associations.

(27)

Grotstein also recalls the detail of some of Bion's interpretations:

Here you are, the most important person you're ever likely to meet in your lifetime, and you're telling me you're on bad terms with this person. That requires evidence.

(29)

Yes, a beautiful interpretation, you say. The snag is that my "beautiful interpretation" was made possible only by virtue of your "beautiful associations". You were so keen on listening to me that you neglected listening to yourself speaking to me.

(29/30)

I have just given you an interpretation about your anxiety, and you seem to feel that it was correct, but in fact we shall never know the source of it. It is not to be known. We can only approximate it—or really, learn what it is not.

(32)

Two features stand out to me and they are testimony to why this book has the potential to be enormously helpful clinically as well as theoretically and historically. The first feature is Bion's emphasis on the patient's relation to themselves and the second is his explicit awareness with the patient of how much isn't known. These features come to life in the detail of Grotstein's discussion of Bion's work that follows.

I will end with a return to the myth of Ariadne's thread. I have suggested that Ariadne's thread reflects Grotstein's own journey in relation to Bion's work. The existence of the thread is hopeful but the darkness of the impenetrable labyrinth is real. "Darkness" is an overused word but in this book one senses that Grotstein's understanding of human nature has been obtained through the darkness, and that the book can be relied on to give a true access to mutative psychoanalytic work.

REFERENCES

Reiner, A. (2016) *Of Things Invisible to Mortal Sight: Celebrating the Work of James S. Grotstein.* Oxford: Routledge.

ACKNOWLEDGEMENTS
AND SOURCES OF INFORMATION

In addition to my reading of all Bion's published works, I am dependent on the following published texts on his works, which I found immensely useful and rewarding: *Introduction to the Work of Bion* by Leon Grinberg, Dario Sor, and Elizabeth Tabak de Bianchedi (1977, 1993); *Wilfred Bion: His Life and Works 1897–1979*, by Gérard Bléandonu (1993); *The Clinical Thinking of Wilfred Bion*, by Joan and Neville Symington (1996); *The Dictionary of the Work of W. R. Bion* (2003) and *Wild Thoughts Looking for a Thinker* (2006), by Rafael E. López-Corvo; Paulo Sandler's *The Language of Bion: A Dictionary of Concepts* (2005); Donald Meltzer's *The Kleinian Development, Part III: The Clinical Significance of the Work of Bion* (1978) and *Studies in Extended Metapsychology: Clinical Application of Bion's Ideas* (1986); *In the Analyst's Consulting Room* (2002a) by Antonino Ferro's, as well as his *Psychoanalysis as Therapy and Storytelling* (1999) and *Seeds of Illness, Seeds of Recovery: The Genesis of Suffering and the Role of Psychoanalysis* (2002b); and Thomas Ogden's *Reverie and Interpretation* (1997).

Although I may seldom refer to works of the above contributors in the text, I assure them and the readers that I have studied all of their works and *absorbed* them—that is, in Bion's unique way of putting it, I "dreamed" their works, disassembled them into kaleidoscopic bits, and reassembled them anew as they spontaneously came into my mind. In short, I have "cannibalized", not "plagiarized", the works of my colleagues and have transformed them as they made sense to me anew. Bion once shared with me the fact that he did the same—as did Winnicott. Consequently, I wish not merely to acknowledge the above authors but to offer them my profound gratitude for their invaluable contributions.

I am deeply indebted to Francesca Bion for her invaluable notes on the manuscript and her gracious permission to quote from Bion himself, and to Oliver Rathbone, Alex Massey, and Christelle Yeyet-Jacquot, my faithful shepherds at Karnac, for their steadfast guidance in bringing this work to publication. In addition, I have consulted other individuals who had been in psychoanalysis and/or in supervision with Bion. In the last category I include myself and my own memoirs and reminiscences of my psychoanalysis with him, which lasted for six years—and the precious bits of information I would get from him during and after sessions and on other occasions. I am especially indebted to Antonino Ferro, Elizabeth Tabak de Bianchedi, Lia Pistener de Cortiñas, Paulo Sandler, Thomas Ogden, Arnaldo Chuster, Lee Rather, Christian Godbout, Rudi Vermote, and Raphael López-Corvo for having read the manuscript in advance and offering their invaluable notes. I am also grateful for conversations and communications with individuals whom I regard as "Bion scholars", including Corbett Williams, members of the "Bion Collective", and members of my Bion Study Group in San Francisco, which includes Enid Young, Lee Rather, Stefanie Nickel-Rather, Zenobia Grusky, Maureen Franey, Jeffrey Eaton, Laurel Samuels, John Schneider, Ivria Spieler, David Tresan, Billie Lee Violet, and Tom Herington, from whom I continue to learn about Bion in remarkably creative ways. I am grateful to Harry Karnac for the gift of allowing his Bion Bibliography to be included in the book. Finally, I would like to give my special thanks to my wife Susan for her wonderful support thorough the many years of my immersion in this book, during which she all too often became a writer's widow. I also should like to thank Anouska Chydzik-Bryson with deepest gratitude for her patience and labour.

Publication acknowledgements

I wish to thank the following for permission to republish earlier contributions from my own work, as well as the work of others:

The editors of the *International Journal of Psychoanalysis* for their permission to republish portions of: Antonino Ferro, "Clinical Implications of Bion's Thought", *IJPA*, Vol. 87 (2006), pp. 989–1003; James Grotstein, "The 'Seventh Servant': The Implications of a Truth Drive in Bion's Theory of 'O'", *IJPA*, Vol. 85 (2004), pp. 1081–101); and James Grotstein, "Projective Transidentification: An Extension of the Concept of Projective Identification", *IJPA*, Vol. 86 (2005), pp. 1051–1069.

Robert Lipgar and Malcolm Pines for their and the publisher's permission to republish "Introduction: Early Bion", in *Building on Bion: Roots: Origins and Context of Bion's Contributions to Theory and Practice* (London: Jessica Kingsley, 2003), pp. 9–28.

Claudio Neri, Malcolm Pines and Robi Friedman for their and the publisher's permission to republish "'We Are Such Stuff as Dreams Are Made On': Annotations on Dreams and Dreaming in Bion's Works", in *Dreams in Group Psychotherapy: Theory and Technique* (London: Jessica Kingsley, 2002), pp. 110–145.

ABOUT THE AUTHOR

James S. Grotstein, MD, was Clinical Professor of Psychiatry at the David Geffen School of Medicine, UCLA, and training and supervising analyst at the New Center for Psychoanalysis and the Psychoanalytic Center of California, Los Angeles. He was a member of the Editorial Board of the *International Journal of psychoanalysis* and was past North American Vice-President of the International Psychoanalytical Association. He has published 254 papers and is the author or editor/co-editor of 12 books. His papers include "The Seventh Servant: The Implication of the Truth Drive in Bion's Theory of 'O'" (*International Journal of Psychoanalysis*), "Projective Transidentification: An Extension of the Concept of Projective Identification" (*International Journal of Psychoanalysis)*, and "The Voice from the Crypt: The Negative Therapeutic Reaction and the Longing for the Childhood That Never Was" (*Contemporary Psychoanalysis*). His books include *Who Is The Dreamer Who Dreams the Dream?: A Study of Psychic Presences* (2000) and *"But at the Same Time and on Another Level . . .": Psychoanalytic Technique in the Kleinian/Bionian Mode"* (in press). He maintained a private psychoanalytic practice in Los Angeles for over 50 years.

Dr Grotstein was the only person to have been in analysis with Bion who has written about him in a major way.

A BEAM OF INTENSE DARKNESS

Prelude and prologue

"So much the rather thou Celestial Light
Shine inward, and the mind through all her powers
Irradiate, there plant eyes, all mist from thence
Purge and disperse, that I may see and tell
Of things invisible to mortal sight."

John Milton: Paradise Lost

WILFRED RUPRECHT BION:
Prometheus bound and unbound, man of achievement, mystic,
and navigator of the "deep and formless infinite"

PRELUDE

Once, following an analytic session of mine, Bion, unusually for him, went to his bookshelf, pulled out a German edition of Freud's correspondence with Lou Andreas-Salomé and translated it for me on the spot. I made instant notes about it moments afterwards: "When conducting an analysis,[1] one must cast a *beam of intense darkness* so that something which has hitherto been obscured by the glare of the illumination can glitter all the more in the darkness." I have come to realize that this was the statement that was to become

DOI: 10.4324/9781003348665-1

1

the Ariadne's thread that would run through Bion's later thinking and is what he surely meant by his now famous exhortation to the analyst to *"abandon memory and desire"* while conducting an analysis—so *as to have Faith in the creative response of his own unconscious.* It was also the hallmark of his ultimate ontological epistemology, transformations in, from, and to "O", the Absolute Truth about an infinite, impersonal, and ineffable Ultimate Reality.

Bion as a "mystic"

The term "mystic" has many connotations, but the one that I mean to suggest is close to Bion's, which is a psychoanalytic and an epistemological, not a religious, one. During the heyday of positivism the analyst endeavoured to become more *knowledgeable* about his analysand. Bion has brought psychoanalysis into the realm of relativity and uncertainty. A "psychoanalytic mystic" is required not only to *know about* his analysand as much as he can—via transformations from O to K (from the Absolute Truth about Ultimately Impersonal Reality to knowledge about his *personal* reality), but also to *"become"* that enigmatic uncertainty and surrender attempts to *know* it. The mystic is not troubled by not knowing. He is a "Man of Achievement" in so far as he is receptive to being influenced by his analysand to the degree that he can allow his own conscious–preconscious–unconscious repertoire of emotions and experiences to be spontaneously retrieved and accessed (reverie, intuition, com-passion).

The mystic does not seek the mystical; he wraps his mind around it and becomes it. The mystic sees the mysterious—the thing-in-itself—in the obvious and the obvious within the mysterious. The mystic is able to disregard illusion and is able to enter mysteries with equanimity. The mystic accepts his *moira*—the portion of Fate that is personally and impersonally dealt him—with equanimity and serenity and recognizes what belongs to him personally and what does not. As we shall see, I believe that the security of the mystic lies in part in his confidence in the intactness of his contact-barrier.

He is at one with O. The mystic is that potential aspect of each of us, of our "higher self", of our *"Übermensch"* (Nietzsche, 1883) that spontaneously allows oneself to experience emotion—*and the Truth that emotion carries as its cargo*—and to become experienced by the experience itself—that is, to become infused with and by O. Thus, one "becomes" the experience, O, bimodally: namely, meeting O halfway, passively and actively, as expressed in the ancient Greek middle voice, which simultaneously reflects both the active and passive voices (Greenberg, 2005; Peradotto, 1990).

Bion has enfranchised mysticism as an invaluable and obligatory component of psychoanalytic epistemology. The twentieth-century science of Freud and Klein was *ontic*, linear, more suitable for the study of inanimate objects. Bion became aware early on that psychoanalysis was an *ontological* science, one whose domain was non-linear, where considerations of being and existence and one's relationship to other beings were in constant jeopardy of emotional turbulence and catastrophic change.

The mystic alone (i.e., the mystic component of us) is qualified to comprehend the non-linear uncertainty that now characterizes psychoanalysis. The evolved human being—the mystic—is capable of "negative capability", the tolerance of doubt, frustration, and uncertainty, but is also able to tolerate the cosmic meaninglessness of being (existence). This evolved individual, the one who has become O, has traversed beyond the depressive position and attained the *transcendent position* (Grotstein, 1999a, 2000a, 2004a, 2004b). He has become an *"Übermensch"*, "higher man". Since Bion, analysts are now mandated to tap into their mystical core. Psychoanalytic training forever afterwards must constitute in part the honing of one's mystical receptivity, one's ability to achieve reverie and be able to contain while patiently awaiting the emergence of the Language of Achievement from within oneself. The task of training analyses has now broadened and deepened. Training analyses will now differ in so far as it is now the training analyst's task to help his analysand-in-training to become a competent mystic.

With regard to Bion's relationship to mysticism, Eigen states:

> Bion pays homage to the mysticism of old—the Changeless Eternal Infinite, the all potential formless Void, O itself. But he also opens to a mysticism of changing moments, a dynamic, restless O. We meet O not simply as peace, but turbulence, even catastrophe. We can not keep up with incessantly evolving O. We work with premonition. And since we are O, part of O, we work through premonitions of ourselves. [Eigen, 1998, p. 20]

PROLOGUE

In the late 1970s a well-known and reputable psychoanalytic book publisher, who had happened to agree to publish a book of mine, commissioned me to write a book on Bion. I decided to undertake an edited work that would include contributions from Bion admirers and scholars worldwide. It was a difficult undertaking for me because at the time I was still in analysis with Bion. The book came to be named *"Do I Dare Disturb the Universe?" A Celebration of Wilfred R. Bion.* The title had to be altered to *"A Memorial"* rather than *"A Celebration"* because Bion died suddenly on 8 November (my birthday!) 1979. In the meantime the publisher had published Bion's four major works—*Learning from Experience, Elements of Psycho-Analysis, Transformations,* and *Attention and Interpretation*—in a single volume entitled *Seven Servants.* The sales of this book were apparently so small that the publisher, thinking that works about Bion would not sell either, cancelled his contract with me. I was disappointed, but I certainly understood. From the commercial publishing point of view he was right at that time to have done so. I then independently published it as the only venture of "Caesura Press". It took me years to appreciate the prescient wisdom of that name. I just broke even financially!

That was then. Today, all one has to do is to pick up any major psychoanalytic journal, particularly the *International Journal of Psychoanalysis,* venture into any bookstore, or go to virtually any psychoanalytic or psychotherapy conference, and Bion is there. His ideas have spread beyond the ghetto of his Kleinian roots to every major school within the psychoanalytic framework. It comes as a surprise to many that he was one of the founders of intersubjectivity. Virtually every mental health worker today is familiar with container and contained, maternal reverie, perhaps even with α-function, α-elements, and β-elements, and certainly with his contributions to group psychology. Those concepts belong to "popularized Bion".

The mental health public, particularly psychoanalysts, now seems more curious for the more recondite Bion, whose ideas still remain below the tip of the iceberg for many. This work is an attempt to bring these ideas to the surface to demonstrate their theoretical and clinical (practical) usefulness—hopefully in a reader-friendly way. I say this in the face of critiques of my previously published works, in which I had been accused of being "Bionian"—that is, "dense"—in my style of writing. I hope the present volume shows that I have taken the "compliment" to heart and have tried to be as explicit and clarifying as I could. One of the greatest legacies Bion transmitted to me in analysis was to be able to find my own voice—to listen to *myself* listening to (and reading) him. This I have done!

Bion was a diligent student of Plato and of the pre-Socratics, particularly Heraclitus. From them and their wisdom he was able to make the most significant paradigm changes in psychoanalytic theory and technique to date. One of their ideas was that of *transience*—or *flux* or *evolution*. Everything and everyone is in flux, is evolving. Yesterday's patient is not today's patient. The same holds true for Bion's ideas: *they too are in flux!* We may come to realize aspects of them that Bion may have presciently adumbrated but never consciously anticipated. Mine is a work in progress (flux) about a grander work in progress (evolution). It is not so much a merely faithful rendering of his ideas as my *digestion* of his work—at *the moment!* If I am right, Bion is more practical and clinically useful than most—including my former self—have realized.

An imagined dialogue between Bion and me

I have become aware of a realization that Bion regretfully foresaw. When readers and scholars do begin to appreciate him, there often is a tendency for them to idealize him. Bion scholarship, in my opinion and I think in his own, has focused on his work almost like an exegetical text, a Bible, as it were, rather than a living, evolving entity containing variables and invariants and probes destined for further explorations by others. Over and over again Bion would remind me that I should be more focused on my own responses to what he said rather than on him and his words. I have decided to take him up in this text on his generous invitation. I firmly believe that Bion wishes and needs to be played with in a spirit of active, respectful enthusiasm. He has to be challenged before he is swallowed: after all, did he not play with Freud's and Klein's works?

The reader will see for himself the degree to which I have done so—with what I believe was pre-arranged permission from Bion.

The scope of the book

The scope of this work is my faithful attempt to synopsize, synthesize, extend, and challenge Bion and his contributions and to present his ideas in a reader-friendly manner—as my digestion of them. Bléandonu has given us an in-depth view of Bion's personal background and an almost encyclopaedic rendition of his contributions as they sequentially emerged. Grinberg, Sor, and de Bianchedi, like the Symingtons, have discussed his major contributions in depth. López-Corvo and Paulo Sandler have approached his works encyclopaedically. I should like to choose a middle ground so as to avoid redundancy. My plan, consequently, is to present what *I* believe is his most important legacy-to psychoanalysis: the ideas that are on the cutting edge of our field that, in my estimation, need to be known by the mental health profession at large. It will be noticed that I have scrupulously avoided discussing Bion biographically. I think for me that would be sacrilegious. He was my analyst, and he left Los Angeles before my transference neurosis was resolved.

In short, I should like to "interpret" ("dream") Bion so as to highlight and define the broader and deeper implications of his works. I should like both to present his ideas faithfully and also to use his ideas as launching pads for my own imaginative as well as reasonable conjectures about directions in which his ideas point. In that category I include especially such ideas as the "Language of Achievement", "reverie", "truth", "O", and "transformations"—in, of, and from it, but also L, H, and K linkages (to show how Bion rerouted Freud's instinctual drives to emotions), "container ↔ contained", Bion's ideas on "dreaming", "becoming", "thoughts without a thinker", the "Grid", his erasure of the distinction between Freud's "primary and secondary processes" and the "pleasure" and "reality principles", "reversible perspective", "shifting vertices", "binocular vision", "contact-barrier", the replacement of "consciousness" and "unconsciousness" with finiteness and infinity, Bion's use of models, his distinction between "mentalization" and "thinking", among many others. In other words, the book is organized according to *my* rough estimation of an approximate order of importance of his theoretical and clinical contributions presented as a synthesis of the whole. The plan that organizes this work is my attempt to cite and then annotate what I believe to be representative excerpts from his principal works. As I have just stated earlier, I wish this text to be a faithful exposition of Bion's works as well as a "dialogue" with him in which I respectfully question some of his ideas and put forward some of my own.

Caveat 1

Unlike most works that aim to be scholarly, this is a very personal text. Bion was and continues to be very important to me personally, intellectually, and professionally. Although he would hate the idea, I believe I am a "Bionian–Kleinian". I have found Bion difficult to read and have therefore perused his works many times. I seek in this work to show I came to understand—a word he hated—and then "became" what wisdom I could acquire from him. The text is the result of my personal ascent of the North Face of Truth, O. *This work*, in other words, *is my own personal diary of reading Bion*. I cite other scholars, each of whom I greatly respect, sparsely: I did not want to lean too much on their points of view and thereby lose my own self-direction.

Similarly, I have cited profusely from the main Bion texts, but have all but ignored citing from his later works. This work, consequently, is to some degree an annotation of his major works. After having read *Bion in New York and São Paulo, Bion's Brazilian Lectures 1* and *2, Clinical Seminars and Four Discussions, Four Discussions with W. R. Bion*, and especially *The Tavistock Seminars* and *The Italian Seminars*, I realized that I had a serious problem. I could have cited the entirety of all of them, so rich and packed with his wisdom were they. Also, by the time I got to them, my text had already become overlong.

Space limitations prohibit my review of Bion's trilogy, *A Memoir of the Future*. That undertaking is a work that is now in progress. All I can say here is all too brief and compact: The *Memoir* is Bion's dreaming of his autobiography, with all its sorrow, horror, and redemption. He warns us of the danger of the mind's demons, which when amplified by the leverage of the group process, can destroy the world. The saving grace is rendering the contending voices into respected vertices and offering them the opportunity for a "disciplined debate".

The reader will also recognize that I have cited many portions of Bion's works, often at great length, thereby rendering major portions of my book into a veritable annotated work on his contributions. I have done this deliberately. I wish to show (1) the rightful provenance and progression of *his* ideas, and (2), as I show in my annotations, how I derived my own sense of what Bion meant. The reader will also note the sparseness of clinical examples. I have found that it was difficult to find clinical examples that would be clear and precise enough. However, I have borrowed from the works of Ferro, Ogden, de Bianchedi, as well as my own in this text to discuss Bion's theories with clinical relevance. On the other hand, when I could, I found myself in another dilemma: the results of my own reverie were often so intimate as to prohibit publication.

Some Bion scholars may be disappointed in what and whom I have selected *not* to list or discuss. This work has been written for a broad reading public. As a consequence, many themes that I considered too recondite have regretfully been left out. Once again I wish to emphasize that this work is the story of how *I* personally came to appreciate Bion's writings—through very hard work and through "dreaming" it. I followed the dictates that I had learned from him in analysis: "Don't try to understand *me*! Pay special attention to *your emotional responses to me!*—which I took to mean that I, by attending to my responses to him, should allow Bion, to open the gates of my infinite self and so become incarnated by my godhead! I know this language may bother some. It clearly bothers O'Shaughnessy (2005, p. 1530). It will become more reasonable as the reader reads on. I close with a koan from John Lennon: "Reality leaves a lot to the imagination"!

Caveat 2

Bion's writings, though fewer in quantity than those of others, like Klein and Freud, are dense, syncretistic, and repetitive in words. He repeats himself over and over again—differently—from different vertices and in different contexts. Furthermore, his work seems holographic. The word "holographic" is used differently depending on the context into which it is placed. My use of it can best be illustrated by an analogy to the chromosome. Every cell of the body contains the genome for the whole body. The stereoscopic effect in art can be remarkable. I myself, though no artist and certainly no Bion, seek to use what I think of as the holographic model for this work. By this I mean that while I attempt to be faithful to Bion's works categorically, I also may seem to repeat myself on numerous occasions. I can only hope that the reader will realize that I know that I am repeating when I do so—as my only way of faithfully expatiating Bion's thoughts.

Caveat 3

In my original plans for the book I had considered using clinical material, my own and others', to demonstrate how "Bionian technique" can be applied. Although I present a few brief case examples of how *I* use Bion, it finally dawned on me that to try to do so in a wider way would be an attempt to concretize or reify Bion's ideas. One can never be a Bionian analyst. One can only be a psychoanalyst allowing oneself to be informed by immersion in reading and "becoming" Bion.

NOTE

1. I learned later upon reading another translation of Freud's letter that Freud had referred to "reading a book", but I am sure I heard Bion say "analysis". Also, he (Bion) later cited this passage as "blind myself artificially to focus all the light on one dark spot" (1970, p. 57).

CHAPTER 1

An introduction

I have been asked to undertake the daunting task of writing a book on Bion that will introduce a distillation and synthesis of his ideas for the general public. Those readers who are already familiar with his works realize how difficult a task that is. Bion's ideas are highly unique and are presented by him with such density at times that it often is difficult to capture his meaning—but that is Bion through and through. As I wrote in another contribution, his published works remind one of solving a picture puzzle, but one in which the configurations change as one is trying to find the right piece, or of reading Borges' (1998) "Book of Sand" or "The Library of Babel" where the pages and the books proliferate to infinity as you begin to read them (Grotstein, 2004b, p. 1081). He hated the idea that he or his ideas would be captured and then imprisoned in static "understanding". Furthermore, as he suggested to me on numerous occasions in analysis, he was more interested in *my response* to what he said than in *my grasp* of *his* interpretations, or, for that matter, his ideas. Likewise, *he* was more interested in *his* inner responses to my associations.

I realized only later that I was being introduced to the *"Language of Achievement"*: the infra- and translingual form of pre-lexical and/ or infra-lexical emotional communication between infant and mother and analysand and analyst. It was only still later that I came to

DOI: 10.4324/9781003348665-2

realize that Bion was introducing us to the foundations of Faith (F) and Truth (T) and their emotional underpinnings. In fact I began to understand that the importance of emotions lay in their cargo, personal truth. In being able to tolerate the frustration of awaiting the arrival of the vanguards of certainty and the relief that certainty offers us when we are needy and *un*certain, we then come to be able to experience apparitions[1] or revelations of the anticipated object from within us, from our inner Platonic/Kantian, numinous reservoir, which allows us to anticipate the yet unknown and yet-to-arrive object by formatting our consciousness, as it were, with "informed" but infinite expectations. Faith lies in our belief that there will always exist a noumenon that corresponds to a potentially realizable object that can always anticipate the arrival of that future object or the return of the erstwhile departed object.

It is my impression that Bion always regretted that all too often his style of presentation, both in his lectures and in his writings, paradoxically resulted in his being admired, adulated, and worshipped as a "genius", which he undoubtedly was, rather than being the mere transmitter of the subject's own inner wisdom. As one reads Plato, one cannot help identifying Bion with Socrates: there, too, Socrates' own humble genius outshone his humility as mere transmitter to his listener of the wisdom within the listener of which the latter was totally unaware. As we shall see later in this work, Bion, following early Freud and later Lacan, even more than Klein at times, came to the true but lost meaning of transference: we transfer our unconscious wisdom to the analyst and then envy him for *his* wisdom as the "one who knows". We as patients thereupon envy our projected wisdom now resident (in unconscious phantasy) within the analyst. Do we miss the analyst over weekend and holiday breaks, and/or do we miss our lost, detached, and transferred unconscious self in the analyst? What I am getting at is this: I believe that Bion, like Socrates, never felt that he was successful in dodging transference and so sadly remained larger than life to almost all who encountered him. Thus, in much of Bion scholarship, including my own, there seems to be little "dialogue" or "disciplined" debate with his ideas. Although I have been guilty heretofore of this tendency, the reader will soon enough see how "Bionian" I have become in questioning some of his now famous assumptions. I shall, on occasion, become a veritable Jacob wrestling with the angel.

Bion's style of writing and communicating

Bion's style of writing as well as communicating—that is, answering questions at conferences—puzzled some. As Francesca Bion writes:

> He believed that "La réponse est le malheur de la question"[2]; both in his professional and private life problems stimulated in him thought and discussion-never answers. His replies—more correctly, coun-ter-contributions—were, in spite of their apparent irrelevance, an extension of the questions. His point of view is best illustrated in his own words:
> "I don't know the answers to these questions—I wouldn't tell you if I did. I think it is important to find out for yourselves."
> "I try to give you a chance to fill the gap left by me."
> "I don't think that my explanation matters. What I would draw attention to is the *nature of* the problem." [F. Bion, 1980, p. 5]

Any reader of Plato's *Dialogues* (1892) can easily spot Socrates, as I have already suggested—but also Freud and the original spirit of psy-choanalysis. The "answer" lies within the questioner: that is, within the unconscious. Many analysts know this and believe it. Bion *lived* it! His works have never yet been satisfactorily translated from the "Linear B" of his elusive yet exhortative poetics. He heralds and in-vokes the mystical, religious, spiritual, aesthetic, and psychoanalytic vertices—for us, not to understand but to *become* as we evolve.

Bion's writings seem to be quite understandable to some and less understandable to too many others. His prose reveals a style of sen-tence structure that reflects an Edwardian public-schooling with im-mersion in Latin and Greek. I recall his use of the word "macilent" in one of his works. I looked it up in vain in a number of dictionaries. Finally, gaining access to a dictionary published in Edinburgh in 1870, I found the word "macilent, now rare, emaciated". "Macilent", inter-estingly, reveals one aspect of Bion's writings: they are "bare bones", in a sense. There is no spare word or idea. Bion's style consequently encompasses complex components, but certainly one of them is his upbringing. Bion leaves you orphaned outside his text for you to seek your own way by your own inherent navigational compass—one you never believed you possessed until you met him. Bion's style of writ-ing is unique, often maddening, without proper markings or guide-posts to help you anticipate the next turn in the road of ideas he has privately charted. Often he seems to speak apodictically, not sharing with the reader the provenance of his thought.

He refused to position himself as the wise man or guru who liked to have disciples at his feet. Like Socrates, he always insisted that he knew nothing or never wrote anything original but that every individual had within him/herself all the potential wisdom he or she would ever need (The Ideal Forms, the noumena). He likened himself, again like Socrates, to a "midwife" to the ideas that were latent within the would-be disciple. In Los Angeles he refused to "supervise". He would only offer a "second opinion". When I inquired about this, he stated that when he fought in the First World War, he came painfully to realize that headquarters, which was located far behind the lines, gave orders that were ill-informed because of their distance from the scene of action. Likewise, any therapist, no matter how inexperienced and untrained, knew more about his or her patient than did a "supervisor" who was not in the actual experience with the patient.

In short, he was humble. Yet this humble man has been able to dare to "disturb the universe" of psychoanalytic positivism and certainty with ideas that issue from the vast sweep of his polymath, autodidact erudition and remarkable imaginative conjectures. These ideas now stand the test of time as worthy rational conjectures and arguably constitute perhaps the greatest paradigm shift in psychoanalysis to date. I pay him the highest compliment when I suggest that he was a "Yeshivabucher activist", a "messiah–genius", a veritable Prometheus, the "doyen of uncertainty", and the "navigator extraordinaire of the deep and formless infinite".

According to Bléandonu (1993):

> Bion's style is a mixture of dazzling illuminations, provocative aphorisms and tiresome digressions. Underscored by contradiction, it obliges readers to choose either timid or risky interpretations, and does so in order to avoid oversimplification, and defy paraphrasing. It could be compared to an uncut diamond, and the reader, in search of illumination of its refracted light, is drawn in to a labyrinth of obscurity. [Bléandonu, 1993, p. 1]

Grinberg, Sor, and de Bianchedi (1977) state:

> We had many doubts before deciding to undertake what seemed a very risky and difficult venture: to write an introduction to Dr. Bion's ideas. On the one hand, we were encouraged by the requests of many colleagues and students who found great difficulty in comprehending the concepts he developed in his books; but at the same time we were held back by the responsibility of having to convey, in a simplified form, certain very complex hypotheses whose deep

meaning has demanded from us long hours of work. [Grinberg, Sor, & de Bianchedi, 1977, p. xv]

Paulo Sandler (2005), in presenting a rationale for undertaking his formidable *Dictionary* on Bion, says:

> This is an attempt to address a fact derived from this author's experience with colleagues around the world for 24 years, namely, that many feel Bion's written work to be "obscure and difficult" . . .
>   It seems to this writer that some of the factors involved in this attributed obscurity fall into the following categories:
> (i)   Lack of attentive reading . . .
> (ii) Lack of analytical experience . . .
> (iii) Lack of experience in life itself . . .
> (iv) A constant conjunction of (i), (ii) and (iii). [Sandler, 2005, pp. 6–7]

Joan and Neville Symington (1996), while not commenting on Bion's allegedly obscure style, do say that

> Psychoanalysis seen through Bion's eyes is a radical departure from all conceptualizations which preceded him. We have not the slightest hesitation in saying that *he is the deepest thinker within psychoanalysis—and this statement does not exclude Freud.* [Symington & Symington, 1996, p. xii; italics added]

According to Eigen (1985):

> In order to read Bion fairly, one must read him closely and, in part, on his own terms. He is one of the most precise, if elusive, of psychoanalytic writers. [Eigen, 1985, cited in López-Corvo, 2003, p. xv]

López-Corvo (2003). In addressing the obscurity, complexity, and elusiveness of Bion's writings, states:

> I have a hypothesis: there is the feeling, when we follow his work sequentially, of a successive tendency toward a greater complication and a more elusive writing style. . . . I feel Bion was obscure with the British, sober with Americans and charming and understanding with Brazilians. [López-Corvo, 2003, p. xvi]

Ogden (2004b) elegantly and poignantly surveys Bion's style of writing and comments that there is (1) in Bion's earlier writings (through *Learning from Experience*) "a dialectical movement between obscurity and clarification which moves toward, though never achieves, closure" (p. 288); and (2) a more evocative form of writing in his later works in which Bion sought to convey his experiences to the reader directly—as the experience itself—as an authentic replication in the latter, without going through obfuscating explanations. Ogden interprets Bion as suggesting that the reader must not only actively participate in the reading of his works, but "he must become the author of his own book (his own set of thoughts) more or less based on Bion's"[3] (pp. 286–287). Above all, Ogden believes, and I concur, that Bion was in effect experimenting with a new form of writing, one that induces the emotional experience and also one that uses familiar words to convey altered meanings.

While reading Hampshire's (2005) new work, *Spinoza and Spinozism*, I learned how Spinoza, the heretic and mystical genius of *his* time, wrote in obscure and elusive Latin in order that his contemporaries would *not* be able to understand him and report him to the authorities. Bion, the heretical mystical genius of his own time, may have done something similar. In his autobiography he documents the effective ban on curiosity that had been imposed by "Arf Arfer", God, as interpreted by his father—and mother—and continuing with his Kleinian family in London (Bion, 1982, 1985). Joan and Neville Symington (1996) seem to confirm the latter part of this statement in their Acknowledgements:

> Sydney Klein has given great encouragement to persevere in investigating our ideas when they have been opposed or challenged. *His independence from group pressures* and ability to see the special contribution of Bion in contemporary analytic theory has been a source of inspiration to us. [Symington & Symington, 1996, p. ix; italics added]

In other words, may not Bion have learned early on to think and speak in code, like his forebear, Spinoza?

One point of view is that Bion, genius that he was, was a poor writer because his prose could not keep up with the expansiveness and range of his thinking. I have another idea, however. My own impression of Bion was that he was very "English" in the sense of being a refined but stalwart individualist. It is my opinion that he maintained his individuality in the Klein group and was to suffer for it. In analysis he insisted that the analysand become an individual in his own right. Consequently, I wonder whether his writing style is his way of distancing readers from projectively—and then introjectively—identifying with him, and leaving them "orphaned" so as to find their own way in the wilderness of new, unprocessed thoughts. Put another way, Bion would not be an ungulate mother who would first chew the food that she would then give to her children. He was the combined parent who had faith that the infants (readers) had the inner resources to chew their own food—and make their own (processed) thoughts.

Perhaps there is another relevant factor that may help to explain some aspects of Bion's writing. He was trained and emerged as an analyst during the "time of the troubles" between Anna Freud and Melanie Klein and their respective followers. On more than one occasion he mentioned how distressed he was over the unscientific nature of the longstanding debates between the two camps and how he was attempting to develop a scientific language for psychoanalysis, one whose very scientific nature would be persuasive to all science-respecting analysts. I believe that that is why, in part, once he had completed his clinical study of psychotic patients, he began a rigorous study of thinking and thinking disorders and applied mathematical analogues or models, in order to become as precise as he could be so as to achieve a veritable psychoanalytic Esperanto—a universal language. Mathematics is unsaturated and can consequently lend itself as a useful analogue to variants and invariants in thinking. Ironically, however, Bion has achieved world fame for his contributions to *intuition*—a part of the newer mystical science that deals with uncertainties and emergence phenomena.

Reading his works and having being analysed by him suggest to me a hypothesis that derives from the above. Bion, the intuitionist, was almost obsessive about achieving *precision* in his ideas. That is why he went to the trouble of invoking so many models associated with mathematics, science, logic, and philosophy. He had become dissatisfied with the problem of communication between analysts about clinical data and was looking for *a universal analogue language*, a unified psychoanalytic field theory, one that was outside psychoanalytic jargon—that is, the "language of substitution"—but could supply a scientific–mathematical precision that all analysts could agree upon. Later, he would come upon the concept of the "Language of Achievement"—the primal language of emotions (Bion, 1970, p. 125).

I should like to proffer yet another hypothesis about why Bion wrote and spoke the way he did. It is my impression that Bion *dreamed* his utterances and his writings—that is, he spoke and wrote in a transformational state of reverie (wakeful sleep) (Grotstein, 2006a). His conception of the concept of O is a continuing testimony to that vision. We see his faith in a scientific–mathematical model ebbing between 1963, when he published *Elements of Psycho-Analysis*; 1965, when he published *Transformations*; and 1970, when he published *Attention and*

Interpretation. Bion had discovered that science and mathematics had their limitations, that mathematical certainty was an illusion, and that the language of science was sense-based, suitable only for *inanimate* objects, not *living* objects. He then turned to Heisenberg's concept of uncertainty and to intuitionistic mathematics (Dutch School), and his language followed suit. His quest for the holy grail of psychoanalytic precision changed to a stoic acceptance of uncertainty, the ultimate result being his psychoanalytic metatheory, arguably the most far-reaching paradigm shift in psychoanalytic history and the most suitable one to date to anticipate the newer era of relativism, probabilism, and uncertainty.

Yet another idea about his style of presentation bears note. Bion, in his zeal for precision in studying an imprecise, non-linear, complex (in the mathematical sense) subject, demonstrated a predilection to speak and write in terms of *models*. He thought and spoke "outside the box", so to speak, rather than inside. I have a notion that this idea may be the most nearly correct one: while reading an interview of Bion by Anthony Banet in 1976, I observed a rare Bion—one whom I came to know only on his last evening in Los Angeles when he and his wife, Francesca, had joined us for a farewell dinner. *He spoke normally.* He was anything but circumspect. He did not speak, then, in models.

Bion was always a very polite but very private man. When one reads *Bion in New York and São Paulo* and *Bion's Brazilian Lectures 1* and *2*, one gets a good picture of how he allows himself to engage and become engaged with others. He rarely answers a question directly. He seems to parry the question and proceed in an unpredictable direction. Let me cite but one example from *Bion's Brazilian Lectures 1*:

> Q.   I would like clarification of the concept of "the future" if we are always dealing with something that is to happen and nothing else, is not the present totally absorbed in that perspective?
> A.   I have been using a concept, and it is one of these situations in which one tends to believe that there is some realisation which approximates to the concept. We are all used to words like "sex" which, if one considers the matter, means nothing. But the word "sex" like "the future", is useful for this kind of discussion. [1973, p. 16]

If one reads the above citation—as well as many like it—carefully, one may be able to begin to detect that Bion is a *magus* and/or a *hypnotist*! The questioner asked about "the future". Bion suggests "sex"—as a model—that distracts from one's focus on "the future". As one reads through *Bion in New York and São Paulo* (Bion, 1980) or *Bion's Brazilian*

Lectures 1 (1973) and *2* (1974), one can begin to detect with increasing certainty that Bion answers his questioners in a way so as to distract their attention, their focus, from what they *believe* they are asking by supplying a novel subject that is seemingly far removed from what the questioner thought he was asking. The effect on the questioner often seemed to be a "deer in the headlights" phenomenon of thinking that Bion was really answering their question when—to me—in fact he was not. He was changing their view from *certainty* to *uncertainty*—so that they could thereupon come to be open to the spontaneously emerging unpredictable answer latent *within them*. Put another way, Bion responds in such a way that the questioner unconsciously *finds* and *becomes* his own answer!

Yet another possibility that occurred to me is that when Bion spoke, conversed, and wrote, he was actively *dreaming* his utterances and writings. By this I mean that Bion may actually have "become" what he was propounding. He was kaleidoscopically dividing all his thoughts (and/or our thoughts), removing thoughts from their original contexts, paring them down to their irreducible elements, and then rearranging them in new contexts so as to highlight some aspects of the thoughts and to place others in the shadows.

When one reads Bion's works in succession, one can detect the beginning of a change in his thinking about psychoanalytic phenomena. Commenting on this putative change, Ogden (2004b) writes the following:

> The experience of reading early Bion generates a sense of psychoanalysis as a never-completed process of clarifying obscurities and obscuring clarifications, which enterprise moves in the direction of a convergence of disparate meanings. In contrast, the experience of reading Bion's later works conveys a sense of psychoanalysis as a process involving a movement toward infinite expansion of meaning. [Ogden, 2004b, p. 285]

Bion introduced a new form of pedagogy in his writings. Perhaps one can say that Bion was all too aware of the propensity of people to idealize and to identify with a leader or a wizard like Freud or Klein and then to surrender their own thinking capacities as they worship at the feet of the guru. Many people who read Bion become frustrated by his prose, deny it, and then identify with and quote him at length—and even become Bion afficionados. Unfortunately, the density and non-linearity of his prose style seems to lend itself either to resentment or to idealization. My South American colleagues have found that reading Bion—especially his trilogy, *A Memoir of the Future* (1975, 1977b, 1979,

1981)—is best done in groups, and I tend to agree. Bion's prose style is exhortative, evocative, and indicative (points to something beyond) rather than iconic and specific, and it demands enthusiastic confrontation, engagement, and participation on the part of the reader—perhaps even meditation—so as to be all the more open to one's *inner* ear and vision.

Bion's fame followed rather than preceded him. In López-Corvo's (2003) opinion his writings were dense at the beginning when he was in London and later in the United States, both places where he initially experienced marginalization and rejection; when he wrote for South American audiences, on the other hand, his writings become clearer and more expressive because of the enthusiastic appreciation with which he and his works were greeted. When he lived and practised in Los Angeles, few knew who Bion was. Some came to him there because they had heard that he was a group therapist. When his four major books were published in the United States under the title, *Seven Servants* (Bion, 1977c), the American publisher lost money on the project and understandably refused at the time to reprint it. However, he did reprint it in 1983 following Karnac's reprinting of these titles. Times have changed significantly since then. Many US psychoanalytic institutes offer courses on Bion but often suffer from a dearth of able teachers to teach his works. Owing to this growing and spreading importance of his ideas, I have decided to compose this brief but hopefully useful work, a synopsis, a synthesis, a perspective, a personal digestion of his ideas.

Before closing this section, I feel compelled to return to my earlier idea about Bion's speaking and writing in terms of models—outside the box.

Bion: the genius

Bion seems to have had to live with the advantages and disadvantages of being accorded the mantle of genius from early on in his professional career—probably because of his unique and highly idiosyncratic but plausible and confirmable observations in the study of groups and then in his observations of psychotic patients and the far-reaching conclusions he drew from these observations. One does not know whether he himself thought of himself as a genius. What is a genius? In my eyes a genius is one who sees patterns, structures, or gestalten in an incipient or incomplete form that ordinary individuals cannot see at first, or at all. Put another way, a genius is one who sees through the camouflage of images and symbols and is in touch, so to speak, with the "thing-in-itself"—a transcendent experience that Bion terms a "transformation in O". It involves the highly cooperative use of the functions of both cerebral hemispheres. Bion was able to observe and to discern patterns that no one, not even Freud or Klein, could detect—similarly with psychotics and analysands generally. Add to genius the quality of intense curiosity and great capacity for focus (observation)—and one has the dimensions of an extraordinary individual. Did he have any negative traits? I don't know, but I have often suspected that his ruthless honesty, discipline, and stubbornness, and his refusal to be political, may have caused him to become marginalized and persecuted all too easily. O'Shaughnessy (2005) suggests that Bion had become "undisciplined" in his later years. I have come to wonder whether the London Kleinians know some things about him I don't know—but, then, perhaps I know things about him (as analysand) that they may not know. It may very well be coming to pass that "undisciplined Bion" will have become Melanie Klein's foremost contribution to psychoanalysis.

I gather that he could be a very good friend but was never "one of the boys".

I have often wondered whether he had become frozen in time as the protective "older-brother" tank commander who must perpetually look out for the safety of his men (and women)—at a respectful distance, true *noblesse oblige*—having been haunted by his comrades-in-arms, those real troops who did not survive. Until recently the concept of trauma has not been emphasized in psychoanalytic thinking generally and in Kleinian thinking specifically. The emphasis was generally on psychosis. One wonders whether, in Bion's analysis with Klein, the latter was really able to deal effectively with the trauma he had suffered—that is, in the First World War—when it was the world that was psychotic ("I died on August 8, 1918 on the Amiens–Roye Road"), his wife dying in childbirth, and so on. In other words, was the Bion some of us "knew" hidden inside a carapace of unspeakable anguish (O)? I recall Francesca Bion mentioning that someone who spoke at Bion's Tavistock Memorial observed that "he was miles behind his face". I put forth this idea in light of Bion's pioneering technical exhortation that the analysand will not be satisfied if he does not believe that the analyst experiences emotionally what he, the analysand, experiences.

"Prometheus bound"

One might compare Bion with Prometheus, the Titan who stole fire from the gods to give to mankind, following which audacious act he was punished by Zeus by being bound to a rock and condemned to have his liver eaten by vultures. Bion often spoke and wrote about the Garden of Eden, the Tower of Babel, the Oedipus myth, and the central link between them—the deity's proscription against man's curiosity. That curiosity will turn out to be, for Bion, the quest for truth—not just truth *per se*, but the Absolute Truth about an Ultimate Reality that is ineffable, infinite, and synonymous with "godhead".[4] Some say that before he came to Los Angeles, Bion's liver was metaphorically eaten by vultures in London after he had become "the pariah of O" in their eyes (Grotstein, 1997a; O'Shaughnessy, 2005). Curiously, he would probably have become the heir-apparent and successor to Klein and highly respected there for his early works on psychosis, the container and the contained, L, H, and K linkages, and communicative projective identification, each of which became standard Kleinian thinking and basic components of the "post-Kleinian" episteme in London, especially as practised by Betty Joseph and her followers.

In other words, following Klein's death, Bion could have easily become the titular head of the Kleinian movement, but the extreme nature of his English individuality as a free thinker, not unlike that of Winnicott, marginalized him early on in the eyes of Klein's Central-European-born followers and those who came after them (Sutherland, 1994; personal communication, 1966). Bion maintained a selective and respectful oppositionality to the group within the framework of a robust individuality: he, the authority on groups, eschewed belonging to groups so as to maintain the integrity of his individuality. He prized individuality more than almost anything and insisted that his analysands should respect their own, and upon entering analysis with Klein he cautioned her to respect and honour his.

Along with Herbert Rosenfeld and Hanna Segal, Bion was one of the few analysts of his time to enter the arena of psychoanalysing psychotic patients. The observations he was able to make about psychotics in terms of Kleinian thinking quickly elevated his prestige. From these experiences he initially formulated his concept of "container ↔ contained", the importance of "maternal reverie", "α-function", and "α- and β-elements", along with a significant extension and revision of Klein's (1946, 1955) concept of "projective identification"—one that he broadened to a normal infantile communicative (intersubjective) mode. It was only when he had "second thoughts" about this work and entered the Promethean domain of the "transformation" of the "Absolute Truth" about "Ultimate Reality", "O", the "godhead", the domains of infinity, and inner and outer cosmic uncertainty that he was placed on the rock and his liver devoured. Over and over again in his work one will find references to myths such as the Garden of Eden, the Tower of Babel, and the Oedipus, from each of which he selected the deity's injunction against man's curiosity—yet he never mentioned the myth of Prometheus. One can add this preoccupation of his to another: the promulgation of a severe, malignant *super*ego, originally an "obstructive object ", which internally "attacked the links" of communication with objects and curiosity itself. It is almost as if Bion's curiosity-phobic background with his parents in India was repeated with his London colleagues. Incidentally, the concept of the obstructive object or negative container constituted a watershed in Kleinian thinking, something to which current post-Kleinians are attempting to adjust: the realization of the prime importance of bad parenting along with—or instead of—primary infantile destructiveness as first cause in the development of psychopathology.

Thus, allegedly, Bion fled to America. His leaving (fleeing?) London had consequences for him. Some of his London colleagues let it be rumoured that he had suffered from strokes or transient ischemic attacks (TIAs) there and had fled to California to seek anonymity.[5] Others spread the rumour that he had become psychotic during his stay there, and they forged a constant conjunction between "California and Bion's psychosis"—a calumny that spread to include those who had been analysed by him in Los Angeles (personal communication, anonymous London post-Kleinian analyst, 2004). He was certainly not psychotic when my colleagues and I knew him here in Los Angeles and had entered analysis with him, but he did suffer two episodes of vaso-vagal syncope while he was here, according to Francesca Bion (personal communication, 2007). His speech and intellect remained unimpaired. I was in analysis with him at the time and could not, transference aside, detect that anything was amiss.

"Prometheus unbound"

His fourth metapsychological work, *Attention and Interpretation* (1970), which continued Bion's inquiry into such concepts as O, the mystic, and the godhead (godhood) and which had been adumbrated in his previous work, *Transformations*, had been written and published while he was in Los Angeles. He had also begun writing his actual autobiography, *The Long Week-End: 1897–1917* (1982), its sequel, *All My Sins Remembered and The Other Side of Genius* (1985), as well as his three-volume fictional autobiography, *A Memoir of the Future* (1975, 1977b, 1979, 1981). Bion's written work and ability to do analysis were no longer respected in London (anonymous London-Kleinian analyst, 2004, alluded to earlier), but as his reputation faded there, it shone all the more brightly in South America, particularly in Brazil as well as in Argentina, where his work continues to flourish, to say nothing now of Spain and, especially, of Italy. For quite some time South American writers, more than any others in the world, have been writing about and discussing Bion. He had been so well received there that he had considered relocating there from London, but he decided against it because of language difficulties. The steady, unremitting course of his recently acquired worldwide popularity augurs well, however, for this Prometheus' becoming unbound at last.

The place that Wilfred Bion will hold in the history of twentieth-century psychoanalysis is still being decided, but his posthumous popularity in twenty-first-century psychoanalysis seems to be certain: it only continues to rise. Analysts and psychotherapists are now discovering or rediscovering Bion. Perhaps this sudden rise in acclaim owes much to the realization of his profound work in reverie, countertransference, intersubjectivity, and communicative projective identification. He has variously been accorded appellations such as genius, maverick, mystic, and psychotic. Some say his contributions transcend even those of Freud and Klein. Certainly, he significantly extended their ideas. As I noted earlier, Joan and Neville Symington (1996) "believe that he achieved an understanding of the mind that has not been surpassed by any other analyst" (p. 26), and with this I agree.

In his personal appearance Bion was always imposing and formidable. He could never escape admiration and awe on the part of most who met him. I have reason to believe that this troubled him because it marginalized him. He would often retort, if asked why he had moved to Los Angeles from London, that he "was so loaded down with honours that he nearly sank without a trace". In his presence one was always impressed by the depth of his mind, the intensity of his focus, and the extraordinary discipline of his thinking, as well as by his graciousness, manners, and accent. He seemed, at least to me, an Englishman of another age—perhaps Edwardian—in manner. He was always polite, but one suspected, as one of his Tavistock colleagues suggested, that "He was miles behind his face". His style in lecturing was interesting. He always spoke without notes. After a gracious introduction by the programme chairman at a lecture for a local psychoanalytic institute, Bion began by uttering: "I can hardly wait to hear what I have to say."

He hinted, suggested, and implied but would never pontificate. In his analytic as well as in his published works one quickly detects his unique capacity for keen observation. It was as if he could see through the camouflage of long-established symbols and icons and detect the deeper and more meaningful substance that lurked behind them. Bion was a psychoanalytic "scout extraordinaire". His capacity to detect the unusual within the usual and the usual in the unusual was absolutely uncanny.

Bion's tools for exploration

Among the tools Bion brought to his thinking were such techniques as: the Language of Achievement, containment, reverie, "binocular vision", "reversible perspectives", "multiple vertices", "abstraction", "common sense", "correlation", "public-ation", "spontaneous conjecture" ("wild thoughts"), and "rational conjecture"—along with his signature injunction to "abandon memory and desire" so as to be able to become meditatively mentally unsaturated and thus open to the unexpected. In terms of the cerebral hemisphere model, Bion was as keen in his rational, logical left-hemispheric thinking as he was in his right-hemispheric intuitive thinking. His use of reversible perspectives was another of his keynote characteristics. He was capable of turning ideas on end and seeing them from many different perspectives (vertices). He often cited the exploits of Field Marshal Slim, who won the Malaysian War against a vastly superior Japanese Army by the technique of shifting perspectives in his strategy against them. Some of his other tools included models like "α-function", "α- and β-elements", and the "gastrointestinal tract" and the "synapse" as two different models for transformation.

Bion may not have sufficiently realized how he had not only revolutionized psychoanalytic metapsychology and brought it back into alignment with nineteenth-century metaphysics and twentieth-century ontology (existentialism), he had also perforated the proud mystique of "objectivity" that had been so sacred to logical-positivistic, deterministic science—the "scientific" Establishment that had so intimidated Freud and with which, in my opinion, he submissively identified. Bion revealed its own mythology in its absolute depend-ence on sense data and reversed the perspective on it and found myths, both collective and personal, to be "scientific deductive sys-tems" (Bion, 1992). Furthermore, he was the first to establish the new "mystic science of psychoanalysis"—a numinous science based on the abandonment of memory, desire, understanding, and a respect for relativity, complexity, and uncertainty.

Bion observed that the normal or neurotic human has achieved the capacity for verbal thought, and the internal thinking couple needs words as the tools for thinking. Yet they also need imagery—the im-agery of the senses that is formed before words as well as afterwards. Musicians think—but not in words. Bion emphasized the importance of (1) the selected fact, (2) the constant conjunction, (3) the reversible perspective, (4) multiple vertices, (5) an absence of memory and desire, (6) the reversibility of progression and regression between PS and D, (7) the importance of binocular vision, (8) reverie, (9) negative capa-bility, and (10) the importance of context, imaginative conjecture, ab-straction, and myth. One can intuit from these that thought originates autochthonously (solipsistically) (Grotstein, 1995, 2000a) as an imagi-native conjecture—but owes its provenance to the impactful presence of the other who both inspires the origin of the imaginative conjecture *and* becomes the object of the conjecture. Together, the other also im-aginatively (autochthonously) conjectures about the subject's conjec-tures. The two conjectures relate to what has been termed, by Jung, Ferguson, Galatzer-Levy, and Ogden, the "third area" and what I call the *"transformational forge"* in the preconscious, where the respective Os of each participant can breed in relationship to the imaginatively conjectured infant of analysis held in mind by both—in association with the virtual analyst–other of the transference. They are invisible "conjoined-twin" effigies.

According to the Symingtons, Bion employs three axes that inter-sect with and interpenetrate each other: (1) Ultimate Reality, (2) the difference between sensuous and psychic reality, and (3) the way an individual comes to know knowledge, and that ". . . the pathway by which such an experience [the mystical] becomes possible is through the close relationship with another" (Symington & Symington, 1996).

He radically and profoundly altered our conceptions of thinking, not only by distinguishing the mind from the "thoughts without a thinker"—the mind's predecessor that inchoately arose in the infant and required a mind to think these virginal, unthought thoughts—but by also revealing to us that these thoughts *and* the mind that thinks them are unconscious: that thinking itself is essentially unconscious. What we nominally call "thinking" could best be called "after-thinking", and our known "thoughts" are best called "after-thoughts.

Whereas psychoanalysis was sacred to Bion, none of its component ideas were. With regard to both Freud and Klein, he had the "Nelson touch": just before the Battle of Copenhagen, the admiral commanding the British fleet realized that the British were outnumbered by the Danish fleet and signalled the captains of his ships to withdraw. Vice-Admiral, later Lord, Nelson put his telescope to his blind eye and uttered that he saw no signal—and went on to win the Battle of Copenhagen. Nelsonic Bion respectfully challenged some of the major canons of Freud and Klein and ultimately fashioned a metatheory of psychoanalysis that extends their work and, at points, significantly departs from it and arguably transcends it. Even more than that, from the rich fund of his polymath and autodidact resources, which included mathematics, philosophy, scientific logic, theology, mysticism, aesthetics, art, history, and mythology, among others, he was able to contemplate the existence of a numinous psychoanalytic subject from multiple vertices and, in so doing, was able to bring the rich lore and acquired learning of Western culture to the psychoanalytic idiom in an astonishing integration and thus restore psychoanalysis to its ancient and ongoing cultural font. Bion brought the Renaissance to psychoanalysis.

I have alluded above to Bion's ability to achieve a remarkable harmony of functioning between his two cerebral hemispheres, which can be equated with the *dreamer* and the *thinker*, respectively. To this idea I wish to append the fact that Bion, though English by heritage, was Anglo–Indian culturally; he undoubtedly brought with him many of the overt and hidden values of that land and integrated them with his later-to-be-acquired English and European left-brain respect for precision.[6] His later venture into O is understandably thought by many to have issued from his Indian transcendental roots.

A Bionic koan might be as follows: *We spend and too often waste a lifetime walking in the shadow of our ultimate unclaimed self.*

NOTES

1. One of the many meanings of "apparition" is "epiphany".
2. Bion borrowed this quotation from Maurice Blanchot.
3. In fact, I overheard Bion describing this idea almost word-for-word to a colleague who had congratulated him on his latest book (*Transformations*)—circa 1965).

4. Bion uses the term "godhead" to designate a Platonic archetype, essence, or Ideal Form, not the deity, "God", as worshipped and quasi-humanized by mankind. The term "godhead" was used by Meister Eckhart, the mystic, and probably originated from the Middle English word "godhood". Its equivalent is "Godliness".

5. In actual fact, according to Francesca Bion, those rumours were ill-founded: Bion suffered from syncope, presumably vaso-vagal syncope (personal communication, 2006).

6. The only times I felt that I really intrigued Bion as a patient were when I informed him that I had sat on the lap of Rabindranath Tagore, the Nobelist translator of the *Upanishads*, when I was four years-old—and that I had learned Hebrew as a child.

CHAPTER 2

What kind of analyst was Bion?

Having undergone four analyses, including one with Bion, I am able to compare him with my other analysts as well as with others in general. Let me begin with a statement of his that I heard second-hand from another colleague. Shortly after arriving in Los Angeles, Bion confided to this colleague that "American analysts actually converse with their patients!" Bion rarely conversed with me. He was the most disciplined analyst I have ever met. His respect for the analytic frame was always obvious. He would never repeat an interpretation, even if I told him that I had not heard it. He would re- mind me that it could not be repeated: the time had passed. On one oc- casion he reminded me of Heraclitus' koan that one can never step into the same river twice. Virtually the entirety of his relationship with me during the analysis was interpretative. He interpreted frequently and often at length. Yet he was always "Kleinian"—but in his own way. I never read any of Bion's works while I was in analysis with him and was therefore surprised later when I read his concept of "abandoning memory and desire". He spoke and interpreted in an active and highly engaged manner; consequently, I don't know when he found the time to "abandon memory and desire". I recall, however, that like a scout, he doggedly tracked the sequence of my free associations. I shall soon share with you some of what he said to me, including his first inter- pretation to me on my first day of analysis with him.

DOI: 10.4324/9781003348665-3   27

I had been in brief "supervision" with Bion prior to entering analysis. He was uneasy with "supervision" and preferred the term "second opinion". He was of the opinion that the therapist, no matter how inexperienced, knew more about the patient that anyone who was not present in that experience. Thus, he could only offer a second opinion rather than a "supervision". It became clear to me that Bion highly valued personal experience over theory and training, though he did not proscribe training, as I shall show later. I also detected something about his views on the power politics of supervision. His second opinions about the case material that I presented to him were always interesting, but I could not always use them—at least so I thought then—partly because at that time I had yet to become immersed in and therefore knowledgeable about Bion's work and Kleinian theory.

Consequently, when I entered analysis with Bion, I was unfamiliar with his published works and had read them only sparingly for the duration of the analysis. Recently, when I was queried at an analytic conference about why I sounded so Kleinian after having been analysed by Bion, I realized that the questioner associated the exclusive use of intuition with "Bionian", not Kleinian, part-object interpretations. Not realizing during my analysis with him that he "specialized" in "intuition", I failed to notice how intuitive he must have been—but, then, how would I have known? What I did experience was that he was very "Kleinian", but with a flourish! He introduced me to part-objects I had never contemplated—consciously.

First, I must reveal a little about why I decided to enter analysis with Bion. A few months prior to that decision, Betty Joseph had visited Los Angeles and presented a paper. I recall even now, so many years later, how deeply depressed I had precipitously become after hearing her present that paper. It was a depression that was utterly beyond words. I then entered analysis with Bion. I was soon to learn that not only was it *beyond* words, it was *before* words. As I entered his waiting room and sat down, I picked up a London weekly magazine that was lying on the stand by the chair. As I glanced at it, I came across an advertisement for "The White House Hotel". Bion then opened the door from his consulting room and welcomed me in. As I stood up to enter the room, I called Dr Bion's attention to the advertisement and mentioned what a wonderful dinner my wife and I had had in the restaurant at the White House Hotel on our first visit to London. Bion said nothing at that moment. I then lay down on his couch, uttered two or three associations, which I have long since forgotten, and then he interpreted the following (to the best of my memory from across the years):

"It is hoped that upon entering analysis here with me you might anticipate having a good meal at *this* White House Restaurant, 'White House' being a way of uniting us, the 'White House' of my native country and the 'White House' of yours, which you are now putting together." [*A Kleinian interpretation—but what a Kleinian interpretation!*]

Bion said quite a bit more in that first intervention, but I can no longer recall it. I do recall, however, how impressed I was that virtually every one of the words in my associations was taken up, used, and rephrased so that I was receiving from him a somewhat altered and deepened version of what I had uttered. It was like hearing myself in an echo chamber or sound mirror in which I was being amplified while being edited. It was dazzling! Then I revealed some details about my depression. I mentioned that I felt that it was "beyond words". He soon reflected back to me that he believed that it was not only "*beyond* words", it was "*before* words" [*Bionian interpretation*]. I presented two persistent visual phantasies to him, one of which harkened back in all probability to my premature birth due to my mother's *placenta abrupta*. The analysis had hit "pay dirt" in the first session. As I mentioned previously, Bion would never repeat an interpretation, even if I had not heard him clearly. He would state, "I cannot repeat it. The time is past. We have to catch it later—downstream—in its transformation."

One could always feel Bion's highly focused attention upon one. Often when I was silent he might say, "That seems to be a meaningful silence." I always wondered how he knew it was "meaningful" (perhaps Bionian reverie?). He was unusually empathic as well as intuitive. I recall how, when I may have appeared "omnipotent" to him, he would interpret to me that I was "*reduced* to becoming omnipotent" because of my feelings of helplessness in a situation I had presented to him.

On another occasion I recall becoming depressed over a situation that had occurred. I shall never forget his response:

"Here you are, the most important person you're ever likely to meet in your lifetime, and you're telling me you're on bad terms with this person. That requires evidence." [*Bionian interpretation*]

Another unforgettable interpretation occurred after I had responded to a particularly effective interpretation by commenting, "That was a beautiful interpretation":

"Yes, a beautiful interpretation, you say. The snag is that my 'beautiful interpretation' was made possible only by virtue of your 'beautiful associations'. You were so keen on listening to me that you neglected listening to yourself speaking to me." [*Bionian interpretation*]

I concluded from that interchange, first, that it was his own unique way of addressing idealization; and, second, that it was his way of helping me, as a patient, to refocus on how *I* experience *my* interactions with him. The traditional Kleinian focus on the object by the infant was shifted to a focus by the infant *on* the infant's focusing on its *experience of focusing on the object*.

As a derivative of this idea, Bion seemed to suggest that the analysand as well as the analyst should *listen to themselves listening to each other*. Bion was clearly a direct descendant of Socrates.

Bion was always essentially Kleinian, however. Because of the recent surge in interest in Bion, many have begun thinking of him and reading him as a guru who was—or who had become—independent of Melanie Klein. My own view from my analysis with him was that he was essentially—and deeply—Kleinian, but with his own unique flourish. I do not believe one can appreciate his works without having a familiarity with Kleinian ideas, such as the relationship between the paranoid–schizoid and depressive positions (P–S $\leftrightarrow$ D), persecutory and depressive anxieties, the archaic part-object Oedipus complex (Kleinian version), greed, envy, and splitting and projective identification. I recall many of Bion's interpretations that were essentially Kleinian part-object interventions. I remember the session, for instance, in which, upon beginning the session, I exclaimed how happy I was. His interpretation was:

"Well, it's felt that you've found the cure. What's missing is the illness." [*Kleinian interpretation*]

What a beautiful way of interpreting the manic defence! It was followed by some reference on his part to urine and faeces, and I knew then I was in a Kleinian analysis. I recall another time when I produced associations that revealed that I had found myself to have been in a state of projective identification with him; his response: "Well, you can't get any closer to someone than to become them."

I remember a time when I regaled him with protests on how badly I had been treated that morning by the psychiatric residents I had been teaching. His response was:

"I hear what you say about how you didn't feel respected by the psychiatric residents, and I have listened to your evidence for that protest. You were there. I wasn't, so I have to accept your version as to what happened. But at the same time and on another level[1] I think you may be referring to a me who is felt to be "resident" within you, criticizing you, having no respect for you in comparison to your respect for me." [*Kleinian and Bionian interpretation*]

It gradually occurred to me that the "residents" comprised a double representation: first, they represented Bion as an enviously critical superego within me; second, they represented the enviously attacking me who was attacking Bion, for whom I stood in the manifest situation. In other words, the residents who were attacking me were a reconstruction of my enviously attacking Bion.

Bion often referred to how dependent on companionship and relationship man is. He would over and over again stress that man always will be a "dependent creature. Man is a dependent creature no matter how autonomous he becomes." He seemed to accord it instinctual status. He also referred to other instinctual longings of man. He often referred to man's "religious instinct", stating that Freud never really understood the power of man's religious instinct—that it may even be more powerful than the libidinal instinct. He also frequently alluded to man's "quest for truth" (see chapter 10), where *I* accord truth the status of an instinctual drive. Along with these ideas, he stressed the *relationship* between self and object and between objects rather than the object itself. Thus, an unconscious attack against an object (old concept) becomes an attack against the *link* with the object.

Yet another unforgettable moment was the session in which I referred to my sister. His reply was:

"Your sister is not a member of your family. She is a member of your father's family. When you were a child and a member of your father's family, you were *rehearsing* becoming a grown-up, the time at which you would find your own family. That is the thing-in-itself. Childhood is the rehearsal." [*A very Bionian interpretation*]

A real "Bion moment" occurred in the following instance: Bion had given me an extensive and thorough interpretation about a worry I was having. I no sooner felt a sense of relief than he said the following:

"I have just given you an interpretation about your anxiety, and you seem to feel that it was correct, but in fact we shall never know the source of it. It is not to be known. We can only approximate it—or really, learn what it is not." [*A quintessentially Bionian interpretation*]

This episode occurred before I had any knowledge of his concept of O or uncertainty and of the "definitory hypothesis" and "Column 2", the latter of which helps one to decide what the definitory hypothesis is *not*. All I could think of as a response at the time were the words of a Hebrew prayer: "The Lord giveth, the Lord taketh away. Hallowed be the name of the Lord."

During the "time of the troubles" in Los Angeles, when the Los Angeles Psychoanalytic Society and the American Psychoanalytic Association sought to expel the Kleinians (I was one), senior Kleinian analysts here and abroad were prevailed upon to write letters in protest. Bion's response was unique. His letter merely stated: "Doctors should not advertise" [*very Bionian*].

On another occasion, following an interpretation, I replied, "I understand." Bion seemed to have been annoyed by my response and exclaimed, "Why didn't you say, 'overstand', or 'circumstand'?" Once again I revealed my ignorance of his metatheory for psychoanalysis and how he viewed "understanding" with a jaundiced eye. Similarly, following another interpretation, I said, "I follow you." He responded with, "Yes, I was afraid of that!" [*very Bionian*].

I recall the time when I was in a negative transference with Bion and became critical of his London Kleinian colleagues. I said something about "perfidious Al*bion*". He asked, "I say, is that a pun?" [*Bionian*]. In the same session I criticized Melanie Klein, after which he asked: "Did you know Melanie Klein? How did you know her?" [*Bionian*]. What a beautiful display that was of his L, H, and K links! How does one really get to *know* another person except by one's emotional response to them—in person? Those are "analytic facts".

Once we were speaking about my interest in Scotland, and I alluded to Mary, Queen of Scots. He replied, "The trouble with Mary was that she believed that she *was* the queen rather than attempting to *become* one. You know, I am not an analyst. I am merely trying to become one" [*this interpretation represents Platonic Bion*].

At times I would feel myself descending into a trance and felt that I was hovering about at the morning of time. When I then left Bion's office, I would instantly feel unusually clear and focused.

I found myself deeply impressed by yet another of Bion's interpretations. Following my associations, which revealed that I had unwittingly become grandiose on an occasion, Bion interpreted:

> "You were *reduced* to becoming omnipotent because you felt you couldn't handle the danger implicit in that circumstance otherwise." [*Very Bionian*]

Being *"reduced"* to being omnipotent was such a precise, technical way of identifying omnipotence as a defence and also identifying the anxiety behind the defence at the same time.

I have saved the best for last. On one occasion, when I was discussing sexual material in reference to my parents, Bion commented:

> "The penis and the vagina are disgusting sexual organs! They deserve each other!" [*Bionian*]

Bion did have a dry sense of humour. I also recall that in a lecture he referred to "a patient who was silent in three languages".

Upon later reflection, long after the analysis was ended, I began to wonder whether Bion was not only an analyst but also a Zen master. Often when Bion spoke I did not understand much of what he was saying—and he said a lot—but I did seem to resonate with it preconsciously. It always had an effect.

On the negative side, a Kleinian colleague who had known Bion in London remarked on how few, if any, remarkable patients had emerged from his analysis in London or Los Angeles—with the exception of Francis Tustin, who seems to have been ambivalent about her analysis with him (personal communication, 1988). None seems to be among the current London post-Kleinians. Time will tell with regard to his American experience.

NOTE

1. I was so impressed by this phrase, which analysts so often use, that I have decided to use it as a title for a textbook on psychoanalytic technique that I am currently in the process of writing.

CHAPTER 3

What kind of person was Bion?

I put forth the question but have no definitive answer. The person who appeared in the interstices of analytic moments ran the range of being distant, withdrawn, disciplined, dedicated, empathic (extremely), personable, warm, interested, friendly—but measured! He did not socialize much to my knowledge with individuals here in Los Angeles, and, reading the accounts of others who worked with him in his "group" days, one gets the impression that his stalwartness and redoubtable individuality may have put people off in England. In public he was quietly but powerfully charismatic. I don't see him as "one of the boys". I have often wondered whether he had any close friends. I often wished that I could have known him post-analytically. The London Kleinians discredit "late Bion": the one after *Transformations* and particularly the one who emigrated to Los Angeles. This pains me enormously, but I cannot help wondering what they knew that I did not; on the other hand, I rather feel that I, having had the benefit of an analytic experience with him, know something that *they* did not, and still do not, know. Bion did not reach out. One had to come to him. This is especially true of his writing. I believe that he was honest and trustworthy to a fault and was quietly adamant in his beliefs but was always the consummate gentleman.

Bion was never dogmatic—except about his ignorance! He was certainly Socrates' descendant.

  DOI: 10.4324/9781003348665-4

At times I had the opportunity to observe him walking at a distance from me. He had a measured gait that seemed almost military to me, thus revealing his self-control. His shoes were always highly polished. His range of emotional expressiveness was narrow. Yet one thing stands out: he was—and is—utterly unforgettable! Had I read his autobiography prior to going into analysis with him, I wonder whether I really would have decided to go ahead. His life was so tragic that one can only empathically grieve while reading about it, especially the entry: "I died on August 8, 1918, on the Amiens–Roye Road."

I recall the dinner my wife and I had with him and his wife, Francesca, at our home on the evening before their return to England. He was quite affable and approachable then. He talked of his war experiences and of other personal matters. He knew, of course, about my affinity for Scotland, so I played some bagpipe pibrochs[1] on my stereo. I recall how deeply involved, almost tearful, he became when the "The Drummer Boy of Mallow" was playing. I treasure that last and only personal moment we shared together.

This chapter is, of necessity, short because I did not get the opportunity to know Bion over time in real time as opposed to analytic time—nor would I mention here the remembrances of him by others. Bion taught me to listen to myself and avoid "gossip": the verdicts and opinions of others.

NOTE

1. I had not realized it at the time, but Bion was very fond of the sound of bagpipes. According to Francesca Bion, "They reminded him of the sound of the 51st Highland Division and the way it lifted the spirit of the troops who had been through such hellish experiences" (personal communication, 2006).

CHAPTER 4

Bion's vision

"... all the unpublished virtues of this earth ..."

Shakespeare, *King Lear*

In 1977 Bion began one of his lectures in New York with:

Well, here we are. But where is "here"? I remember a time when I was at an address—some seventy years ago—which I called "Newbury House, Hadam Road, Bishops Stortford, Hertfordshire, England, Europe. Another small boy said to me, "You have left out 'The World'." So I put that in to too. Since then I have been told by the astronomers that we are part and parcel of a nebular universe, a spiral nebula to which our solar system belongs. ... According to the astronomers the spiral nebula, of which our solar system is a part, is itself rotating; it is a long way from one side to the other and a long time ... before we are at the same spot again—something like twice ten to the power of eight million light years—so far indeed that if we look towards the galactic centre there is nothing to see excepting the remnants of the Crab Nebula which is still in process of exploding. To us it looks immense because we are such ephemeral creatures. [1980, pp. 9–10]

It is my impression that this citation expresses Bion's vision of the triune universe, which includes the internal (the unconscious) and

DOI: 10.4324/9781003348665-5

external (consciousness) worlds, and the Unknown, which is beyond us externally *and* internally. Gerald Edelman (2004) reflects this cosmic dimension in the title of his new work, *Wider Than the Sky: The Phenomenal Gift of Consciousness*. Bion's view of O can only be non-sensually approximated by our concept of an ultra-universe that presents itself first to consciousness and the unconscious and then exclusively through the latter. His vision of our task is for us "to become our O" or, more properly, to have our O, our godhead (which I shall deconstruct later), incarnate us as we are in the act of fully and authentically feeling our passions (emerging emotions)—that is, become united with the ever-evolving O that has intersected[1] with our inner and outer universes—to *become*[2] it by allowing O to become us—knowing all the while that that task would require an infinite number of lifetimes and would still not succeed because O evolves more rapidly than our becoming it.

Whereas Freud and, particularly, Klein, steeped as they were in positivism and in "mechanisms", drives, and phantasies, seemed to view the unconscious as a seething cauldron of negativity and destructiveness, Bion proffered a vastly different view—one that was characterized by emotions and infinite imagination. Bion had uncovered a different "bipolar man" from the one Freud had. He uncovered "infinite man", who was also an incomplete man, one who, though infinite, longed to be realized in and by real human emotional experience: O as inherent pre-conception → conception—in the act of accepting (feeling) O as one's rightful emotions. Put another way, Bion would have finite man accept and allow infinite man to become he (incarnate), as best as he can at each moment, all the while realizing the hopelessness of completing that teleological task. If this seems too dense at the moment, I promise to clarify it as I proceed. I only wish here to give a preview of the "Bionic revolution" for psychoanalysis and for Western thought.

Bion, the transcendentalist

Many Bion scholars and other theorists emphasize Bion's now famous concept of container ↔ contained and his alteration of Klein's conception of projective identification from an exclusively unconscious, omnipotent phantasy to a realistic pre-lexical communication between infant and mother and between analyst and analysand. As a result of these ground-breaking discoveries Bion has been accorded the role of the one who introduced *intersubjectivity* (the indivisibility of the two-person relationship) into Kleinian, as well as general, analytic thinking. What is often lost sight of is *"transcendentalist[3] Bion"*. My reading of Bion and my experience of having been in analysis with him convince me that the importance of analysis was not only its role in facilitating healthy object relations: its more important role was in facilitating the *infusion* of the ego by the Ideal Forms (things-in-themselves) in the crucible of self-acknowledged suffering.

Plato's Ideal Forms or Kant's noumena (things-in-themselves), O, inescapably happen and indent our very being with their intrusive, confrontative surges and fluctuations. The analyst ("who could not be less important or felt to be more important"—Bion, personal communication) is the conduit or link between the ego and consciousness of the patient—through the analyst—to the patient's own unconscious, the ultimate object of the patient's envy. In other words, one of the main values of object relations is the realization that we inescapably need others to establish contact with our inner self or, better yet, to allow our inner self to become us. In this way we evolve as an *"Übermensch"* ("higher man").

A brief note on the differing psychoanalytic aims of Freud, Klein, and Bion

At the risk of the accusation of overgeneralizing, I think the following constitutes a fair summary of the differences in Freud's, Klein's, and Bion's psychoanalytic aims. Freud, I conjecture, would have analysands work through their infantile neurosis (Oedipus complex) and the infantile sexuality that subtends it to enable them to love and to work more efficaciously. Klein would have analysands transcend the paranoid–schizoid position and attain the depressive position, presupposing that their infantile psychosis *and* neurosis have been worked through, including the withdrawal of projective identifications, the undertaking of mourning for the lost object, and the conduction of reparations—in other words, the infantile portion of the personality must renounce its hatred, envy, greed, and omnipotence. Bion, while still including the preceding, would have analysands attain the faith and discipline of "negative capability" so that they can accept and become O—that is, can transcend even the depressive position and be at one with their emotions—so as to keep their rendezvous with their infinite creative self. Of the three, Bion's aims are the more ontological as well as epistemological and phenomenological—to say nothing of hopeful.

Having studied psychoanalysis in a classical Freudian institute and having had four analyses (the first orthodox Freudian, the second Fairbairnian, the third by Bion, a Kleinian–Bionian, and the fourth with a traditional Kleinian, occasioned by the fact that Bion left Los Angeles while I was in the middle of my analysis with him), I have been able to identify some significant differences between Freud and Klein and between them and Bion. In my orthodox Freudian analysis (my analyst had been analysed by Freud) I felt that I was on a pilgrimage to recover buried memories and to keep my rendezvous with my acknowledgment of my repressed libidinal drive. In my Fairbairnian analysis my pilgrimage was mainly with buried memories in terms of objects. In my traditional Kleinian analysis my pilgrimage was with my destructiveness: that is, my death instinct, which hampered my ability to love. With Bion, my pilgrimage was to acknowledge, with reverence and awe, the majesty and enormity of my mind and to recognize how cut-off I was from it—and how my anxieties and symptoms were but intimations of my inner "immortality" and infinite resources. As I discuss later, Bion's discovery of O and its transformations resulted in the primacy of importance of the drives in general and the death drive in particular becoming marginalized. Bion shifted the focus from drives to emotions and restructured the drives as L, H, and K emotional linkages between self and objects and as emotional categories for these links—a revolutionary development!

Where Bion differs from Freud: Freud and Bion on dreaming

Bion read Freud closely, particularly his *Interpretation of Dreams* (1900a) and his "Two Principles of Mental Functioning" (1911b); he then extended and reconceptualized Freud's work on dreaming by hypothesizing that we dream by day and by night and that everything we perceive consciously must be taken into the unconscious via dreaming. Put another way, Bion believed that dreaming is directed as much towards one's daily experiences (day residue) as towards the products of the internal world, and that the analyst must "dream" the analytic session, much as the mother must "dream" her infant's experiences. Behind this idea is Bion's belief that the *experience* of dreaming constitutes unconscious thinking and is directed, in conjunction with α-function, its *model*,[4] towards the processing of β-elements produced by the intersection of evolving O.

Freud believed that dreaming was in the service of the pleasure principle. Ferro (2002a), in his reading of Bion, assigns α-function to the transformation of β-elements into α-elements for sensory dream images and dreaming and for the harvesting of these dream images into narratives. The initial stage of transformation may be called "mentalization", whereas the subsequent stage may be called "thinking". Bion believed that dreaming was in the service of a "joint venture" of the reality and pleasure principles to transform the raw ore of the Absolute Truth about Ultimate impersonal Reality into tolerable personal emotional reality as a mid-stage prior to thinking and objectification. In other words *impersonal* O becomes transformed into *personal* O: that is, the subject *claims* impersonal fate as his portion—*moira*—to accept and to live out.

Where Bion extends, and differs from, Melanie Klein

> "I must leave Ireland and create in the smithy of my soul the uncreated conscience of my race!"
>
> Stephen Dedalus, in James Joyce's (1916) *Portrait of the Artist as a Young Man.*

Bion had lived through, had suffered, traumata (he was keenly aware of the difference between "enduring" and "suffering") that Klein's psychoanalytic positivistic reference-base may have been inadequate to contemplate. Her earth was comparatively flat in comparison to his and ended at the life and death instincts. Bion needed not only the third dimension of roundness but also infinite dimensions to embrace, countenance, or grasp the inner cosmic uncertainty that plagued him all his life and the ghastly, traumatic "black holes" into which his fate had placed him. In short, Klein was probably more competent at analysing the "infantile psychosis" than the nameless dread of trauma and its inescapable "black holes". I say this not to demean Klein. She was arguably the finest or one of the finest analysts, clinically, of the last century. Passages in Bion's autobiography (1982, 1985) and in *A Memoir of the Future* (1975, 1977b, 1979, 1981) seem, however, to hint at something that was missing in his analysis with Klein, and I cannot help wondering whether he spent the rest of his career trying to chart the unknown landscape of inner and outer cosmic uncertainty that he felt his analysis should have explored.

Bion, in fact, extended Klein by adding O, the Absolute Truth *about* Ultimate Reality,[5] supraordinate factors that marginalized and subordinated the life and death instincts as well as the epistemophilic instinct—to say nothing of the positivism that subtended them. He added the infinite dimension to Kleinian—and Freudian—thinking. He extended projective identification from an exclusively unconscious intrapsychic phantasy to a normal, realistic, intersubjective form of communication. He reconceptualized Klein's theory of the succession of the paranoid–schizoid and depressive positions into a higher dialectical dimension in which they occur simultaneously and mediate one another (P–S ↔ D) in the triangulation of O. He added an interpersonal, adaptive, attachment dimension to Kleinian thinking with his concept of container ↔ contained and the absolute necessity for the inclusion into the psychoanalytic equation of the real (external) mother's importance and her state of reverie. He added the concept of reverie to the analyst's toolkit.

Finally, with O, he moved Kleinian analysis from its basis in certainty to "*post*-post-Kleinian" uncertainty",[6] complexity, and infinity. Bion distinguished "countertransference" from "reverie": according to him, the former always represents the analyst's unresolved infantile neurosis, whereas reverie predicates the analyst's resonance with the patient.

Bion also differed from Klein in certain other areas. Some writers have speculated that Klein did not approve of Bion's interest in the study of groups (Sutherland, 1985, p. 54; and personal communication). They also seem to have differed in terms of Bion's notion of inherent pre-conceptions, which he had derived from Plato and Kant. Klein, however, did believe that the knowledge of parental intercourse *was* inherited, but it is my understanding that that was the only exception (Klein, 1960). They certainly differed on the therapeutic importance of the analyst's emotions as a valuable analytic instrument in the analytic session. Klein and Paula Heimann came to grief and parted from each other on this issue. Bion persisted, and now his concept of the analyst's reverie has become an analytic tool used by virtually every school of analysis and taken for granted by psychotherapists everywhere. Not only did he seek to normalize projective identification as communication; he also sought to normalize the paranoid–schizoid position as "patience" and the depressive position as "security".

The difference between Klein and Bion lies in the expansion of the analytic worldview from one restricted to involving the internal world of the analysand to the one we now see practised by the modern London post-Kleinians, one in which issues of intersubjectivity are manifest. In the excellent and informative new monograph, *In Pursuit of Psychic Change: The Betty Joseph Workshop* (Hargreaves & Varchevker, 2004), we can sense that Bion's ghost is unmistakably the "elephant in the workshop". This change in worldview is of considerable importance. We come away from Freud and Klein with an internal worldview that is stoic: the instinctual-drive aspects of the analysand must become tamed (civilized). *We come away from Bion with a more epicurean expansiveness: the internal domain of the infinite is our oyster!*

Another way of thinking about the differences between Klein and Bion involves a philosophical one about the patient. Klein, and even post-Kleinian analytic thinking, emphasizes the infant's relationship to the object, and this relationship(s) *defines* him. In other words, the infant is destined or doomed to become what he believes he has done to the object. Furthermore, Kleinians and post-Kleinians believe that the conflict between the life and death instincts constitutes a first cause (fundamental), with special emphasis placed on the latter with regard to its destructiveness. Because of their belief in the supraordinate position of the death instinct, Kleinian and post-Kleinian analysts seem to become veritable religious missionaries whose task it is to save the infantile portion of the analysand from sin.

As Meltzer (1986) maintained, Kleinian thinking is very religious: it even may seem Calvinistic (I believe this, yet I am Kleinian as well as Bionian). When I reflect upon my analysis with Bion, I can feel how Kleinian he was—even with regard to his derivative references to the death instinct and to his emphasis, especially, on the importance of one's dependency on an object—yet he viewed the patient as an individual in his own right, separate from the object. The hope for the Kleinian and post-Kleinian patient is to come to peace with his vulnerability and dependency but also with his antagonists, omnipotence, envy, hate, and greed—so as to be able to relate to his objects in a reciprocally loving way. He will have been saved from primal sin. Bion's patient becomes heir to the legacy of his infinite self, his "godhood" ("godliness").[7] In order to do this, the patient must be analytically contained and thereby be able to *suffer*, not blindly *endure*, the pain of emotional experiences. Each time an individual *feels* (suffers) his *emotional* pain, he becomes reunited with his godhood self, his infinite self (the Ideal Forms, the noumena), and thereby *evolves*.

NOTES

1. Bion uses the term "intersection" with regard to O rather than "impingement" or "intrusion" in order to achieve more scientific (mathematical) precision.

2. I am using "become" in the way Bion (personal communication) explained to me that Plato did: "That which is is always becoming." In other words, becoming is never completed: it is always evolving.

3. Kant (1787) distinguishes between "transcendental" and "transcendent". The former refers to what Freud (1915e) refers to as the "unrepressed unconscious", which houses Plato's Ideal Forms and/or Kant's noumena and primary categories. The latter connotes speculative attempts to achieve a more lofty status.

4. I discuss what I believe is the relationship between dreaming, the *experience*, and α-function, the *model*, further on.

5. The reader will notice that I arbitrarily reconfigure Bion's conception of O as "the Absolute Truth *about* Ultimate Reality". Unlike Bion, I believe that Truth → truth lies within the self, whereas Ultimate Reality lies both within *and* beyond the self.

6. I explain why I say "*post*-post-Kleinian" as I proceed.

7. It is my impression that Bion's use of "godhead" is not to designate "God" as mankind thinks of and worships (deifies) "Him". It is meant to convey the Platonic archetype or Ideal Form of the one whose consummate wisdom is inclusive of the Forms. "Godliness" would be closer to that usage. "God*hood*", the more ancient English term for it, seems to be a more felicitous term for "god*head*".

CHAPTER 5

Bion's legacy

Overview

W hen Rabbi Hillel was commanded by a Roman general to reveal the essence of the Hebrew Bible while standing on one foot, he said: "Do not do unto others what you would not have them do unto you." While I cannot be quite so brief in epitomizing the work of Bion, I will try to summarize it. Bion pulled the positivistic psychoanalysis of Freud and Klein into the new, uncharted realms of *uncertainty*: from the strictures and prison of verbal language to a realm beyond and before language. Here one experiences the dread of O, the Absolute Truth about an Ultimate, infinite, ineffable, always evolving, uncertain,[1] and impersonal Reality that supplants the putative dread of the positivistic drives. We are born as fateful prisoners to the quality of the maternal—and paternal—container that (who) initially contains our raw dread of O.

Analysts, like mothers and fathers, must be able to descend into reverie so as to be optimally receptive to "becoming" the patient's anguish—as if by exorcism—and to be able to detect the "name" of the anguish by becoming an "analyst of achievement" who is conversant with the "Language of Achievement", the ancient and primal pre-lexical/sub-lexical language of body emotions prior to their being felt by the mind as feelings. Emotions (α-elements), which are transformed

DOI: 10.4324/9781003348665-6

proto-emotions (β-elements derived from the impact of evolving O on one's emotional frontier), are the vehicular carriers of Truth. The recipient of Truth must undergo a transformation of self in order to accept, accommodate to, become, Truth by rendering it first *personally meaningful* through α-function and dreaming and then *objective* through an advanced form of α-function and dreaming—that is, wakeful dream thinking (Bion, 1962b), as contrasted with dreaming while asleep.

Bion's views about
container ↔ contained and α-function

Bion believed that in the container ↔ contained situation the infant projects, for instance, its fear of dying, among other proto-emotions, into its mother-as-container, who, in a state of reverie and with the use of her own α-function, absorbs, defuses, transduces, detoxifies—that is, "dreams"—her infant's projections. During this "exorcistic dreaming" she sorts out the nature and content of the projections: what they *are* and what they are *not* (as if using a Grid). After many successful iterations of this protocol the infant introjects mother's α-function capacity as well, perhaps, as the legacy (memory) of the successful experience. Now the infant, newly equipped with α-function of its own, is able to project internally its proto-emotions into its own α-function and sort them out. *This event, according to Bion, is the beginning of the infant's capacity to think.* If we stop to think about the protocol that Bion puts forth in his conception of container ↔ contained, the medical model of *dialysis* comes to mind as an analogue model.

My own views about
container ↔ contained and α-function

I should like to proffer an alternative protocol to Bion's. While I certainly believe that Bion is correct in his conception, I consider that, side-by-side-with it, another protocol takes place. I posit that the infant is born with rudimentary (inherited) α-function with which it is prepared to generate pre-lexical communications and to receive prosodic lexical communications from mother (Norman, 2004, and personal communication, 2002; Schore, 2003a, 2003b; personal communication, 2006; Trevarthen, 1999, and personal communication, 2004). I believe, in other words, that the infant is born with the emotional counterpart to, or equivalent of, Chomsky's (1957, 1968) "transformational generative syntax". In other words, the infant is born as a semiotic entity in his own right and can communicate with signals and signs (Salomonsson, 2007). He is a capable semiotic individual, one who can generate and receive communications, the latter of which should, I believe, be distinguished from projective (trans-)identification, which "comes online" when communication fails. Mother's task is to affirm and confirm the infant's emotional experience and to facilitate the maturation and development of its capacity for α-function.

Moreover, in my opinion the infant projects not only the fear of dying, because of insufficient containment of its death instinct, but also its fear of "unassisted living"—the unbidden thrusts of its ever-evolving entelechy (the activation of its potential self-to-be and to become), that is, the feared premature arrival of its future. This latter idea, that of entelechy, prompts me to suggest the following: in *my* opinion, the Ideal Forms generate the infant's own rudimentary (yet to be further transformed) α-elements, which conjoin with the pre-processed sensory stimuli (Bion's "β-elements") to form what I, along with Ferro, term "balpha-elements" ("βα", or really, "αβ": Ferro, 1999, p. 47). The whole point here, I believe, is that (a) "α" precedes "β"; (b) the α-element may have an earlier beginning in the Ideal Forms, have already been conceived by a hypothesized Intelligence or Presence (Bion's and Meister Eckhart's "god"), and exist on a gradient of transformational sophistication as it proceeds. The term "β-element" should, according to my reading of Bion, be reserved for pre-processed sensory stimuli. I am fortified in my assumption about the secondary rather than primary (temporally—i.e. position in succession) status of the β-element by a comparison with Bion's (1970) conception that the liar is closer to the truth than are others *because* he knows the truth that he cannot tolerate and therefore has to lie about it.

Bion's analogic thinking

Unlike most analytic thinkers, Bion was able to extricate himself from the closed loop of analytic thinking by using analogic thinking—that is, models. For instance, α-function is an imaginative analogue-model for dreaming, a putative transformational process that orders emotional life. When our physician informs us that our blood pressure is "120/80", we concretize the number as an absolute rather than realizing that that pressure reading is but an arbitrary *analogue* to the unknown and unknowable pressure in our brachial artery at the time. By stepping outside the domain we are studying, we gain a more objective perspective of the subject of inquiry. The binocular perspective (e.g. observation and use of models) allows one to regard any phenomenon from at least two points of view (vertices).

Bion's conception of thinking

Thinking itself is, according to Bion, essentially unconscious. What we nominally call "thinking" might better be called "after-thinking" or "secondary thinking", and what we call "thoughts" might better be called "after-thoughts" or "secondary thoughts". Bion brought psychoanalytic metapsychology into alignment with metaphysics and ontology. He found myths to be useful clinically as "scientific deductive systems" in their own right; he also found science to be a myth because it was "sense"-ibly based.

Freud's conception of the relationship between the Systems *Ucs.* and *Cs.* was linear and conflictual and therefore one-dimensional. Bion, in applying a binocular perspective, allowed for the relationship between them to be not necessarily one of *conflict* but one of binary (cooperative) *opposition*—that is, System *Ucs.* ↔ System *Cs.* Furthermore, he states: "The differentiating factor that I wish to introduce is not between *conscious* and *unconscious*, but between *finite* and *infinite*" (Bion, 1965, p. 46). The same applies to the relationship between the paranoid–schizoid and depressive positions. Klein conceived them to be conflictual, linear, and hierarchic (privileging the latter). Bion conceived of them as operating simultaneously and functioning in a cooperative binary opposition (P–S ↔ D). Ultimately, Bion reconfigured the unconscious as *infinity* in contrast to the *finiteness* of consciousness.

These are just hints at Bion's remarkable agility in deconstructing and reconfiguring existing psychoanalytic models; there are more to follow.

Bion's psychoanalytic protocol: "abandon memory and desire"

Following a suggestion of Freud's, Bion—eschewing the use of the language of the senses (the language of substitution: images or representations)—sought a way for the analyst to approximate the meditative-like stance (reverie) of the infant's mother—to shut out all stimuli from within the analyst (memory, desire, preconceptions, understanding) in order to be optimally receptive to the subverbal emanations of the emotional being-in-flux of the patient. He consequently exhorted the analyst to abandon memory and desire as well as preconceptions[2] and understanding, the derivatives of sensation, so as to avoid being misled by images or symbols that, though they *represent* the object, *are not* the object experientially. Only then can the analyst, with much patience—the patience of tolerating uncertainty and doubt—be qualified to *become*[3] the analysand, or more precisely, become the analysand's state of mind. In this state of reverie, the analyst has thus become the container of the analysand's projected mental content (contained).

"Exorcism" as the model for "becoming"

Although Bion never employed the term, it seems to me that he is, among other things, describing the mystical act of *"exorcism"*, whereby demons are transferred from analysand to analyst (or infant to mother). Where his ideas differ is that in the religious practice of exorcism the direction is unilateral: from sufferer to deliverer. The model is crucifixion with absolution. In psychoanalysis the trajectory is bi-directional: from patient to analyst–container, who then returns them as detoxified. The analyst, as the mother does for her infant, absorbs the analysand's pain by *"becoming"* the analysand/infant (specifically "becoming" the latter's emotional state of mind) and allowing it to become part of him/herself. In his reverie he then allows his own repertoire of personal experiences to be summoned from his own unconscious so that some of them may be symmetrical to or match up with the analysand's still unfathomable projections (β-elements, O). Eventually, the analyst sees (feels) a pattern in the material, the experience of which is called the "selected fact"—that is, the pattern becomes the selected fact that allows the analyst to interpret the intuited pattern (create a permanent constant conjunction of the elements presented—that is, give them a name that binds them). If I read Bion correctly on this subject, the analyst does not *really* become the analysand: he becomes his own autochthonously created *version* of the analysand's distress, the components of which have been harvested and summoned from within the known as well as unknown repertoire of his own emotional experiences (Grotstein, 2005).

Projective identification, interpersonal communication, and beyond

Bion's conception of container ↔ contained, along with his communicative extension of Klein's conception of projective identification, is generally thought of as constituting a two-person intersubjective system. While I believe this to be accurate, I should like to add what I believe occurs on a deeper level. From my personal analysis with Bion and from my reading of *Transformations* (1965) and *Attention and Interpretation* (1970), especially the sections that deal with "incarnation" by the godhead" (1965, pp. 139, 149, 153; 1970, pp. 77, 88), I should like to offer yet another level to the functioning of container ↔ contained. First, I should like to develop the background to my theme. Hegel suggested than man does not need an object: he needs the object's desire. *I* say that, strictly speaking, man does *not* need an object *per se*: he needs *experiences* with objects, which he needs to value and/or devalue (L, H, and K evaluations).

What an infant needs from its mother, or an analysand from his analyst, is, among other things, a "consultation" with his mother/analyst as to who he (the infant/analysand) is and what he needs in order to fulfil himself (to mature, evolve). In analysis, the analysand projects his unconscious (System *Ucs.*) into his analyst; consequently, he expects the analyst to be omniscient about him. In fact, the analysand is communicating with himself (his unconscious) by speaking to the analyst. The analyst has become a *channel* of communication between the analysand and his own unconscious. A derivative of this idea is that envy, particularly in analysis, is directed towards the analysand's own unconscious, with which he cannot communicate, but *it* communicates with *him*, through the analyst as channel (the truest meaning of "transference"). This is what I believe Bion meant when he conceived of α-function and container ↔ contained.

The seamless interrelationship between container ↔ contained, the Grid, α-function, and contact-barrier

The analyst's function as container seamlessly blends, in my opinion, with Bion's notions of α-function, the contact-barrier between Systems *Ucs.* and *Cs.*, and the Grid in so far as each of these processes helps to mediate, isolate, differentiate, distinguish, define, and categorize incoming data, thereby establishing constant conjunctions (names). The α-function intercepts the β-elements (sensory impressions of O and pre-conceptions) of raw, unfertilized experience and transforms them into α-elements, which are suitable for memory and thoughts (feelings)—but also for reinforcing the contact-barrier and contributing necessary dream elements for dreaming. The sturdier the contact-barrier, the more the analysand can learn from his experience because he is better able to think—*because he is able to dream*—thanks to the contact-barrier's capacity to maintain a selectively permeable boundary between Systems *Cs.* ↔ *Ucs.* Thinking, for Bion, follows thoughts that first arrive as "wild thoughts" (1997; López-Corvo, 2006) or "thoughts without a thinker" awaiting a dreamer–thinker (a dreaming–thinking mind) to dream and to think them. Mother's reverie, with her α-function and dreaming, is the infant's first dreamer–thinker. Once the infant has introjected the mother's α-function (Bion's idea), he is then able to dream and think his own thoughts. Thus, the better the container with its (his) α-function, the better the analysand can feel and experience his emotional thoughts.

Further on I argue that α-function, contact-barrier, the Grid, container ↔ contained, transformations, and L, H, and K emotional linkages are all cognate—that is, overlapping views of the same phenomenon from differing vertices—and are components of what I term the *"dream ensemble"*. Put another way, all the above-mentioned Bion models comprise a *hologram*. Just as the chromosome of every individual cell of the body contains the genome for the whole body, so Bion has uncovered the mind's chromosome. Thus, I am proffering a model in which a living entity—dreaming—conceptually absorbs Bion's proposed models. They all do the same thing from different vertices.

Bion's epistemology

The *first* form of thinking is "becoming", which devolves into dreaming (phantasying), much of which is involved in reinforcing the selective permeable contact-barrier, dream-thoughts, and memory. The better the containment by the object or the self, the more effective is the selectivity of the contact-barrier in its capacity to define, refine, and guard the frontiers between *Ucs.* and *Cs.* and selectively allow "wild thoughts" (inspired) through from *Ucs.* to *Cs.* and irrelevant thoughts through from *Cs.* to *Ucs.* and to facilitate dreaming. Dreaming, in other words, reinforces the function of the contact-barrier, and conversely the functioning of the contact-barrier reinforces the function of dreaming.

The *second* form of thinking is Cartesian (cognitive) and is characterized by abstraction, reflection, correlation, publication, and shifting of perspectives. The second form of thinking can be seen in Bion's Grid, which is a polar-coordinated table in which the left-hand column, the genetic column, designates, from top to bottom, the progressive sophistication and abstraction of thoughts, and the column headings across the top designate thinking itself: how the thoughts are being thought about—that is, to what use they are being put. One of the key components of the Grid, Column 2, represents both *negation* and *falsification*, capacities upon which rational thought fundamentally depends. I personally believe that the Grid is apposite for and extends into the unconscious as well. In other words, all thinking, conscious or unconscious, requires sorting into categories. Column 2 designates *negation* for secondary-process thinking, *fictionalization* or *wish-fulfilment* for dreaming and/or phantasying, and *falsification* and/or *lying* for the individual who does not respect the truth. In other words, Column 2 represents what in Aristotelian logic is termed the "excluded middle": that is, if a person is a man, he cannot be a woman.

Interpenetrating Bion's ideas about the first and second forms of thinking is his notion of the contact-barrier and its flexible function of dividing and reuniting different elements. He refers to this in his formula, P–S ↔ D, where the former divides (differentiates) and the latter unites in improvisational combinatorial wizardry. I spoke of Bion's idea that thoughts require a thinker to think them. These thoughts undergo an epigenesis from the union of sense impressions and preconceptions to become realized as a conception and then a concept, and α-function conjoins the pre-conceptions with the sense impressions (the two sides of O that initially present as a β-element). Thinking itself undergoes an epigenesis from the concrete to the abstract (P–S ↔ D) application of L, H, and K linkages, and from primitive forms of α-function (primary process) to more advanced forms (secondary process).

The pursuit of truth

In his biography and in-depth survey of Bion and his contributions, Bléandonu (1993) separates the latter's work into four periods: the study of groups, the "psychotic period", the epistemological phase, and the mystical phase. Yet one can detect Ariadne's thread running through the entirety of Bion's work from beginning to end. That thread can be thought of as the search for and proscription against the acquisition of *truth*. In another contribution I put forth the notion that beneath the hidden order that runs through the entirety of Bion's works lies the concept of a *truth drive* and that all the ego's defence mechanisms are principally counterposed to the irruption of unconscious truth rather than of libido and aggression (Grotstein, 2004b). The human being, in other words, is really a truth-seeking and/or truth-avoiding individual, and psychopathology (symptoms) reflect a predisposition to the latter, while a healthy state reflects the former.

The role of the "infinite" and "incarnation" in Bion's thinking

Bion was a psychoanalytic cosmologist in so far as he valued the vastness and infinite resourcefulness of the unconscious, which he was ultimately to rename "infinity". His aim was to acquaint man with the awesomeness and wonder, rather than the dread, of the ineffable Otherness within and beyond him and to lead him to respect the truths that constantly evolve from it. Bion's analytic stance is to encourage man to allow himself to become incarnated by his ineffable, infinite reservoir of cosmic being. He discovered man's ontological (affective) epistemology and helped lay the groundwork for the nature of his phenomenology. I recall being transformed and transfixed by these ideas when I was in analysis with him. Bion's cosmic (internal and external) thinking was in marked contrast to that of Klein, whose episteme emphasizes dread (death instinct as first cause).

Godbout (2004) clarifies Bion's concept of the *incarnation*:

> To use Bion's expressions, he can only "become" it, "*incarnate*" it, be "at one" with it or, more accurately, "it" can only become, "it" can only *incarnate* itself in the person of the analysand. Bion insists on this subtlety, the change of "direction" from the analysand consenting to *incarnate* his "godhead" to the "godhead" consenting to incarnation in the person of the analysand, in order to differentiate what would pertain to mental health (the latter) and what would be closer to insanity (the former). [Godbout, 2004, p. 1133; italics added]

One of Bion's most complex concepts is that *of "incarnation"* (1965, p. 139; 1970, p. 77). He distinguishes between the status of Plato's Ideal Form and that of the state of incarnation in the first citation and clarifies it somewhat in the second citation when he speaks of the *mystic* and the latter's relationship to the group. I have conferred with a number of Bion scholars on this matter, and the consensus from most of them is that the act of incarnation does really apply to the transformation of an Ideal Form (inherent pre-conception, noumenon) to a conception through becoming an experienced realization and thus a phenomenon, but from others that Form and incarnation are distinct from one another. After being considerably perplexed about Bion's meaning in regard to this matter, I have come up with the following imaginative → reasonable conjectures about Form versus incarnation:

A. We must distinguish between: (1) the ordinary, *finite,* human-being aspects of ourselves; (2) our *infinite* (but incomplete) self representing the Ideal Forms and the noumena; and (3) the latent, if not actual, mystic or potential mystic, within us, the one that is distinct from the Forms and springs from a separate part of the psyche, the "god" part.

B. In the case of the infinite self, the Ideal Forms or noumena become *realized* by becoming transformed into conceptions → phenomena, which belong to the "*K link*", knowledge (about our emotions).

C. In the third case, the separate potential "god" portion of ourselves becomes incarnated as our realized mystical self as we "become O", bypassing the K route, and thereby ascend to transcendence in (becoming) O (Grotstein, 1999a, 2000a). This "God" is conceived by Bion, following Meister Eckhart, as an "immanent" god, one who dwells within us (Fox, 1981; McGinn, 1994, 1996).

D. Perhaps we may think of "godhood" (godhead) as the mystical, numinous essence of our godliness as a result of this incarnation. We will never *be* or *become* God; we can only become "godly" (godhood).[4]

E. Perhaps, additionally, we may think of "god" as the container of O, the contained.

F. Finally, the emergence of the mystic may correspond to transformations in O and our achievement of becoming an "*Übermensch*" (higher man) and also the "Man of Achievement".

It would seem that Bion's "godhead" represents the homunculus or demon who "knows" or who has "become" the composite potential wisdom of the other domain, the unconscious, infinity. Laplace's "demon" serves this function for mathematicians and physicists

(M. Schermer, 2003). He (it) is the one who knows all conceivable mathematical formulas and computations. Perhaps we could accord this construct an alternative title: the "Librarian of Plato's Ideal Forms and Kant's noumena, the only one who has access to the names of the 'memoirs of the future'". In another contribution I termed him the "ineffable subject of the unconscious" and the "dreamer who dreams the dream" and the "dreamer who understands the dream" (Grotstein, 2000a).

Bion:
the ontological and phenomenological epistemologist

Bion's contributions to epistemology are unique. For him, first of all, epistemology is irreducibly ontological (the study of the experience of being, of existence) and phenomenological (emotional). Second, he uniquely and brilliantly distinguished between *thoughts,* which are primary (as emotions), and *thinking,* which is secondary and had to arise in order to think (feel) the "orphan" "thoughts without a thinker" (López-Corvo, 2006). Next, he transcended Cartesian thinking, in which thoughts and mind are separated, to posit the concept of *"become",* which he apparently borrowed from Plato. "Become" in Plato's works has two meanings: (1) "That which is, is always becoming" (i.e. always evolving, in flux, never achieving), and (2) the percipient (perceiver) must "become" the percept, which represents a transformation in O prior to a transformation from O to K—the analyst's interpretation to the patient. "Become" does not implicate the analyst's fusion of personalities with the analysand. It means something quite different. According to Bion, the analyst, in response to and in resonance with the emotional outpourings from the analysand, must allow himself, in a state of reverie, to become induced into a trance-like state in which his (the analyst's) own, native internal reservoir of emotions and repertoire of buried experiences can become selectively recruited to match those he is experiencing resonantly from the analysand's inductions—and then *become* them (transformation *in* O) (Grotstein, 2004b). Then the analyst ponders over his experience, thinks about it, and then interprets it (T O → K).

Bion made two significant contributions to the field of general epistemology. First, as alluded to earlier, he noted that thoughts ("thoughts without a thinker"), which are released with each emotional moment, emerge before a mind exists to think them, and that a mind must be developed that has the capacity to think them. The model for the mental process that has to be created he arbitrarily terms "α-function", a topic upon which I shall elaborate later. This function has much in common with the Krebs cycle for the intermediary metabolism of carbohydrates in physiology. In other words, α-function constitutes the model for an intermediary cyclic process of transformation in which the raw Absolute Truth about Ultimate Reality—and the emotional sense impressions (β-elements that release them) must be subjected to the "digestive enzymes" of the mind so as to be converted into humanly tolerable emotional truths about outer and inner reality.

Second, he rediscovered a form of epistemology first propounded, I believe, by Plato in *Theaetetus* in which the percipient (perceiver) must *"become"* the percept in order for perception to take place. "Become" will turn out to be a major Bionian concept that suffuses his ideas about maternal and analytic reverie and intersubjective projective identification. Bion's differs from Cartesian thinking in so far as the latter form of thinking, the one we take for granted, does not presuppose from the outset that a difference or separation must exist between the perceiver (subject) and the perceived (object) or the thinker and the thought.

Bion often mused over the irony, as I have already suggested, that psychoanalysis was a verbal form of treatment about phenomena that occurred *before* words were understood and would remain forever *beyond* words. In fact I first consulted him for analysis for persisting difficulties that putatively originated at, if not before, my premature birth. I now wish to reiterate something that I stated earlier. I recall an instance of my analysis with Bion when he gave me a satisfying interpretation about a deep anxiety that I had at that moment. He followed his interpretation with the following comment, which I recall from across the years: "I have given you an interpretation about your distress, and you appear to regard it as correct, one that reasonably addresses the situation you present. Yet we shall never know the origin of your anxiety. It is not to be known. It is ineffable. We can only roughly approximate it, know *about* it." The real answer to the origin of my anxiety, I concluded, would remain in a constant state of uncertainty and ineffability.

Models versus theories

Bion was fond of using analogic models that he could apply to the mind's transformative functioning but which would exist outside the actual functioning. All we can know is that the analogous (analogue) variation in a model is external to, but matches, the experience. The models he uses are analogic in order to give as much precision as possible. In order to understand Bion's penchant for models over theories, one has to understand where Bion was coming from, so to speak. Bion eschewed ordinary spoken and/or written language because it was sense-derived, meaning that it was *representative* of the object (object representation) but did not *reveal* the human vitality of the object in a state of flux or evolution. All living organisms, including the human being and most especially the infant and the analysand, are radiantly expressive semiotic beings whose individual, unique personalness is utterly *indivisible*—and is at the beck and call of any willing receiver. In summary, the very use of words that psychoanalysis has extolled since Freud is utterly useless in comprehending the living, ever-changing, indivisible human being—thus, the need for models.

We all live in a world of transferences in which we confuse our image (representation) of the object with the object (individual) himself. Bion may be likened to the patriarch Abraham, who eschewed idol worshipping in favour of an invisible, ineffable, inscrutable deity—who is One—who/which is utterly beyond the reach of our senses, our capacity to understand, comprehend, or grasp and whom/which we are compelled, with faith, to experience through the blindness of our emotions. Bion was not religious, but he saw the advantages of religious metaphors (models) and thought that at times they were superior to the psychoanalytic models in addressing that quintessential mystery known as man.

The model is an arbitrary analogue, a separate but parallel system whose observable variations seem somehow to correspond to the more mysterious variations in the ineffable subject. The use of models may, consequently, be thought of as corresponding to Bion's concept of the Language of Achievement. Bion may be thought of, in this regard, as an analogue not only of the patriarch Abraham, but also of a painter or sculptor who wishes to use his aesthetic capacities (Ehrenzweig, 1967) "to capture the light"—that is, the shadow—of the living being in a state of flux.

Bion's models include, in the main, α-function, α- and β-elements, caesura, the Grid, contact-barrier, and L, H, and K linkages. To these Ferro (2006) adds "selected fact" and "negative capability" (p. 51). Bion also uses the model of the digestive processes of the alimentary canal for his conceptualization of transformation, to which I add: (1)

the model of the immune system (as in dreaming and/or α-function), and (2) the explanatory model of the Krebs cycle for the intermediate metabolism of carbohydrate. Another Bionian model is that of the neuronal synapse. That model seems to apply to his conceptualization of the activity of the contact-barrier between the unconscious and consciousness (Bion apparently did not find the idea of the mental apparatus useful) or, later, between infinity and finiteness. This model is of enormous help in understanding his communicative form of projective identification (what *I* call "projective *trans*identification", Grotstein, 2005).

First, the contact-barrier is defined as being selectively permeable—that is, an intelligence can be imputed to it that is able to select whom or what to let in, whom or what to let out, and whom or what to retain and not to retain. Second, the synapse model implies that the pre-synaptic membrane is separate from the post-synaptic membrane and any communication between them across the synapse must take place with the help of a third entity, one that is extraterritorial[5] to each—namely, the chemical neurotransmitters, which, after becoming affected and thus altered at the pre-synaptic membrane, are then able to "prime" the post-synaptic membrane to become sensitive to the new neurotransmitter message. What this means for the phenomenon of communicative projective identification is that the subject does not project directly into the object. It means that the subject projects into his *image* of the object, and the object is receptive to and primed to respond with its counter-image of the subject.

The next step is as follows: the subject's image, analogous to the pre-synaptic membrane, primes—that is, affects—the object's image of the subject *and* the latter's self-image, following which the object selectively recruits those images, ideas, emotions, memories, or whatever, from within his own unconscious, infinite resources and capabilities and responds with their own inherent corresponding (symmetrical) analogous possibilities (Grotstein, 2004a). Just as the neural impulse has to cross many synapses before it reaches its final destination, so must the emotional impulse in projective transidentification have to cross synapse equivalents to reach the object with verisimilitude. In short: Bion's psychoanalytic epistemology is ontological and phenomenological and accounts for the transformation (epigenesis) of the phenomenon of *experience* to the *notation* of experience. Bion contrasts models with theories. Models are *analogues* that are independent of the contextual field in which they are employed, whereas theories are defined within the contextual field in which they are used. Evolution is a theory about the origin and development of all species, whereas α-function is a model that constitutes an analogue to the mysterious processes of mental/emotional transformations.

In *Learning from Experience*, Bion states:

> The "selected fact", that is to say the element that gives coherence to the objects of the paranoid–schizoid position and so initiates the depressive position, does so by virtue of its membership of a number of different deductive systems at their point of intersection. . . . *The analyst has to concern himself with two models, one that he is called upon to make and the other implicit in the material produced by the patient. . . .* [1962b, p. 87; italics added]

I understand this passage to mean that the model of the *selected fact is bimodal*: One aspect lies in the analyst's capacity to be patient while awaiting the arrival of the selected fact because he has faith in his intuition that a pre-conception of the selected fact exists potentially within him. The second inheres in the patient in terms of his free associations—that is, this aspect of the selected fact inheres in the patient's material, but the analyst needs to tolerate the frustration of not knowing and to have faith that a selected fact exists until it seems to have arrived. Another way of looking at this complex problem is to suggest that the selected fact resembles the original conception of the *symbol*, the components of which had erstwhile become scattered and await reunion with one another in order to become the restored, integrated symbol. Later in this text I suggest that since the selected fact exists before it is detected, the whole concept of O—especially in terms of "uncertainty"—is challengeable. Put another way, if the selected fact (the "strange attractor" of chaos theory) is always already *a priori* present, then uncertainty does not exist: only our conscious experience of O is uncertain. O is Certain within itself.

Bion says:

> The model makes it possible to find the correspondence between the patient's thinking and the main body of psycho-analytic theory [the analyst's pre-conceptions—JSG] by interpretations that are related closely both to theory and the statements and conduct of the patient. *Model making thus increases the number of contingencies that can be met and decreases the number of psycho-analytic theories that the psycho-analyst needs as his working equipment. . . .* [1962b, pp. 87–88; italics added]

I gather from this citation that in the analytic situation models are more versatile than theories. The analyst is armed with a body of theories (i.e. the Oedipus complex, P–S ↔ D, etc.) that constitute the supportive background for the analyst's thinking. Models, on the other hand, like the selected fact, α-function, etc., have more versatility in addressing the immediacy of the analytic situation moment by moment and ultimately linking a realization with an already known theory.

In summary, Bion believed it was important to distinguish models from theories in order to sharpen his precision in approaching psychoanalytic phenomena. My own feeling is that models are *"ad hoc" instruments* that lie outside the phenomena with which they engage and with which they probe the personality and analytic associations, whereas theories are within the loop of the phenomena and offer basic explanations for them.

What is a "β-element" really?

Bion conceived of α-function and β- and α-elements as models for the epigenesis and evolution of thoughts and thinking. The analogies between α-function and dreaming, on the one hand, and Freud's (1911b) combined primary and secondary processes on the other, seem clear. For Bion, α-elements seem to be the transformed version of β-elements. But what is a β-element? Is it the same as O? Bion seems to suggest as much when he associates the β-element with O as well as with the noumenon and the Ideal Forms as well as with godhead (Bion, 1962b, p. 84; 1965, pp. 13, 139; 1970, pp. 14, 58)? When placed contiguously, Bion seems to intimately *associate* but does not formally *equate* the following: O, Absolute Truth, Ultimately Reality, the thing-in-itself or noumenon, Ideal Form, godhead, β-element. My version of what Bion really meant was that the β-element is *not* O; it is O's proto-emotional descendant—that is, the β-element is the emotional sense *impression* of O: the ghost of O ("ghost of departed qualities"—Bishop Berkeley, *The Analyst*, 1734).

I should like to suggest the following alternatives:

A. When Bion speaks of the "Absolute Truth" and "Ultimate Reality", I prefer to restate it as "the Absolute Truth *about* Ultimate Reality", which conveys that *truth always resides within the individual as a potential or actualized verdict that the individual renders when exposed to*

Ultimate Reality and prompted by the "truth drive" (Grotstein, 2004b). Ultimate Reality is located within the confines of the self and is everywhere external and may even lie beyond System *Ucs.* internally as "internally Other", the "Unknown", as distinct from the unconscious—that is, the domain of the numinous.

B. Beta-elements (1) constitute the *sense impressions* (on "consciousness, the sense organ receptive to psychical qualities") that evolving O creates as it intersects the individual's emotional frontier; they thereby constitute O's *shadow* or *imprint* (impression)—in other words, they are not O. They represent the initial *sense impression* of O's intersection of our emotional receptors—our affective sentinels who are on watch. "Friend? Foe?" They also (2) are representative derivatives of the Ideal Forms, the noumena or things-in-themselves, which present as inherited and/or acquired pre-conceptions.

C. Beta-elements become transformed by α-function one way or another, *irrespective of whether or not they are accepted for mentalization.* The β-element is O's bimodal derivative and represents the indifference, neutrality, or impersonalness of evolving O. Once the β-element contacts the individual's emotional frontier and its α-function, it becomes automatically transformed into an α-element in Bion's episteme—that is, a now *personalized* transformation of O. Then α-function, which is in charge of encrypting (encoding and transforming) the β-element, may decide that this is "too hot to handle" and may then reject it—*but now no longer as a β-element.* Put another way, when a β-element *seems* to be refused alpha-beta-ization by α-function, as happens in psychosis, *I* believe it does not remain a β-element but becomes transformed into a *rejected* and *degraded α-element* (victim of denial) or even a bizarre object. My assumption presupposes that α-elements of differing degrees of maturation occur from the beginning. Thus, the β-screen constitutes a *degraded α-screen* that menacingly hovers around the projecting subject awaiting the recognition that had been denied it. Having renounced it, one must reclaim it. We have a fated rendezvous with it, since our initial renunciation of it was a renunciation of our personhood in our initial contact with it.

I have arrived at this hypothesis for the following reason: When Bion (1962b) speaks of the "β-screen" (pp. 22–24), he describes it as an enclosure comprised of the agglomeration of untransformed β-elements that imprison the psychotic patient. Brown (2005, 2006) and I (Grotstein, 2005) hypothesize that the pathological organization known as the "psychic retreat" (Steiner, 1993) applies to the post-traumatic stress disorders as well as to psychotics and is comprised of these rejected β-elements as an imprisoning enclosure. The very fact that they seem to cluster around the patient so menacingly conveys to me that they *are proclaiming their personal connection to the patient, which the latter is denying.* The β-element (really, "degraded α-element") becomes an encapsulating screen because it belongs to the individual, like Tausk's (1919) "influencing machine".

D. Beta-elements may only be "β" to us: they are the projected results of our attempts to mystify them into what is to us the "dark matter" of the "deep and formless infinite". To them, however, they are in their own right not only descendants of the Ideal Forms but also intimations, echoes, and adumbrations of all their future recombinant possibilities of their own and our imaginative conjectures—looking to become real-izations. *The real and most important difference between a β-element and an α-element, consequently, is that the former connotes the impersonalness of Fate (O), whereas the latter, the α-element, indicates that the subject has attributed personalness to the experience and personally claims it as his own.* Put another way, β-elements represent unclaimed elements, and α-element claimed ones. Bion thought of β-elements as the initial sense impression made by incoming stimuli (O) and thought they were *physical* (physiological) in nature, in contrast with α-elements, which were *mental*. I believe that if one makes a distinction from the psychoanalytic vertex between mind and body, then Bion is correct in his assumption of β-element (physical) → α-element (mental). However, if we also assume from the psychoanalytic vertex that a differentiation between mind and body is an illusion (Aisenstein, 2006; Bion, 2005a; Grotstein, 1997a), then the issue becomes more problematic. Bion (2005a) states:

> In saying that, I have made an entirely artificial separation; I have talked about the body and the mind as if they were two entirely different things. I don't believe it. I think that the patient whom you see tomorrow is one, a whole, a complete [irreducible—JSG] person. And although we say—obeying the laws of grammar—that we can observe his body and mind, in fact there is no such thing as a "body and mind"; there is a "he" or a "she". [2005a, p. 38]

E. I believe, consequently, that β-elements may be reconceptualized as follows: When O intersects our emotional frontier and makes an impression there of its presence, the initial response is the formation or appearance of an α-*element* (personal). It may either continue in its transformational course into dream elements, contact-barrier, and memory, or come to be rejected by the mind and degraded *after the fact* into "β-elements" and thereby remain "impersonal", "unclaimed" in the "dead post office" of the mind. May not Bion have also thought of this idea when he selected "β", which *follows* "α" in the Greek alphabet? Moreover, α-elements are, in my opinion, continuations of their *Anlage* as "thoughts without a thinker" that have been thought all along by "godhead" ("godhood") or demon "god" (Bion, 1992, p. 305)!

F. Emotions are the vehicles that *transmit* β-elements and then α-elements, which signify the Absolute Truth about Ultimate Reality. The dread of emotions is due to the nature of the cargo (Absolute Truth about Ultimate Reality) that they carry in their hold, O. This conception marginalizes the role of emotions as *vehicles* of Truth, not Truth itself.

G. Using Bion's concept of reversible perspective, we may see Bion's transformational schema thus: it may *not* be α-function that transforms β-elements into α-elements, but, rather, it is *we* who become transformed—it is *our subjective perception* of β-elements that really undergoes transformation. In other words, our perception of the experience of the β-elements becomes transformed, not the β-elements themselves. From this vertex (perspective), α-function and/or dreaming furnishes us with a subjective, personalizing filter so that we may be protected from the blinding glare of O while we transform ourselves so as to experience it. In this way we can imagine ourselves, albeit unconsciously, to be manipulating what and who enters us, rather than acknowledging that we are passive subjects of Fate (O) . Put another way, *Truth cannot be transformed*; only the *perceiver* of the Truth can be.

H. Beta-elements now replace Freud's drives as the irrupting *repressed* from the unconscious. The content of the repressed (dynamic unconscious), in other words, thereupon becomes chaos (complexity) and/or infinity represented as β-elements and/or "thoughts without a thinker": that is, the "unborns"; β-elements represent the noumena or inherent pre-conceptions, which are "unborns" awaiting realization in experience as phenomena (conceptions).

I. Bion defines β-elements as being similar to the "proto-mental system" inclusive of basic assumption (resistance) groups (Bion, 1961, p. 108).

J. "The β-elements are characteristic of the personality during the dominance of the pleasure principle: on them depends the capacity for non-verbal communication, the individual's ability to believe in the possibility of ridding himself of unwanted emotions, and the communication of emotion within the group" (Bion, 1992, p. 190).

K. Bion describes β-space:

> I shall suppose a mental multi-dimensional space of unthought and unthinkable extent and characteristics. Within this I shall suppose there to be a domain of thoughts that have no thinker. Separated from each other in time, space and style, in a manner that I can formulate only using analogies taken from astronomy, is the domain of thoughts that have a thinker. This domain is characterized by constellations of α-elements. These constellations compose universes of discourse that are characterized by containing and being contained by terms such as, "void", "formless infinite", "god", "infinity". [1992, p. 313]

L. I am coming to believe that α-elements, rather than being considered the absolute opposite of β-elements, should really be thought of as existing as a gradient or spectrum of inchoate → sophisticated α-elements corresponding to a similar gradient for the effective activity of α-function.

*   *   *

I end this section as I began it, by asking: "What is a β-element really?" The "jury is still out", but I ask the reader to conjecture why Bion arbitrarily decided to start in reverse order: β- before α-? Or did he realize—and are we now catching on—that α *is always before* β!

NOTES

1. I shall take up the issue of "uncertainty" later when I proffer an alternative understanding of it.

2. Bion distinguishes between "preconception" and "pre-conception" in that the former is a saturated thought, whereas the latter is an Ideal Form or thing-in-itself. (See chapter 7.)

3. As I mentioned earlier, Bion uses "become" in the Platonic sense of becoming: "that which is is always becoming"—that is, always in flux (Bion, personal communication, 1977).

4. It must be remembered that for "godhead" we should understand "god-hood"—the Ideal Form or the thing-in-itself.

5. Perhaps this third entity is what Bion, following Meister Eckhart and other "heretical" mystics, meant by the concept of the "immanent god" within us, one who is extraterritorial to the Forms, stated earlier.

CHAPTER 6

Bion's metatheory

I n discussing Bion's metatheory, Paulo Sandler (2005) says that:

> Bion displayed a distinct preference for developing *observational theories* [italics added] for the psychoanalyst's use, rather than for creating new theories. . . . One of the few exceptions, which would remain unpublished during his lifetime, was a paper entitled "Metatheory". It was an attempt to describe *scientifically* some elementary basics of psycho-analysis. One of its terms is "Breast". Like "penis", "splitting" and "violent emotions" it was devised as a "class of interpretations". . . . The *"interpretation breast"* is made in conjunction with the *"interpretation penis."* He treats the "name given to the word 'breast', as a hypothesis, following Hume's view "that a hypothesis is the expression of a subjective sense that certain associations are constantly *conjoined, and is not a representation corresponding to an actuality."* [P. Sandler, 2005, p. 91]

Sandler has here grasped the essence of Bion's enterprise in creating a psychoanalytic theory that was not only based on clinical observation but also included metaphysical concepts: literally, the metaphysical concept of the *hypothesis* of a breast or penis: in Plato's terms archetypal Ideal Forms, essences, or in Kant's terms, noumena or things-in-themselves—that is, not sensible to perception. Of importance also is Hume's concept of the *"constant conjunction"*, finding a pattern in which two objects or thoughts become thought of as belonging together. This could apply to the *name* "breast" becoming affixed to the *hypothesis* "breast", It is also applicable to the idea of "pattern", being able clinically to discern a pattern in the patient's free associations.

In my own thinking, I believe that Bion's metatheory might have been his attempt to affix (constantly conjoin) psychoanalytic theory and the clinical observations obtained in psychoanalysis with a metaphysical theory of *a priori* hypotheses—that is, hypotheses that are older than we are. The term "meta-" also suggests Freud's (1915e) concept of "metapsychology", which originally included a genetic, a dynamic, and a structural perspective (p. 181). The concept of metapsychology represents what Hume would call a constant conjunction—an enclosure that includes the entirety of the psychoanalytic landscape. I think that Bion's metatheory ultimately constitutes a more expansive metapsychology than Freud's. In what follows I arbitrarily treat the entirety of Bion's works as components of his metatheory.

Bion lists the items in his metatheory as follows: frustration, denial of frustration, modification of frustration, concern for truth and life, violent emotions, the breast, the penis, and splitting (Bion, 1992, pp. 244–254). I have dealt here with these items only briefly. They deserve a more detailed perusal in Bion's works. The manner in which the infant relates to frustration, either through denial or through modification of it, becomes decisive for mental growth and determines—as well as is determined by—his embrasure of truth and authentic life. The breast and the penis are the sought-for links to important objects—mother and father, respectively. Violent emotions constitute the passions of caring about the unpredictable caprices of needed objects, one of the reactions against which would be splitting.

The capacity of the mind depends on the capacity of unconscious *negative capability,* the capacity to bear negativity and withstand its persuasions to abandon a task. Inability to tolerate empty space limits the amount of space available. Bion's concept of container ↔ contained became his answer to why individuals had difficulties in tolerating frustration, but, to my knowledge, he never formally connected the two phenomena. What Bion seems to be emphasizing is how to develop the capacity of the mind and receptivity to deal with O, "thoughts without a thinker", the inexorable "noise" that relentlessly confronts our inner and outer senses. Bion states:

> The paranoid–schizoid and depressive positions are related to a part of the domain of thought, that part of it in which *there exist thinkers corresponding to the thoughts awaiting someone or something to think*

them. The thinkers might be likened to objects sensitive to certain wave-lengths of thought, as the eye or radio telescope is sensitive to a particular range of electromagnetic waves. *Such thinkers can be impinged upon by thoughts that are too powerful in relation to the sensitivity of the receiving apparatus.* Or they may be unmatched by a reciprocating thinker.

The human being, despite similarities to other human beings, *may not,* through over- or under-sensitivity, *have an apparatus adequate to thinking the thoughts.* He becomes aware of these thoughts usually through the medium of what is ordinarily known to him as *religious awe,* and is variously expressed as *incarnation, evolution of godhead, platonic forms, Krishna, mystic experience, inspiration,* and the like. *Thus the source of emission of the received or evolved thoughts is felt as external, God-given....* The fate of the thought and the thinker is to follow one of the paths I have indicated as peculiar to ♀♂, or some variation. In some circumstances the impact is incandescent, growth-producing, and then the individual thinker becomes an emitter or intermittant. A chain reaction is set up, as I have already described it in terms of the *messianic thought, mystic,* etc. The problem is whether one is to regard this model, ♀♂, ... as a model for a configuration that underlies certain groups of particular instances, or is it simply a way of regarding meaningless, incoherent, unrelated phenomena, and making them appear to have coherence and a meaningful pattern? Does it in fact matter which it is? Do facts arrange themselves in this pattern, or is it a peculiarity in the individual that he finds it necessary to discern this or similar patterns in the facts he observes? *The craving for validation may then be a wish to localize the emitter in God, universe, person, conscious and unconscious, by instruments that are micro- or macro-scopic and appear to confer authoritatively the guerdon of truth.* [1992, pp. 304–305; italics added]

The above citations certainly do not embrace all the ideas in Bion's metatheory, but they do express that aspect of it that is related to that arm of O which mysteriously springs from the inherent noumenal hardware, the Ideal Forms and the things-in-themselves, located, putatively, in the unrepressed unconscious. The individual who lacks an apparatus to think (dream) the thoughts may either project them elsewhere as untransformed β-elements (degraded α-elements, in my opinion) or regard them as religious or messianic epiphanies. St. Paul's vision on the Road to Damascus comes to mind.

Bion's metatheory includes his concept of container ↔ contained, communicative projective identification, the transformation of β-elements into α-elements by the process of α-function, the reconfiguration of L (love), H (hate), the Grid, and K (knowledge) from drives into interrelated emotional links between self and objects—all within the context of considerations of Truth. The α-elements are mentalizable by and for the mind, unlike β-elements, which are somatic and inchoate emotional sense impressions. Alpha-elements constitute the elementary alphabet of thoughts. They proliferate to form larger and more complex meanings, are routed to the contact-barrier for reinforcement of its functioning as a mediator between Systems *Ucs.* and *Cs*, are taken up by dream work to be used as dream thoughts, and are stored for memory. Underlying all the above processes, which are expressed in the vocabulary of *models*, are Bion's (1965) concepts of transformation and of dreaming.

Bion's whole theory of mind rests in part on the concept of transformations. By this, he means that mental elements—that is, β-elements → α-elements[1]—undergo an epigenesis from the concrete to the abstract so as to allow the mind to achieve progressively greater sophistication. The process of thinking begins inchoately as the newborn infant, unknowingly afraid of its imminent premonition of dying, communicates this anxiety to its container–mother, in whose reverie she is able to employ her α-function to absorb, detoxify, and make sense of the infant's emotional communication. Following this, she is enabled to respond to her infant in innumerable appropriate ways. After many iterations of this process, the infant introjects mother's α-function as well as the legacy (memory) of its bimodal operation (infant → mother; mother → infant). Once this mode of communication has been introjected by the infant, it thereafter functions within the infant as the process of thinking: that is, the projective identification of "wild thoughts"—emotions, "thoughts without a thinker", β-elements—into a newly installed infant container. Through this the infant is enabled to become an autonomous thinker.

Dreaming—as we see further on, when I discuss the subject at greater length—seems for Bion to be the all-embracing factor, the *sine qua non*, an ensemble of processes (perhaps for Bion the actualization of the his model, α-function, etc.) whereby the subject's mind, acting like a filter or lens throughout the day and night, alters the perception ("does something to . . .") sensory stimuli both from within the internal world and from the external world—so as to render the stimuli mentally and emotionally tolerable. The ultimate source of the stimulus lies in Bion's (1965, 1970) concept of O—the Absolute Truth, Ultimate Reality, infinity, godhead. Put another way, α-function, the hypothetical model, and/or dreaming, the living process in actuality (to which I refer as the "dream ensemble"), screens and transforms raw intersecting impression from O (as β-elements) and, as stated above, transduces and "translates" them into information (thoughts) and appropriate responses.

Bion (1977a) also conceived of a Grid as a mathematical model for the categorization of thoughts and their development on the vertical axis and the progressive processing of thoughts on the horizontal axis. Bion, the epistemologist, realized that thoughts are primary and seek a mind to think them.[2] The thoughts are on the vertical (genetic) axis, and the mind that thinks them is on the horizontal axis. The basis for this Grid is Freud's (1911b) concept of two mental functions: the primary and secondary processes. Bion's "definitory hypothesis" corresponds to the former and the secondary process to the latter. Bion united the two under his concept of α-function. It must be remembered that Bion was ultimately an ontological epistemologist. He was concerned with how we come to know what we know. The ontological (existential) and epistemological problem in psychoanalytic treatment is for the analyst to find the analytic object (the maximum unconscious anxiety, O) within the patient (the patient's symptoms) by experiencing, in a state of reverie (waking dream thoughts), his own version of O from his unconscious resources that match up with the patient's experience. Altogether, the analyst must employ sense (the totality of his observations of the patient), myth (the conception of the patient's unconscious phantasies and the analyst's phantasies about them, in the context of the underlying myth that subtends them), and passion, the analyst's capacity for emotional representation—that is, his ability to *feel* his *emotions,* which are triggered by, are in response to, and are in resonance with those of the patient. This is a brief epitome of Bion's works.

The origins of thinking

In laying down the groundwork for a psychoanalytic ontological epistemology, Bion had first separated mind from thoughts, believing that the latter precede the former genetically. Then he laid the groundwork for the origin of thinking as well as for thoughts. The mind had to be created in order to accommodate the emergence of "thoughts without a thinker"—in order to "mind" (bind) them into constant conjunctions: that is, thoughts with names.

What is essential to the capacity to think is the ability to tolerate frustration—and thereby be able to tolerate the breast's absence. This capacity to tolerate frustration enables the infant to contemplate the existence of an empty space where the breast once was—and to which hopefully (with faith) it will return. This tolerance allows that hallowed space to become an unsaturated spatial signifier-container that corresponds and is dedicated to the object-thought that belongs there. The infant must hold the space in reserve for the return of the object as its part of the covenant with the object and, in so doing, *thinks*.

In *Transformations*, Bion states:

> Cs. (A1) [definitory hypothesis—β-element—JSG] is of the nature of tropism. It involves ψ(ξ) [ψ represents the mind as a constant and ξ the unsaturated element—JSG] in which (ξ) seeks saturation. This "consciousness" is an awareness of a lack of existence that demands an existence, *a thought in search of a meaning*, a definitory hypothesis in search of a realization approximating to it, a psyche seeking for a physical habitation [real-ization—JSG] to give it existence, ♀ seeking ♂. [1965, p. 109; italics added]

The mind, ψ, is the psycho-geometric-space constant (whether in analyst or patient) that is associated with unsaturated "no-thought", ξ, which seeks saturation by definitory hypothesis. Consciousness, sensing both mind, ψ, which is associated with the unsaturation, seeking-saturation of ξ, *and* the "unborn pre-conceptions" seeking realization as conceptions (thoughts), arranges the rendezvous between them. Put another way, the mind needs a geometrically formatted space in which to think its thoughts. Thoughts need to be anticipated by an expectant ("unsaturated") "no-thought", which has to summon its yet unborn counterpart, a "thought without a thinker" (Ideal Form, noumenon, thing-in-itself, "memoir of the future") with which to keep a rendezvous.

Bion gives us another hint as to why he insists on using mathematical metaphors and imagery:

> The idea implicit in the theory of transference is that the analyst is the person onto whom the analysand transfers his images. The theories of Melanie Klein already show that such a medium is not adequate for Tp β in what I have called projective transformations. In particular, it does not help the analyst to recognize the elements of projective identification as they appear amidst clinical symptoms and material. The analyst must be able to detect signs of projective identification in a field which, relative to that which obtains in classical theory, is, as it were, *multidimensional. The analytic situation requires greater width and depth than can be provided by a model from Euclidean space. A patient who, in my view, is displaying projective transformations* and requires the use of Kleinian theories for comprehension, also

uses a field which is not simply the analyst, or his own personality, or even the relationship between himself and the analyst, but all those and more. [1965, p. 114; italics added]

Bion seems to be distinguishing between classical transference, which he associates with Euclidean space ("rigid motion transformation"), and Kleinian transference: that is, projective identification, which he terms "projective transformation", a phenomenon that he also associates with "–K space" (p. 115). In the final analysis, he seems to be defending the need to transcend what he believes are the limitations of classical theory by using geometric and post-geometric analogies. Perhaps this idea may become clearer if I use a concept from ego psychology. Jacobson (1964) distinguishes between *object* representation and *self* representation. In the classical transference the object representation becomes displaced (not projected) *onto* another object representation, the analyst. In Kleinian thinking it is the self-representation that becomes projected *into* the object representation, the analyst. I infer that Bion believes that extreme states of projective identification become a more radical type of transformation that involves a loss of self and therefore approximates, if not actually achieves, –K, α-function in reverse, the psychotic state. Bion defines –K space as follows:

To make a step towards definition of this space we consider it to be a –K "space" and contrast it with K "space"—the space in which what is normally regarded as classical analysis takes place and classical transference manifestations become "sense-able". . . . –K "space" may be described as the space where space used to be. It is filled with no-objects which are violently and enviously greedy of any and every quality, thing, or object, for its "possession" . . . of existence. . . . –K "space" is the material in which, with which, on which, etc., the "artist" in projective transformation works. [1965, pp. 115]

So much for –K space, now for saturated "no-things":

[I]t will be remembered that in a system in which β-elements dominate, "thoughts" are "things", and I pointed out that β-elements do not lend themselves to use as column 4 elements [attention—JSG] do because they are already saturated; there can be no pre-conception (Row D) that can be *used* as a pre-conception, awaiting the realization that produces a conception, because the β-element is already saturated. We can now see that the defects of the no-thing are precisely these—the "absent" or "non-existent" object occupies the space that should be vacant. [1965, p. 118]

To demonstrate the above Bion presents a clinical example in which the "patient occupies the couch because he is determined that no one else should" (p. 118). He aims to saturate the session in a way that prevents Bion from working effectively. Furthermore, no one can take the patient's place. He uses words that once had meaning but the meaning has now been destroyed or stripped away so that the words mark the place where meaning formerly was. "This absent meaning (that is nevertheless present) will not permit any meaning to take its place" (p. 118). Consequently, O cannot be represented.

Bion then goes on to state:

> I [use—JSG] the point (·) to represent the "place where" a something (as contrasted with a no-thing) could be, and the line (———) as the locus of a point or the place where a point is going. . . . I shall try to make it more suitable for thought by considering point (·) and line (———) to represent a relationship thus: the point (·), "place where", stage, must be conceived of as pertaining to the genetic axis: the line (———) must be conceived of as pertaining to the horizontal axis. A preconception, represented by · is a stage of development (a seed, so to speak, is a tree at [a] particular stage of its development: so is a tree). A pre-conception represented by a line (———) is a use (such as D4). [1965, p. 119]

It may help to know that Bion's use of these geometric models has to do, among other possibilities, with attempting to chart the vectors of a relationship—for example, the point is where the breast once was, the line is where breast went, and so on. Continuing this line of development, Bion states that Euclidean geometry referred to the experience of space and that the intrapsychic origin of "the space" is, as suggested earlier, the place where a feeling, emotion, or other mental experience has once been. Here is how Bion now precisely formulates it:

> The rules governing points and lines which have been elaborated by geometers may be reconsidered by reference back to the emotional phenomena that were replaced by "the place (or space) where the mental phenomena were." Such a procedure would establish an abstract deductive system based on a geometric foundation with intuitive psycho-analytic theory as its concrete realization. The statements (i) the resumption by the psyche of an emotional experience that has been detoxified by a sojourn in the good breast . . . and (ii) the transformation of the emotional experience into a geometric formulation as the counterpart of a concrete realization for a geometrically based, rigorously formulated deductive system (possible algebraic), may now be regarded as the (i) intuitive psycho-analytic and (ii) axiomatic deductive representations of the same process. . . .

The intuitive statement lends itself to the representation of genetic stages: the axiomatic formulation lends itself to the representation of use. [1965, pp. 121–122]

This last citation is perhaps the clearest and most succinct statement Bion has ever made about his view of the relationship between geometry (plane, solid, and algebraic) and emotions, including intuition. As I have stated earlier, what Bion seems to have been pursuing was a *notation system* as an analogue or model that, unlike words, is utterly free from a penumbra of distracting associations—and also one that would, because of its mathematical–scientific rigour, appeal to science-respecting colleagues in all schools of psychoanalysis (personal communication):

Distinction between the "geometric" and "arithmetic" developments can be made thus: the geometric development of points and line are primarily associated with the presence of or absence, existence or non-existence, of an object. The arithmetic development is associated with the state of the object, whether it is whole or fragmented, whole object or part object. ... The geometric development is associated with depression, absence or presence of the object: the arithmetic development is associated with feelings of persecution, the Kleinian theory of a paranoid–schizoid position. [1965, p. 151]

Bion, the avowed Platonist, was undoubtedly following in the latter's footsteps when he chose geometry as his medium of exposition of metapsychological (metaphysical?) ideas. Let me cite a portion from Lawlor's (1982) *Sacred Geometry*:

For Plato, Reality consisted of pure essences or archetypal Ideas, of which the phenomena we perceive are only pale reflections. (The Greek word "Idea" is also translated by "Form"). These Ideas cannot be perceived by the senses, but by pure reason alone. *Geometry was the language recommended by Plato as the clearest model by which to describe this metaphysical realm.* [Lawlor, 1982, p. 9; italics added]

Conclusion: the analyst must be able to tolerate frustration (as must the developing infant) in order to be receptive to "Ideas", which are ultra-sensory and can only be contemplated through reason (intuition).

"Thoughts without a thinker":
Bion's "unborns"

Bion (1992) created the concept of "thoughts without a thinker" (p. 326). What he seems to mean by this is that unthought thoughts are primary, emerge from the two arms of O (inherent pre-conceptions and sensory data of emotional significance), and seek a thinker (mind) to think them. The ramifications of this epistemological nuance are of enormous importance, not only to psychoanalysis, but to epistemology generally and to religion. In short, Bion is suggesting that the unconscious and the sense organs feel incomplete and need a transforming container to mediate them. It also suggests that the unconscious, in psychoanalytic theory, and "God", in religious dogma, seek a mind or soul to real-ize them—that is, to *complete* them. Put another way, God needs man to incarnate him, which is most apparent in Catholicism but also in Judaism and Islam. Put yet another way, primal thoughts are like Wordsworth's unborns looking for earthly assignment.

Thoughts without a thinker seem, in particular, to be those aspects of the unrepressed (inherited) unconscious, Plato's Ideal Forms, and Kant's noumena or things-in-themselves, which are summoned by the subject's experience as the impact on his sense organs of imping-ing data of emotional significance. The Forms and/or noumena seem to function as infinite *formatting* strategies to protect the subject from being overwhelmed. They are "memoirs of the future", as Bion suggests. They "remind" us of the general category of the stimulus that is new to us but not to it. They constitute "emergent thoughts" that are summoned by desire and/or by experience. In terms of desire, one may think of summoning the muse to help with a creative task—as I am doing at this moment. In terms of experience, they seem to be summoned by our sense organs and emotions. Most often we do not know what summons them. They are also known as free associations in analysis and as random or "wild thoughts" (Bion, 1997). Bion extols them and encourages analysts not to ignore them (Bion, 2005a, 2005b). He alludes to them as the content of "Definitory Hypothesis" in Column 1 of the Grid.

The concept of thoughts "without a thinker", or "wild" thoughts, is problematic (López-Corvo, 2006). We all know what Bion means. His terms are the counterparts to Freud's (1905d) instinctual drives, which are thought of as comprising a "seething cauldron". Moreover, the unconscious functions in a different dimension than consciousness—that of the zero dimension of infinity (Grotstein, 1978) and of progressive dimensions of symmetry (Matte Blanco, 1975, 1988). These dimensional factors present as *chaos* to consciousness and give it its fiendish and cataclysmic reputation. That is why α-function or dreaming is neces-sary: to mediate O's infinite, absolutely symmetrical nature. Thoughts without a thinker or wild thoughts are never not thought. There is no randomness in either the cosmic or the psychological universe.[3] They are thought by an internal ineffable presence, gnomon, or "demon-God", which/who organizes them and presents them to the analyst as free associations. They are the hidden *order* of thoughts without a thinker. The Muse is its other name.

Bion's Taming Wild Thoughts

> In case one of these strays comes along, I think I shall try to be prepared for its reception by arranging certain categories that might be suitable for *placing the stray in a temporary—"box"*. The first box I am thinking of is really not suitable for anything so ephemeral as what I usually call a thought, namely something that is physical;[4] I shall call it a "β-element". . . . There is something a bit more sophisticated: a similarly physical creature, but one that arouses in me primordial thoughts or feelings, something that is sort of a prototype of a mental reaction. These I shall call "α-elements". . . . There have been . . . those occasions when I have . . . fallen into the prevalent idea of saying that I had a dream, but I can only say that I felt physical pain—my arm ached.; . . . That is the kind of thing . . . that I should like to put in this category. . . . There is another one in which I am nearly awake and nearly asleep; there I have certain ideas that are comprehensible to me when I am fully awake and of which I can tell you exactly in terms of *verbal formulations of visual images what I say I dreamt or saw in my sleep.* [Bion, 1997, pp. 29–30; all italics added]

After first defining the gradual differences in the experiencing of β- and then α-elements, and pictorial images, Bion then places them into the first (left-hand side) vertical column of the Grid. He then goes on to "capture a number of strays" from his meditative free associations, applies *speculative imagination* to them, and finally seeks the ultimate pattern that organizes them by *speculative imagination* or *imaginative conjecture*:

> Free associations—sometimes we hear of analysis in such a way that we think what a wonderful time we are all having, wandering about amongst the weeds, plucking the wild and beautiful flowers, admiring the brambles, the bushes, and not getting anywhere near to disturbing the sleep of the sleeping beauty—the wisdom that lies fast asleep somewhere in the thickets; somewhere buried. . . . Is that voice in any way audible? [1997, p. 37]

Here, Bion highlights the importance of free associations and their *ultimate* connection to important pieces of emotional residue from past or present experiences. We must be patient as we listen to the "sleeping beauty" within the analysand or within ourselves in order to await the emergence of the raw nugget of meaning and significance.

In *The Italian Seminars* Bion (2005a) also describes wild thoughts, which are the equivalent of Michelangelo's "prisoners" or "unborns":

> If you can be wide open, then I think there is a chance that you might catch some of those wild thoughts. And if you allow them to lodge in your mind, however ridiculous, however stupid, however fantastic, then there may be a chance of having a look at them. That is a matter of daring to have such thoughts—never mind whether you are supposed to have them or not—and keeping them long enough to be able to formulate what they are. [2005a, p. 44]

Bion, the Promethean, thus initiates the *"psychoanalytic Renaissance"*!

Godhead (godhood) as the "thinker" of the "thoughts without a thinker"

Here, and elsewhere in the book, I proffer an alternative idea with regard to Bion's concept of thoughts without a thinker looking for a thinker to think them with the suggestion that, even though it makes sense consciously and phenomenologically, there can really be no such thing metapsychologically. These thoughts without a thinker or "wild thoughts" (López-Corvo, 2006a, 2006b) *seem* to come to be understood when the selected fact appears, which finally and at last reveals their coherence. Yet the very (factual) existence of the selected fact before it arrives to be intuited or observed by the analyst strongly implies that it has an earlier—an *a priori*—existence. I think that this means they (the "thoughts without a thinker") have never lacked coherence or certainty in their own original domain in psychic reality—and thus have always had a "Thinker".

That "Thinker" goes by the name "godhead" ("godhood"), elaborated by Bion (1965, 1970). Consequently, if godhood ("selected fact") is the thinker of the thoughts without a thinker, order always occurs and continues to occur in the universe (the unconscious). *Thus, "uncertainty" is uncertain only in the proximal domain of consciousness. In the unconscious "uncertainty" (O) is quite certain!* This idea emerges when one uses Bion's tool of *"reversible perspectives"*.

What appear to be incoherent "thoughts" (β-elements) from the vertex of consciousness can be seen as coherent thoughts from the vertex of the unconscious. In seeking transformation in order to qualify for entrance or admission to the domain of consciousness, they may *appear* to be unruly orphans, but they have been *thought* all along by the "Ineffable Thinker Who Thinks the Thoughts without a Thinker" (Grotstein, 2000a)—none other than Bion's designation *"godhead"* ("godhood" or "godliness" in the Platonic archetypal sense), *the Infinite Presence that is at one with O*, the archetype of the mystic. I have elsewhere also named it the "Ineffable Subject of the Unconscious" or the "Dreamer Who Dreams the Dream", the "Dreamer Who Understands the Dream", and the Muse (Grotstein, 2000a). In other words, we *phenomenologically* believe that we first experience a random assortment of incoherent, "wild thoughts" and must await the arrival, with patience, of the selected fact to appear, which seems to give them coherence. *Metapsychologically*, however, we get a different picture: the thoughts without a thinker have never lacked coherence, meaning, and a Thinker in their own original domain, psychic reality.

In seeking transformation in order to qualify for entrance or admission to the domain of consciousness in which realizations of the latter by the former can occur, they may *appear* as unruly orphans, but they have been *thought* all along by "godhead" (godhood), the "Ineffable Thinker Who Thinks the Thoughts without a Thinker", aka the "Ineffable Subject of the Unconscious" or the "Dreamer Who Dreams the Dream". It is a matter of perspective (stereoscopic, binocular vision) and also of the act of transferring the already thought thoughts from the "Thinker" (godhood) to a more humble one who believes *he* is the "thinker".

Postscript

In reading Bion on the concept of transformations, I have come to the following conclusions, the first of which I have already frequently adumbrated:

A. Since Truth and Reality cannot be transformed, *it must be the subject himself who experiences them who must become transformed*—that is, *accommodate to* Truth and Reality. T $\beta \rightarrow \alpha$ thus becomes our illusion, our rationalization (our manic defence) about what happens from this vertex of thinking (reversal of perspective).

B. In reading Bion one gets the impression that he both extols the majesty of the inner world of the archetypal Forms and noumena reached only by imagination, intuition, and painful realizations, upon which circumstances one becomes incarnated by them, but he also treats them as *primitive* or *inchoate* in their immediate offspring, the β-element. Yet he extols the Language of Achievement over the language of substitution. Might we now say, consequently, that the term *"transformation"* should be reserved for the manner in which the *subject adjusts himself* to *accommodate to the Absolute Truth about Ultimate Reality* and *"translation"* should be reserved for the mediation of the Language of Achievement and its pseudonym, "thoughts without a thinker", as it is rendered into the language of substitution, the "α-language", the human "vulgate"?

C. As I have also mentioned earlier, I believe *godhood* (aka "godhead") to be the "ghost-writer" of the "thoughts without a thinker".

The "contact-barrier"

Bion took Freud's old concept of the "contact-barrier" from his "Project for a Scientific Psychology" (1950 [1895]), which Freud (1915d) later replaced with the "repressive barrier". Bion then uniquely reconceptualized the contact-barrier as acting like a neuronal "synapse"—that is, functioning as a selectively permeable membrane between the unconscious and consciousness (and the reverse) in order to preserve the integrity and autonomous functioning of each domain so as to permit selective interchange between them. [It is *my* imaginative conjecture—not Bion's—that the quality of selectivity of this membrane may be due to the functioning of a *numen*, an ineffable threshold "presence" who/which vitalistically decides what (and who) enters and departs either way through the conscious ↔ unconsciousness membrane. This Presence's *nom de plume* is "godhead" (godhood)]. Freud held that repression defends consciousness—later the ego—against the unconscious—later the id—but not the other way around. Bion, applying "binocular vision" and a "reversible perspective", allowed for the repression of both and for selective interaction between them. Freud (1950 [1895]) thought of the contact-barrier as the equivalent of the neuronal synapse. Bion likewise uses the idea of the synapse but metaphorically as a model for transformational junctions.

System Ucs. ↔ System Cs
$$\nwarrow O \nearrow$$

With the application of reversible perspectives and binocular vision, Bion was able to reconfigure the relationship between Systems *Ucs.* and *Cs.* in yet a different way. Now that he had propounded O as the source of ontological and epistemological experience, he reconfigured the relationship of these two systems, first as an *inter*relationship, as stated above, and as a triangulation of O (System *Ucs.* ↔ System *Cs.* triangulate O). Bion did the same with Klein's concepts of the paranoid–schizoid and depressive positions: P–S ↔ D triangulate O. One may understand his binocular triangulation model as an application of the structuralist model known as "binary opposition" (Lévi-Strauss, 1970).

Emotional truth, O, as first cause
and the re-categorization of the drives as emotions

More notably, Bion's episteme shifted Freud's—and even Klein's—emphasis on the life and death instincts (drives) to that of *emotional truth, O*, as first cause, thereby rendering what heretofore were the libidinal and destructive drives, along with the epistemophilic drive, into L, H, and K emotional categories and linkages between objects and between self and objects. In another contribution I put forth the notion of a "truth drive" that consists of evolving O and the internal sense organ, "attention" (intuition, unconscious consciousness), which is sensitive to the relentless evolutions of emotional truth from the internal world (Grotstein, 2004a, 2004b). (See chapter 10.)

α-function and dreaming
versus primary and secondary processes

One of Bion's most innovative reconceptualizations of Freud's contributions was his application of binocular thinking to Freud's notion of the primary and secondary processes. It is of such importance that, in order to elucidate it, I feel the necessity to take a detour through Matte Blanco's (1975, 1988) concepts of symmetry and asymmetry. Matte Blanco hypothesized that human beings use two incompatible forms of logic: formal Aristotelian logic (i.e. Freud's secondary [realistic] process) for consciousness, which he calls "bivalent logic", and "bi-logic" for the unconscious (corresponding to Freud's primary processes). He also conceived of an antinomy between symmetry and asymmetry, the former being more characteristic of the unconscious and the latter of consciousness. However, Matte Blanco also believed that the system of logic of the unconscious, while predominantly symmetrical (everything is equated with everything else; there are no contradictions), also consists of some representations of *a*symmetry (of differences) in a binary-oppositional structure known as "bi-logic".

Thus, what Freud termed the "primary processes" characteristic of unconscious thinking can be understood from Matte Blanco's mathematical rendering as a system of varying relationships between symmetry and *a*symmetry, with a predominance of the former over the latter. The secondary processes (bivalent logic), on the other hand, are characterized predominantly by *a*symmetrical thinking but also include symmetrical thinking for comparisons and differences. Thus, each form of thinking, symmetry and *a*symmetry, is doubly represented, in the unconscious primary processes and in the secondary process of consciousness, but bi-logic is mediated by the Principle of Symmetry (pleasure principle), whereas bivalent logic is mediated by the Principle of Asymmetry (the reality principle).

Now, how does this apply to Bion? Bion (1962b, p. 4), in effect, erased the differences between the locations of the primary and secondary processes by stating that each was represented on both sides of the contact-barrier, one facing internal reality in the unconscious and the other facing external reality in consciousness. Thus, α-function (which itself includes both the primary and the secondary processes as binary-oppositional structures) is doubly represented, in consciousness and in the unconscious. It is a model for a transaction[5] that transforms β-elements, the sensory stimuli of emotional experience (O's imprint on the emotions), into α-elements that are suitable for mentalization—that is, for notation (memory), repression, for reinforcement of the contact-barrier, and for a continuing supply of dream elements for dreaming.

Despite the fact that Bion seems to imply that there is a difference between dreaming and α-function, he seems to speak of their functions as overlapping. However, Ferro (2002b), to whom I have alluded above, helps us out by assigning the function of dreaming to the later assortment of already-processed α-elements into dream narratives. My own view is that dreaming is the realistic *experience*, and α-function is its *model*. Thus, dreaming is *within* the loop of the experience, and α-function is *outside* the loop. (See also Paulo Sandler, 2006a)

Bion has put forward a profound paradigm change for psychoanalytic theory and practice—that the first cause in the psyche is not the traditional drives, the libidinal and destructive, but the Absolute Truth about Ultimate Reality, O. These former drives now provide modifying affect-categorical attributions to the object relations that partake in

O. Put another way, *how one feels about an object is primary*. The former drives, now reconfigured as L, H, and K emotional linkages, help to instruct him how they are being affected along with α-function and/or dreaming.

NOTES

1. I would represent this process as β-element ↔ α-element, as I have previously explained.

2. That the unthought thoughts—that is, "thoughts without a thinker"—actually *seek* a thinker may be more than poetic phantasy. Who, then, is the "thoughts" seeker? I have much to say about this paradox further on.

3. The idea of wildness or randomness is not only the conscious subject's initial impression of O's infinity and absolute symmetry, it is also a holdover, I believe, from German Romanticism, which emphasized the preternatural wildness of Mother Nature. These background ideas helped to contextualize the theories of Freud and Klein, and even Bion at times.

4. Yet Bion (2005a) also states that there is no difference between body and mind (p. 38).

5. It is extraordinary how similar this transformational process is to the ancient Hebrew religious custom of money-lending: exchanging secular money for holy money in the temple with which to purchase sacred lambs for ritual slaughter—a practice against which Jesus railed. It also parallels Freud's injunction that psychoanalysis cannot treat a psychoneurosis; it can only treat a transference neurosis that that has been transferred from an infantile neurosis.

CHAPTER 7

Bion on technique

B ion's contributions to psychoanalytic technique are complex, innovative, profound, and worthy of intense and repeated study. I do not think that I exaggerate when I state that his formulations on technique constitute the most radical paradigm change in psychoanalysis, yet one must acknowledge, as does Paulo Sandler (2005), that some of Bion's ideas on technique do have Freud's concepts as their provenance. Psychoanalysis prior to Bion was, however, largely a left-hemisphere technique (text as opposed to process), in spite of Freud's (1915e) hints about unconscious-to-unconscious communication during analysis. Bion, a keen observer (left-hemisphere: "observation", "sense"), described a right-hemispheric analytic technique ("attention", "reverie", "intuition")—a state-of-the-art process that continues to impress the world of psychoanalysis and psychotherapy.

Bion's recommendations on technique

Very succinctly, Bion offers five suggestions in relation to technique:

A. Use sense, myth, and passion when conducting an analysis. Sense refers to the use of keen observation by any and/or all the senses. Myth refers to the particular mythic template that may be found to organize and join together the analytic object, the O of the session,

DOI: 10.4324/9781003348665-8

which in Kleinian terms is the maximum unconscious anxiety. Bion (1992) suggests that the analyst search for and store myths as the equivalent of a scientific deductive system with regard to psycho-analysis (p. 238). Myths also subtend conscious and unconscious phantasies. Passion designates the analyst's fluctuating emotional state in resonance with the emotions of the patient. As we shall see, *Bion recommends the use of two forms of observation by the analyst: emotional and objective*—that is, intuition and attention.

B. Abandon memory, desire, understanding, and the use of precon-ceptions. Each session constitutes the first day—again—of the anal-ysis. Do not remember previous sessions. Let them remember you spontaneously. Do not desire to cure the patient.

C. Descend into a state of reverie ("wakeful dream thinking") so that you can be optimally receptive to your (the analyst's) unconscious emotional resonance with the patient's emotions and be able op-timally to recruit them. The analyst must not proffer an interpre-tation that he does not feel. The patient will know. Furthermore, the analyst must not repeat an interpretation. Every interpretation should be a surprise both to the analyst and to the patient (personal communication over the years of my analysis).

D. Freely employ speculative imagination and speculative reasoning.

E. The analyst must "dream" the analytic session—that is, he must "dream" the patient's as yet undreamed or incompletely dreamed emotions (O at large).

Bion's exhortation to the analyst to *eschew* (*abandon*) *memory and desire* (1970, p. 30) has become his hallmark, but it was prefigured by Freud (1912e) in his lectures on technique. What it presages is the analyst's capacity for reverie, for "becoming" the analysand, a technique ad-umbrated by Freud but explicated far more fully by Bion. What Bion means by this is for the analyst not to confuse his imaginative creation of the image of the analysand with the real analysand—and be able to help the latter to do the same with him.

Night-time vision as a model for wakeful dreaming

As one reads Bion's works, particularly his recommendations for the analyst's stance in experiencing his patient, one gets the impression of the use of a mental counterpart to night-time vision. During the night the rods of the retina, rather than the more proximal cones, become the effective receptors of light, and they lie off-centre in the eye. In night-time vision, consequently, the subject is compelled to look somewhat to the side of the object (stars, for instance) that he is gazing at. I suggest that this phenomenon constitutes an analogue model for Bion's suggestion to "cast a beam of intense darkness".

Sense, myth, and passion

Bion believes that during the analysis the analyst must use sense, myth, and passion (Bion, 1963, p. 11). By "sense" he means perception or observation. By "myth" he means the apposite unconscious phantasy and its mythical template. By "passion" he means the experience of emotional suffering. This troika of psychoanalytic tools is used by the analyst to fathom what is transpiring in the patient. Thus, the analyst must observe the patient and conceive of the relevant phantasy and then myth—all with his left-hemisphere listening. He must then experience his own internal version that corresponds to the patient's emotional suffering—with his right-hemisphere attention. Then the analyst interprets. As soon as the analyst has intervened appropriately, the patient experiences the result of the analyst's use of sense, myth, and passion and now feels safe enough to experience his emotion. If it is safe for the analyst to detect and experience his version of the patient's emotional experience of O, then this act vouchsafes the patient the ability to experience his own O. That is what is meant by container ↔ contained, reverie, and the analyst "becoming" the patient and "dreaming" the session.

Technique as philosophical prescription and proscription

Bion's suggestions on technique are interesting from another perspective. They are more than suggestions for technique; they are philosophical *pre*scriptions as well as *pro*scriptions about psychoanalysis and life. Today, the concept of philosophy is quite different from what it was in ancient days (Brunschwig & Lloyd, 2000). Now we generally think of philosophers as university professors or consultants or contributors to prestigious literary journals—discussing highly recondite ideas. In ancient Greece, in contrast, philosophy constituted a way of life, a recipe for practical living, whether a person was a Stoic, an Epicurean, or whatever. Followers of a philosophy often lived together. The word "cult" is too strong, but the ways of life practised by cults today approximate the ancient Greek idea but without the narrow rhetoric. Bion's episteme constitutes, in my view, largely a Stoic way of life, both professionally and personally: one should love truth and accept its unpredictable and tragic nature as manifested (realized) in its ambassador, emotion. The reward for doing so is to become heir to one's "divine" (numinous), infinite, and infinitely imaginative, creative self, which, when realized, allows us to evolve as a self.

Speaking on technique, Bion, says:

> What does the psycho-analyst do? He *observes* a mass of "elements long since known but"—till he gives his interpretation—"scattered and seemingly foreign to each other". If he can tolerate the depressive position, he can give this interpretation; the interpretation itself is one of the "only facts worthy of one's attention" which, according to Poincaré, "introduces order into this complexity and so makes it accessible to us". The patient is in this way helped to find, through the analyst's ability to select, one of these unifying facts. [1992, p. 5; italics added]

These ideas represent the quintessence of Bion's technique: the analyst must have *patience* while he continues to *observe* and allow a mass of seemingly *random or chaotic associations* to settle in his mind. Patience means the *ability to tolerate frustration*. This and the *faith* that a *coherence exists*[1] allow the analyst to await the emergence of *the selected fact* (Poincaré, 1963), the veritable "strange attractor" (chaos theory) that gives pattern, coherence, and meaning to the hitherto scattered elements. The selected fact inheres in the analysand's complex associations, but the analyst seems to possess his own inherent and/or acquired version of it, which resonates with that of the patient. I believe that Bion also hints that the selected fact is bimodal in so far as it lurks both as a pre-conception within the analyst and as an entity inherent within the patient's associations. In other words, *two coherences are dialoguing with one another*.

On the relationship between technique and dreaming, Bion states:

> I think the *fear of dreams must contribute to making the patient anxious to avoid the dream-work of the conscious state*. Should it simply be introjection that is avoided? No: because according to me the process of introjection is carried out by the patient's "dreaming" the current events. Introjection–Dreaming, would be the formula. . . . [1992, p. 43; italics added]

In studying psychotics, Bion found that they either did not dream or were afraid of dreaming. When they did dream, this was by expulsion—that is, projective identification—whereas non-psychotic patients dream introjectively—that is, they accept the emotional truths implicit to the dreaming. The psychotic is afraid to dream for fear of encountering the Positions—particularly the depressive position, where psychic reality looms so powerfully:

> Anxiety in the analyst is a sign that the analyst is refusing to "dream" the patient's material: not dream = resist = not introject. . . . I mean that the conscious material has to be subjected to dream-work to render it fit for storing, selection, and suitable for transformation from paranoid–schizoid position to depressive position, and that unconscious pre-verbal material has to be subjected to reciprocal dream-work for the same purpose. *Freud* says Aristotle states that a dream is the way the mind works in sleep: *I* say it is the way it works when awake. [1992, p. 43]

Here in this representative excerpt the reader may catch some of the most radical of Bion's ideas. The analyst must not shrink from the anxiety of *his duty* to *dream* the analytic session. Furthermore, *all stimuli from within and without—that is, "the sensory stimuli of emotional experi- ence"—must first be dreamed by the analyst so that they can become uncon- scious—and unconsciously processed by α-function so as to be rendered into mentalizable elements (α-elements).*

> [T]he *analyst must have a view of the psycho-analytic theory of the Oedi- pus situation.* His understanding of that theory can be regarded as a transformation of that theory and in that case all his interpretations, verbalized or not, of what is going on in a session may be seen as transformations of an *O that is bi-polar. One pole is trained intuitive capacity transformed to effect its juxtaposition with what is going on in the analysis and the other is in the facts of the analytic experience that must be transformed to show what approximation the realization has to the analyst's preconceptions—the preconception here being identical with Ta β as the end-product of Ta α operating on the analyst's psycho-analytic theories.* [1965, p. 49; italics added]

Many readers who are only casually familiar with Bion's recommen- dations to use intuition by eliminating "memory and desire" may not be familiar with "left-hemispheric" Bion, the psychoanalytic ob- server par excellence and disciplinarian who also recommends that the analyst should be so well versed in the Oedipus complex (both the Freudian *and* the Kleinian versions), as well as with Klein's concepts of splitting and projective identification and the movement from the paranoid–schizoid to the depressive position, that he can take them for granted. In addition, it becomes important to realize that the analyst's thinking about and applying his theoretical knowledge involves a *transformation* (personalized version) of those theories.

Bion also reveals that O is bipolar—that is, that it is implicit to the sensory stimuli of emotional experience (from within and without) on the one hand, and to the unconscious inherent pre-conceptions in the unrepressed unconscious on the other. The human being is existentially trapped between the two arms of O. The reader will also note what is left unsaid but implied: that the first cause is no longer Freud's or Klein's drives—bipolar O is now the first cause. Consequently, all psychopathology and/or mental health now issues from how well one is able to tolerate, countenance, contain, dream the irruption of the truth drive which reveals the emotional truth of O.

Bion continues:

> Part of the equipment of observation is pre-conception used as pre-conception—D4 [pre-conception–attention—JSG]. It is in its D4 aspect that I wish to consider the Oedipal theory; that is, as part of the *observational* equipment of the analyst. . . . The analyst's theoretical equipment may thus be narrowly described D4, E4 [conception–attention—JSG], F4 [concept–attention—JSG]. [1965, p. 50–51; italics added]

The terms "pre-conception" and "preconception" need clarification. "Pre-conception" (with hyphen) refers to the inherent template of ideas—what Plato called the Ideal Forms, Kant the noumena, things-in-themselves, "memoirs of the future", the transcendental analytic. It anticipates forthcoming O so as to become O's realization as an actual conception. "Preconception" (closed up), on the other hand, designates a saturation of the observer–container function—even an unexamined prejudice about something or someone—or the constituents of the body of pre-formed knowledge that the analyst must know as he is listening to and observing his patient, thereby foreclosing the analyst's mind to further spontaneous reverie for discovery. Bion then lists the theories related to the Oedipus complex that the analyst needs: projective identification, splitting, intolerance of frustration, envy, greed, part-objects, the theory that primitive thought springs from the experience of a non-existent object (the place where the object is supposed to be but is not), and the theory of the violence of primitive functions:

> These theories, as extensions of the oedipal situation, must be present in the analyst's mind in a form that enables them to be represented in a wide range of categories. [1965, p. 51]

The use of the Oedipus complex and assigning it to E4 is of interest. Originally Bion had titled Column 5 "Oedipus", but later called it "Inquiry". He often conjoined the faculty of curiosity and Oedipus' alleged arrogance in relentlessly inquiring about the truth. He now assigned "Oedipus" to Column 4, Attention–Observation, as the successor to the more passive Notation (Memory).

> The analyst's theoretical equipment may thus be narrowly described D4, E4, F4, but the state of mind in which the theories are available in the session should cover a wider spectrum of the Grid. With this proviso in mind I propose to limit to the following description of theories to statements that fall in the categories E1, E3, E4 and E5. I mean to employ the following theories:
>
> (1) The theory of projective identification and splitting; mechanisms by which the breast provides what the patient later takes over as his own apparatus for ♀♂ function.
>
> (2) The theory that some personalities cannot tolerate frustration.
>
> (3) The theory that a personality with a powerful endowment of envy tends to denude its objects by both stripping and exhaustion.
>
> (4) The theory that at an early stage (or on a primitive level of mind) the oedipal situation is represented by part objects.
>
> (5) The Kleinian theory of envy and greed.
>
> (6) The theory that primitive thought springs from experience of a non-existent object, or, in other terms, of the place where the object is expected to be, but is not.
>
> (7) The theory of violence in primitive functions.
>
> . . . I shall now consider phenomena that the state of expectation represented by these theories might be expected to reveal. One difficulty, of those to which I referred. . . . concerns the communication of material from an experience that is ineffable; the scientific approach, as ordinarily understood, is not available and an aesthetic approach requires an artist. [1965, p. 51]

The analyst should function in D4, E4, and F4, which designates his successive stages of observation—pre-conception → conception → concept—from the initiation of observation to the attention to the selected fact to the formulation of the interpretation and its ultimate abstract significance. As one looks at the Grid—D4 to E4 to F4—one can track the progression of the analyst's *thinking* from *"attention"* about the relevant *"pre-conception"*, through its becoming realized as a *"conception"* and then into a *"concept"* (abstraction). This protocol circumscribes the analyst's processing of the analysand's associations. Bion then describes the onset of the use of α-function. In the beginning the infant must borrow mother's α-function, which helps it to split off bad persecutory objects from good ones and allows it to project the former into mother as container. He also alludes to "bandits" on the path of progression: for example, intolerance of frustration, envy, greed, archaic oedipal (persecutory) part-objects, the dread over the absence of the object, and the dread of the violence of one's unmitigated emotions. Thinking and maturation (learning from, and through, experience) require the subject's ability to tolerate frustration (which allows one's attention-receptor (container) to remain open.

Bion lists projective identification, splitting, intolerance of frustration, envy, greed, archaic (part-object) Oedipus complex, the ability to experience the non-existent object (symbolic representation), and violence as the principal components of the analyst's requisite knowledge of obligatory preconceptions, as mentioned above. He also adds that for him psychoanalysis does not conform to what is commonly known as "science", which is the study of inert objects; rather, it can be known only by an ineffable approach from the aesthetic vertex. I believe that Bion means that the "science" that is appropriate for psychoanalysis is a *mystical science*—one that is non-linear and deals with complexity, infinity, and indeterminacy, one that emerges principally from the aesthetic vertex, by which he implies dreaming: that is, imagination, fiction, creativity.

> If psycho-analysts can abandon themselves to analysis in the psycho-analytical sessions, they are in a position when recollecting the experience in tranquillity to discern their experience as part of a greater whole. Once that is achieved, the way is open for the discovery of configurations [patterns—JSG] revealing yet other and deeper groups of the theory. . . . [1992, p. 285]

I think that here Bion is alluding to a common theme of his—that the more one enters the depressive position, the more the information to be garnered seems to expand by geometric ratios, leading to epistemic dismay and greed. Bion (2005a) states elsewhere: "We now know so much we can't be wise" (p. 66).

> I should explain that I regard the psycho-analyst's capacity to *observe and absorb as much of the analysand's material as possible* as important for the following reasons:
>
> 1. It will enable him to *combine what he hears with what he has already experienced from the patient* to give an immediate interpretation in the circumstances of the actual session.
> 2. At the same time he will observe features that are not comprehen-

sible to him but will contribute at a later stage to the comprehension of material yet to come.

3. There are still other elements of which the analyst will not even be conscious but which will build up an experiential reserve that in due course will influence his conscious views about the patient's material on a specific occasion.

Reason 1, although apparently leading to the operative interpretation, is of less consequence than 2 and 3 because the interpretation is merely setting a formal seal on work that has already been done and is therefore no longer of much consequence.

Reason 2 is of great importance because it is part of the dynamic and continuing process on which the whole viability of the analysis depends. The more the psycho-analyst is open to these impressions, the more he is prepared to participate in the evolution of the analysis. [1992, pp. 287–288; italics added]

Bion believes that the analyst should immerse himself in the material with quiet abandon—and will be rewarded. It is as if the analyst is preconsciously developing a "tree of imaginative inference" for future blossoming, which allows for the evolution of the analyst, analysand, and the analysis itself:

Indeed I believe that it is very important that the *analyst should retain his freshness of outlook so that he never falls into the mistake of treating any session as if it were the repetition of a previous session.* Even in instances where it appears to be almost indistinguishable. . . . [1992, p. 290; italics added]

Bion treats each psychoanalytic session as if it were the first. This is why he exhorts the analyst to abandon memory and desire—so as to maintain a "fresh outlook" on the new idea. Note also his reference to Klein's positions. Bion was very Kleinian despite his radical emendations.

I have found it important to regard every session, no matter how familiar the material may seem to be, as if one were scrutinizing the elements in a *kaleidoscope* before they shake into a definable pattern. . . .

I suggest that for a correct interpretation it is necessary for the analyst to go through the phase of "persecution" even if, as we hope, it is in a modified form, without giving an interpretation. Similarly, he must pass through the depression before he is ready to give an interpretation. . . . [T]he change from paranoid–schizoid to depressive position must be complete before he gives his interpretation.[2]

> *On the whole I am more satisfied with my work if I feel that I have been through these emotional experiences than I do if the session has been more agreeable. I am fortified in this belief by the conviction that has been borne in on me by the analysis of psychotic or borderline patients. I do not think such a patient will ever accept an interpretation, however correct, unless he feels that the analyst has passed through this emotional crisis as a part of the act of giving the interpretation.* [1992, pp. 287–291; italics added]

The first italicized citation is typical of Bion, the mystic, the one who kaleidoscopes (scatters) what appear to be understandable associations and allows them to gestate and reconfigure recombinatorially of their own accord unconsciously and independently (unconscious mentalization). What is unseen in the obvious is Bion's desire to uncover. The second italicized citation constitutes Bion's legacy to psychoanalysis. The analyst must *become* the analysand's *passion* (emotion) and overcome it by *dreaming* it. He must *experience* it and *transcend* it—evolve from P–S to D.

Additional concepts on technique

The analyst's interpretation finds the analysand's personal experience of O through detecting the L, H, and K linkages between analysand and analyst (infantile dependency; two-person relationship) and linkages between objects and between them and himself (oedipal triad).

The analyst's analytic instruments include *sense, myth,* and *passion. Sense* occupies a binary-oppositional structure with *attention* (intuition, reverie). The former constitutes the function of sensory *observation* of the analyst's behaviour and the analyst's impressions from scanning and parsing the analysand's free associations—and also the analysand's observation of the analyst. The latter constitutes a function of *passion,* the analyst's submersion into his own subjectivity to locate matching experiences and emotions that resonate with the analysand's emotional experience and convey credible patterns and configurations. *Myth* is the unconscious template towards which the thus uncovered unconscious phantasies lead—for example, the Oedipus myth.

Ferro (2005) emphasizes Bion's technical concept of "waking dream thought" (Bion, 1962b, p. 8). Bion states that the analyst must "dream" the analytic situation, which is tantamount to dreaming the analysand, or, in my opinion, facilitate the completion of the analysand's uncompleted (therefore still symptom-causing) dream. Ferro speaks of the effects of this wakeful dreaming: (1) it provides a constant monitoring of the analytic field, including the fate of his interpretations; (2) the only concern for the analyst is his wakeful dreaming of the analysand's unconscious narrative derivatives; (3) "it shifts the analyst's attention from the content to what generates the dream itself". Ogden (2003) discusses Bion's theory of dreaming from the vertex of a patient's inability to dream.

In addition, however, I would add to Ferro's keen summary of Bion's recommendations the left-hemispheric approach—that is, "parsing" the analysand's associations. I know that Bion did that with me when I was in analysis with him. As I recall, he would, in fact, pay very close attention to the *sequence* of the associations and bring them to my attention.

Bion has repeatedly emphasized that the infant employs projective identification into mother as container. I have distinguished between projective identification and projective *trans*identification, the former referring to Klein's (1946, 1955) concept of it as an omnipotent unconscious phantasy, and the latter referring to what Bion (1962a, 1962b) meant by communicative projective identification (Grotstein, 2005). Since the publication of that contribution, I have altered my views. I have now come to believe that the infant is born with the rudiments of α-function and generates α-elements, albeit primitive, immature, and non-lexical ones. Schore (personal communication, 2006) confirms this hypothesis. It is only when there is a disruption or breakdown in their communication that the infant is reduced to having to use projective transidentification (heightened emotional display) with the not-so-containing (at the moment) container–mother.[3]

Ferro also adds another player to Bion's dialectic ensemble: the oscillation between negative capability and selected fact, where the former optimally leads to the latter.

Again, I must repeat that the analysand, like the infant, is not necessarily projecting β-elements. I have come to believe (as I stated in chapter 6) that there may be no such a thing as a β-element *per se*, only a degraded α-element. The β-element is an already prejudiced term employed by consciousness and/or the ego because of a premonition and then, as a result, the issuing of an interdiction to the acceptance of an *already known* difficult-to-bear α-element. In other words, as soon as O intersects with the subject's emotional frontier, an α-element is born by virtue of the instantaneous activity of α-function. "β-element" is a disapproved-of α-element by default. These have to be denied, split off, and projected. They are α's scapegoat. *Caveat:* I remind the reader that these views are idiosyncratically—but I hope not heretically—my own. I am fortified in postulating them because of Bion's placing the "β-element" before the "α-element", which is counterintuitive.

Psychoanalysts and psychotherapists are well advised to read Bion's (1976) "Evidence": in this he reveals how the analyst should patiently acquire evidence for his interpretation, and how he personally does so. Patience must be joined with emotional and objective (sensible) observations, with the use of imaginative conjecture and imaginative reason.

Bion's modifications and extension of Kleinian technique

Bion's contributions to Kleinian technique are subtle, profound, and far-ranging. They constitute significant modifications and extensions, as well as continuations of Melanie Klein's original technique. Despite all the variations he improvised, however, it must be noted that Bion—as I as well as those of his other analysands whom I interviewed experienced him—was first and foremost *Kleinian* in his technique. Thus, Bion's innovations can be considered to be "variations—and innovations—on a theme by Klein". The "ghost" of (early and middle) Bion haunts, pervades, and utterly defines the technique currently practised by the London "post-Kleinians", especially Betty Joseph and the participants in her long-standing workshop on technique, as I shall show.

Bion's first major innovations were perhaps his best-known concepts of communicative projective identification[4] and container ↔ contained, the latter being the outcome of the former. This idea carried along with it many important derivative ideas. (1) Bion believed that normal projective identification took place between the infant and its mother as a form of communication rather than merely being evacuation, thereby transforming the concept and operation of projective identification from an exclusively unconscious, omnipotent, intrapsychic mechanism to a normal intersubjective form of communication by extending the unconscious phantasy into an intersubjective reality. (2) The container ↔ contained concept expanded Klein's one-person conception of psychoanalysis by emphasizing the prime importance and irreducibility of the infant's *relationship* to its mother and, by extension, the analysand's irreducible relationship to his analyst. In other words, Bion introduced the intersubjective[5] approach into Kleinian as well as classical psychoanalysis (Bion, 1959). In this model the mother enters into a state of reverie and absorbs and processes (attunes) her infant's emotional displays and experiences with her (3) α-function in preparation for her corrective intervention with her child. (4) His emphasis on emotions rather than on drives constitutes another derivative. (5) His concept of transformations, particularly the analyst's transformation of the O^6 of the analytic session into K, from the ultimate unknowable to the known, thereafter became the mainstay—but most anonymously—of the post-Kleinians in London. The impact of these ideas on the technique employed by the London post-Kleinians and others is to shift the focus of the analyst's awareness from the *content* of the free associations to the unconscious *process* transpiring between the analyst and analysand.

Prior to Bion's contribution, Kleinian analysts emphasized—though not exclusively—the anxieties that the analysand developed between sessions. After the introduction of this idea about transformations in O and from O to K, Betty Joseph and her followers began to highlight the ongoing "here-and-now" in the ever-evolving transference–countertransference situation in the analytic session. They cited Bion's concept of container ↔ contained but seem rigorously to avoid any reference to transformations in and from O, presumably because of the alleged mysticism with which they associate O. One has only to read recent works by London post-Kleinians to realize that they include Bion's theory of transformations without mentioning O. In Betty Joseph's *Psychic Equilibrium and Psychic Change* (1989), or particularly *In Pursuit of Psychic Change: The Betty Joseph Workshop* (Hargreaves & Varchevker, 2004), one can observe first-hand how closely and effectively, but anonymously, they apply Bion's (1965) theory of transformations in and from O. It must also be pointed out, however, that they also utilize Joseph Sandler's (1976) concept of role-responsiveness in conjunction, the emphasis being on what role the analysand is trying unconsciously to impose on the analyst to ensorcell the latter into enacting.

There are other derivatives of Bion's container ↔ contained model. One of these is his concept of dreaming. Bion, unlike Freud, believed that we dream by day as well as by night and that we dream O, the Ultimate Reality that impinges upon our sensory-emotional, intersubjective frontier. This Reality may result from an external or internal stimulus to which we must adjust or accommodate. Dreaming is our way of rendering the experience unconscious and allowing selective aspects of the experience back into our conscious awareness through the selectively permeable contact-barrier (Grotstein, 2002). In terms of the analytic situation, according to Bion (1992, p. 120), the analyst must dream the analytic session. The idea that the analyst should "dream" the analytic session—by "abandoning memory and desire"—became

an important extension of his intersubjective theory of projective identification and a critical modification of the concept of countertransference as an analytic instrument.

Yet another derivative of the model is Bion's (1962, p. 54) concept of "binocular thinking", which he applied in a number of ways.
Container ↔ contained was itself an example in so far as it involved
the interaction of two individuals, where the roles of container and
contained could be switched. Another example is Bion's idea that,
rather than being in conflict, as Freud suggests, consciousness and the
unconscious are in binary (cooperative) opposition in triangulating
O. In addition, he postulates something similar for the relationship
between the paranoid–schizoid and depressive positions, P–S ↔ D
(differentiation ↔ integration), which also cooperatively triangulate
O. The following is one way this new configuration can be seen clinically: The analysand may present material that clearly reveals persecutory anxiety typical of the paranoid–schizoid position. Yet if we pause
for a moment, we begin to realize that the *paranoid–schizoid aspects* of
the analysand are being presented by the *cooperative aspect* of the analysand who is in the depressive position all along.

As Ferro (2005) points out, for Klein wisdom comes from the breast.
For Bion, wisdom comes inside *through* the breast and/or penis.

Bion as a "post-post-Kleinian"

A diligent reading of all Bion's works up to the very last clearly reveals how Kleinian he was. Over and over again, he invokes splitting,
projective identification, envy, greed, hatred, paranoid–schizoid and
depressive positions, the Oedipus complex (Klein's view, part-object),
as well as others. He actually suggests that the analyst's technique requires knowledge of the foregoing so as to be able to supply the requisite phantasy and myth for the clinical situation. This knowledge that
the analyst acquires in his training must be so well known by him that
it can be forgotten (suspended preconceptions) so that he can employ
reverie—by abandoning (suspending) memory, desire, understanding,
and preconceptions. The paradox is that the analyst must first learn
them (and become them) in order to forget them, whereas they, ideally, will not forget him. Thus, Bion was very Kleinian—but in his own
unique and creative way.

O'Shaughnessy (2005) has recently revealed how contemporary
"post-Kleinians" regard Bion. They seem to think highly about his
clinical work and theoretical contributions, up until the mid-1960s.

She praises his invoking the concept of an epistemological instinct and his interesting conceptualization of K. However, O'Shaughnessy, and apparently the post-Kleinians, do not approve of O and its transformations. She describes his moving to O as a lapse in his "discipline" (p. 1524) and therefore, presumably, in his credibility. She implies that Bion's *A Memoir of the Future* trilogy (1975, 1977b, 1979, 1981) was non-scientific. Consequently, "Kleinian–Bionian" means one thing in London among the "post-Kleinians", but virtually everywhere else in the analytic world "Kleinian–Bionian" means the whole of Bion's contributions as well as those of Klein. It is for these reasons that I nominate Bion as a *"post*-post-Kleinian" and the concept of O (Truth, uncertainty) as first cause, as distinguished from the life- and death instincts (positivism) as first cause. I believe that this idea constitutes the defining caesura between the two schools from the vertex of the London Kleinians but not for Bionian–Kleinians. The model that comes to mind is that of the conjoined twin where sameness and difference coexist.

The shift from positivism to ontology, epistemology, and phenomenology: transformations in and from O

Arguably, however, one of Bion's most radical departures from Klein, though not explicated by him directly, was the ultimate implication of O for psychoanalytic theory and practice. For Freud, the critical content of the repressed against which the ego defended was the libidinal drive, although he later added the death drive. For Klein the death drive became the more important of the two repressed drives and the ultimate explanation for psychopathology. Bion, while never formally repudiating the prominence of the death or the libidinal drive, instituted the notion of "evolving O", which I have interpreted as "ever-evolving *truth*"—that is, a "truth drive", which exerts pre-eminence as the content of the repressed (Grotstein, 2004a). By "truth", both Bion and I mean "emotional truth". Thus, the analyst is always searching for the analysand's hidden emotional truth in every analytic session, with the death drive in a secondary position—as defensive armament that is mobilized or recruited by anxiety to attack one's awareness of and links with his dependent relationships on objects that are the occasion for the pain of emotional truth in the first place. According to this reasoning, consequently, *the death instinct is always secondary, never primary*, and is defensive against the awareness of mental pain at the cost of the consciousness of relationships. It attacks links with objects that inaugurate the pain.

When one begins to contemplate that O is the fundamental organizing principle and views the life and death instincts as its positive and negative mediator, respectively, one can perceive a profound psychoanalytic paradigm shift from traditional *positivism* (the primacy of the drives) to *ontology* and *phenomenology* (the primacy of O, Impersonal Existence, the Absolute [Emotional] Truth about Ultimate Reality— that is, "raw", untamed, unmentalized experience). The old task was to acknowledge one's unconscious destructive impulses and rivalry towards the object. The new task is to become evolved enough to be able to allow for the acceptance of Truth as truth, by which I mean the transformation of impersonal Truth into personal truth.

NOTES

1. When Bion states this, he is saying more than he consciously thought, I believe. If there is already a pattern, a selected fact has always already been there to give coherence to the "thoughts without a thinker". So there has always been a "thinker" for the "thoughts without a thinker" (Grotstein, 2000a). This "thinker" is "godhead" (godhood). I develop this theme in chapter 6.

2. It is this passage, which I read a long time ago, that led me to create the idea of the "transcendent position", a position beyond the depressive position (Grotstein, 1993a, 2000a).

3. I hope that my newly developed suggestive revision of the concept of β-elements as misbegotten α-elements will not seem confusing. Despite my respectful departure from Bion on this issue, I shall respect his nomenclature as I proceed.

4. As I have earlier stated and shall expand on later, I now see fit to separate off the act of "communication" from projective identification (transidentification) *per se*. The latter, I now believe, is a breakdown default when the former fails.

5. It must be borne in mind that Bion's intersubjective approach was only part of his communicative contribution; ultimately, the object communicated with is a bridge between the patient and his unconscious.

6. O is Bion's arbitrary term for the existential or ontological moment, generally between two—or more—individuals. It represents the raw, unmentalized experience of the Absolute Truth about Ultimate Reality occurring in each and between each.

CHAPTER 8

Clinical vignette encompassing Bion's technical ideas

The patient is a 32-year-old screen and television writer who is married, childless, and currently he and his wife are planning to have a baby.[1] He brings the following material on a Monday session (he is in analysis four times per week). He is worried about his mother, who is living in a foreign country with an allegedly unscrupulous man. She is suffering from a progressive dementia, presumably Pick's Disease. He is also worried about work in his industry. He himself is suffering from Crohn's Disease, a chronic auto-immune inflammation of the bowel. He had just had a colonoscopy that revealed a slight worsening of his condition.

> ANALYSAND   I don't know what I'm most concerned about, my mother, my Crohn's, my career, or having a new baby—and the cost of that. I called my mother over the weekend but couldn't reach her. I'm really worried about her. Oh, yeah, I had a dream last night. I was in the jungle with my wife, L, and suddenly encountered a large, menacing snake. I was initially frightened but then recalled my Boy Scout training. I located a forked branch of a tree, tore it off, and carefully applied it to the snake's head so as to impale it. I then felt more confident in myself and in my power to cope with danger.

          DOI: 10.4324/9781003348665-9

His associations were as follows: (1) concern (a) about money now that he and his wife are trying to have a baby; (b) about what to do with regard to the "greedy psychopath" who lives with his mother, who has control of her, and who wants more money from her trust fund; (c) that he may have to go either onto steroids or a very expensive drug to contain his Crohn's Disease; (2) he is upset and anxious about being passed over by the producer with whom he had an interview two weeks ago: "Maybe I should change agents?"

While listening to him, I felt uneasy, felt my own gut wrenching, and suddenly, out of nowhere, had a picture of an umbilicus.

I interpreted that he was suffering from feeling that he felt himself to be an inadequate man who could not take care of his present and future family because he still felt umbilically tied to his mother, strangling or impaling her—like her unscrupulous lover. The umbilicus that has remained too long and therefore injures mother is represented by his worsening Crohn's. How can he become an adequate, capable, grown-up person when he still feels umbilically tied to mother? Perhaps he experiences me, because of my giving this interpretation, as a father whom he resents for trying to pull his greedy, infantile snake-self off mother. Perhaps he also fears that the snake-doctor–me is making him physically worse by subjecting him to psychoanalysis (separation).

> ANALYSAND [*he is quiet for a moment and appears to relax*]:   "I don't know why, but I'm suddenly thinking of my fascination with computer games. Does that mean I have to give them up too?"

> ANALYST [*I immediately thought of St. Paul's "First Letter to the Corinthians", in which he says something about "giving up childish things"; he had been too close to his seductive mother growing up, which apparently evoked father's anger*]:   "I think that my leaving you over the weekend has been equated with the producer passing you over. Also, when you ask about giving up computer videogames [*to which he has been almost "addicted"*], I think that you think that a father–me is taking back your rights to be Mummy's baby and is thrusting you into maturity and responsibility."

> ANALYSAND: "Are you saying it's my turn now to go out there in the concrete jungle? L. is very critical of me for spending so much time on the video-games. But you know, the guys I play with are real productive dudes. J. is a professor at CalTech; B. is a successful movie producer; and R. is a doctor."

ANALYST [*as the analysand began to speak, I thought he was confirming my interpretation, but subsequently I felt he had unconsciously become a teenager who was appealing to a strict father-me to allow him to stay up later and play with his friends; I could feel the pressure of his plea*]: "By telling me about the status of your fellow players, I wonder if you're not trying to persuade me that playing video-games is alright. I wonder also if it isn't a compromise formation. You seem to be saying, 'O.K., I'll grow up. I'll go out into the world and make a living for me and my family—but only if I can keep my toys and play with them so as not to deprive my child self.'"

ANALYSAND [*long silence*]: "You mean I can't go home again. I feel sad."

The session was over, but he seemed greatly relieved—and confirmed his positive reaction the next session. In my estimation the interpretation allowed him to evolve from P–S to D.

Analysis of the session

The *analytic object* (the unconscious analytic symptom or conflict) was detected by me both through my preconscious experience of the *selected fact* (the image of the umbilicus, which became the "wild thought" and an "imaginary conjecture"—which ultimately became my "definitory hypothesis"—about what constituted the maximum unconscious anxiety in the patient's material). I employed sense, myth, and passion in order to formulate the nature of the analytic object. The threatening snake I sensed as father's penis inside mother threatening to attack him as the unscrupulous interloper. The myth was the Oedipus complex, particularly Klein's early version of it, which transpires inside mother's body. I experienced the following passions: (1) empathic identification with his travail in life and with regard to his worsening physical condition; (2) feeling, via trial introjective counteridentification, a sense of responsibility and guilt for this unfortunate trend; and (3) a feeling of concern that we were closing in on the O of the session, which he would have a hard time in tolerating: that he was the unscrupulous would-be lover of his mother's insides who psychically caused her to suffer dementia—that is, "holes in the brain"—and that his Crohn's condition is his introjective confirmation of this unconscious awareness. The problem is whether or not he can feel relieved by the snake–doctor-(caduceus)–me, who might have been a deadly persecutor in the dream. In the myth of the labyrinth, am I the helpful Ariadne, or am I the dangerous penis–father, the minotaur who eats innocent children?

It is my impression that I functioned as a container for the patient's unknown O, the contained—which consisted of "wild thoughts", "thoughts without a thinker", "beta-elements". I ultimately understood them as definitory hypotheses (intuitions) and facilitated their transformation from O → K, first within me and then in the patient. While listening to the patient, I was in a state of reverie and was able to "dream" the patient's psychoanalytic object by transposing his literal associations into the mythic register of a specific unconscious phantasy—and was thereby able to put the patient into contact with his personal emotional truth. The image of the snake constituted an ideogram (a visual image).

The interpretation expressed the common denominator between the patient's three worries: about his medical condition, about making a living, and about his mother. My experience of my activity was that of binocular attention and observation—that is, right-hemispheric (intuitive: using symmetrical analogues as models), and left-hemispheric (the sequence of the signifiers in the narrative).

The transference–countertransference situation included, first of all, the analysand's transference (projective identification) into the analytic text (his free associations) and then his transference into his behaviour with me—that is, the plea to let him remain a child.

NOTE

1. This case is also presented in another work (Grotstein, 2007b).

CHAPTER 9

Bion, the mathematician, the mystic, the psychoanalyst

R eading Bion's works chronologically, one notes several por-
tentous trends. Even his graduation paper (from the British
Psychoanalytic Institute), "The Imaginary Twin" (Bion, 1950),
was an exceptional, if not highly recondite, contribution, but one written in the classical Kleinian mode. It would not be long before Bion's
uniqueness expressed itself. In "Differentiation of the Psychotic from
the Non-Psychotic Personalities" (Bion, 1957b) we begin to see an intrepid, redoubtable, and highly intuitive as well as observant psychoanalytic explorer and voyager, one who has discovered—or perhaps
re-discovered—the pathological counterpart to what normally could
be called the "divided self" or the self as "conjoined twins". What I
have in mind here is his later excursion into the division of the personality into a normal, conscious, *finite* self and the *infinite* self of O,
of "godhood". The reader of his early works can also not avoid noting
Bion's unusually keen capacity for clinical observation.

It was in "On Arrogance" (1957a) and "Attacks on Linking" (1959)
that Bion, with his keen powers of observation joined to his equally
unique powers of intuition, noted that his psychotic patients, as infants, seemed to have been deprived of the *normal opportunity* to employ (interpersonal, communicative) projective identification with an
appropriately containing mother. What emerged from that intuition

    DOI: 10.4324/9781003348665-10

and observation were the following: (1) Klein's concept of projective identification as an exclusively unconscious omnipotent phantasy was broadened to its new conception as normal emotional communication between infant and mother. (2) Bion uncovered the key "pathogen" for psychosis (and trauma) in his formulation of the "obstructive object", which in his later works was to become the murderous, hyper-moralistic *super*ego. This toxic, chimerical object consisted of the infant's initial hostility towards mother, then its heightened rage at her for not being a containing mother, the image of mother as hating the infant, and the image of her as projecting in reverse.[1] (3) Bion hypothesized that alongside the toxic influence of the "obstructive object", the psychotic patient, as an infant and carried forward to adulthood, was unusually intolerant of frustration and therefore concretized and filled his mental space of maternal absence with a "no-breast" as a negative realization and as a hateful internal object instead of being able to allow the space of the "no-breast" (yet) to remain open to expectation. (4) The concept of "container ↔ contained" emerged as a landmark and endowing conception that served as a guarantee that every infant is entitled to proper emotional containment—analogous to Bowlby's (1969) concept of attachment and bonding. For Bion, however, it was the cornerstone of his foray into ontological epistemology, which began with his "A Theory of Thinking" (1962a), the distillation of his observations and the resulting conclusions. In short, Bion discovered that—and why—psychotics could not *think* or *feel*: because they could not allow themselves to suffer emotional pain. He was later to ponder why they also could not *sleep* and therefore were unable to distinguish between sleep and wakefulness and between consciousness and the unconscious.

Bion, the mathematician

Now that he had made these landmark discoveries, Bion began to turn his full attention to the *scientific* aspects of thinking: One reason for doing so was that it was part of his nature, as it was part of Freud's, to attempt to bring scientific respectability to psychoanalysis. Another was his deep regret about experiencing so much dissent between the various psychoanalytic schools (personal communication, 1972). He attributed the dissent to the fact that psychoanalytic theory had not been standardized (scientifically). Thus emerged Bion, the mathematician. In his next three works, *Learning from Experience*

(1962b), *Elements of Psycho-Analysis* (1963), and *Transformations* (1965), the mathematical Bion emerges boldly but reconditely. He speaks of "elements", "functions", "constant conjunctions", "realizations", "factors", "rigid motion transformations", and so on. One feels one is back at university, taking a course in higher mathematics. What Bion seems to have been doing was using *analogic* concepts that can match up with emotional changes in the analytic subject. His designation "α" was useful to him because it was unburdened by any fixed meaning or penumbra of associations. He linked it with the mathematical concept of "function":

> "Factor" is the name for a mental activity operating in consort with other mental activities to constitute a function. Factors are deducible from observation of the functions of which they, in consort with each other, are a part. . . . The word used to name the factor is employed *scientifically* and therefore *more rigorously than is usual in conversational English*. [1962b, p. 2; italics added]

The italicized aspect of the citation says it all: that is: "scientifically", "more rigorously than in conversational English". Bion was seeking scientific rigor for a field of inquiry—the emotions—which, he would later say, needed a new kind of science to embrace them: a *mystical science*, an *emotional science, a non-linear, intuitionistic science* capable of tracking chaos, complexity, and emergence, newer mathematical models that Bion's work prefigured and anticipated. Bion was one of the first, if not actually the first, psychoanalyst to see the shortcomings of traditional science in its applicability to human emotions. Science, as Bion would later say, was applicable only to inanimate objects, not to animate ones.

> The function I am about to discuss for its intrinsic importance also serves to illustrate the use to which a theory of functions could be put. I call this function *an α-function so that I may talk about it without being restricted, as I would be if I used a more meaningful term, by an existing penumbra of associations.* [Bion, 1962b, p. 2; italics added]

Again, what is included in the italicized portion of the citation clearly demonstrates Bion's penchant for clinical (observational) precision. Thus, his virtual obsession to achieve precision drew him into "pushing the envelope" of the materialistic science he knew (he was extraordinarily well informed in science and the philosophy of science). His interest in mathematics ran parallel with that in science and also in logic. In fact, it was a sense of precise logic that he was trying to achieve through his use of mathematics. He began using initials as icons—L for love, H for hate, K for knowledge, I for ideas, R for reason, F for faith—as well as α for alpha, and β for beta, the way scientists and mathematicians do. The term "function", mathematical in its origin, is used by Bion to express a *living articulation* (similar to joint articulations) between different aspects of the personality and between the individual and external personalities. (I discuss other aspects of Bion's use of mathematics in chapter 19, where I explicate his use of points, lines, circles, and tangents.)

Bion, the mystic and bearer of the "messiah thought"

In *Transformations* (1965) we begin to see what appears to be a radical change in Bion's episteme, yet it had been gestating in his mind since his earliest days. In setting out the various kinds of mental transformations, he listed "transformations in and from O" (p. 46)—and with this entry and its succession, Bion crossed the Rubicon. The book was published just before Bion left London for Los Angeles. His contributions up to that time had come to be highly regarded by London Kleinians, and Bion began to be mentioned in hyphenation with Klein. However, starting with *Transformations*, his contributions were considered heretical and non-main-stream Kleinian or even Kleinian–Bionian. O marks the formal beginning of Bion as the mystic—that is, a mystical analyst. To this very day many are unclear about what Bion meant by O. His mystical turn had much in common with a mystical side of Freud, and Bion acknowledges his ancestry there. He does not, strangely, acknowledge the mystical contributions of Winnicott, Lacan, or Jung, whereas he does respect those of Buber. Those he mainly refers to are the pre-Socratic Greek philosophers, especially Heraclitus for his concept of "flux", Plato, Meister Eckhart, and Isaac Luria. Why did he take this right turn in his journey?

Implicit in Bion's earlier conception of container ↔ contained (1962b) was a subtle but profound change in the way he advocated listening to the patient. Earlier on, he had demonstrated that he listened to the *content* of the patient's associations. With container ↔ contained we witness a paradigm shift whereby he advocates listening and feeling what you, the analyst, are experiencing at any precise clinical moment, irrespective of content—that is, *process*. As he interpreted to me once when I was in analysis with him, "The analyst, rather than listening to the patient, should listen to himself listening to the patient!" This is how Bion first introduced the *mystic vertex* into psychoanalysis—as a new form of technique.

O, the "messiah thought", and the hidden order of mysticism

There was more to be gleaned from the mystic vertex, however, and that was in terms of theory. This bring us back to O. What is O? O can be defined as that Ultimate Reality always in flux, that is free of representations, images, or symbols. O was chosen by Bion because, I conjecture, it constitutes a circle and thus an enclosure or containment. Yet it is also an unsaturated icon that is ever ready to address our speculations. Bion (1965, 1970) defines O as the Absolute Truth [about] Ultimate Reality, but he also associates it with infinity, β-elements, the Ideal Forms, noumena or the things-in-themselves, and *godhead* (godhood). While O constituted a general concept, Bion used it mainly in the context of the infant–mother and analysand–analyst relationship. This aspect designates the "sensory stimuli of emotional experience", the external manifestation of O. If one reads Bion carefully, one detects another more mystical source of O—the unrepressed unconscious itself and its numinous denizens. Here is where mystical Bion intuited the messiah aspects of O. The mystic does not mystify. He finds the mysterious lurking within the obvious and, conversely, detects the obvious within the mysterious. That was Bion!

O as godhead (godhood or godliness)

Something else happens within the above analytic scenario of sense, myth, and passion: In the very act of the patient's *"re-becoming"* his own hitherto unaccepted emotion, he is re-becoming himself—*and* something else. His very acceptance of the hitherto barred emotion suddenly opens the door of his unrepressed unconscious, and the whole panoply of the Ideal Forms (inherent and acquired pre-conceptions, "memoirs of the future") and the noumena or things-in-themselves springs forth to join up selectively and appropriately with the newly reaccepted emotion, which was, in retrospect, the key to the unlocking of the former. But why is O depicted by Bion as "godhead"? The unrepressed unconscious is characterized mathematically as being *infinite* and absolutely *symmetrical* (Matte Blanco, 1975, 2005). The human individual, according to Bion, is born with a religious instinct, predisposed to experience "reverence and awe" in relation to deities imaginatively created to accommodate the need to worship (Bion, 1992, p. 284; personal communication, 1979). Thus, the analytic subject may unconsciously phantasize the existence of a godhead who is, as infinite, symmetrical, and omniscient, a veritable "Librarian Extra-

Ordinaire" for the Library of the Ideal Forms. This entity has been variously known as "Descartes' Demon" and "Laplace's Demon", the latter being the one who knew all possible mathematical computations. But there is another quality of this godhead that bears scrutiny.

Stitzman (2004) calls attention to Bion's theme of O when he reminds us that Bion first addressed the mystical domain of psychoanalysis in *Transformations* (1965) by referring to the analyst's need to "become" the patient, whereas in *Attention and Interpretation* (1970) he states that what is to be sought is the restoration of god as the mother and the evolution of god (the formless, infinite, ineffable, non-existent), which can be found only in a state in which memory, desire, understanding, and preconceptions[2] are absent. O in this case is Ultimate Reality arriving as Absolute Truth.

I cannot leave the subject of godhood without reiterating my opinion that godhood is the "thinker" of the "thoughts without a thinker" and the prime generator of α-elements—without a detour with β-elements except in default (see chapter 8).

The mystery behind "incarnation"

When the patient becomes again his lost, split-off, and projected self by re-owning his hitherto unbearable emotions, he inwardly unconsciously proceeds from "pre-conception" to "conception", which transformational act can be equated with a *realization* of an object in reality. This sense of realization is conjoined with yet another phenomenon, the "incarnation" of the "god-container" of O into the potential and potentially evolving mystical self within us. Stitzman has wisely understood Bion on this matter.[3] The patient does not incarnate the godhead—that would constitute mania or psychosis. The godhead must *choose* to incarnate the patient. But who is the god who must choose man to incarnate *him* or *her*? The overtones of the Christ myth are striking. The god (God?) who alone must choose to incarnate mankind represents man's wish for an incomplete and mute god to seek incarnation with human beings in order to incarnate him as a realization. This seems to be a Darwinian god. The payoff for the patient in analysis, however, is that he becomes not only more himself from reclaiming his lost emotions. He becomes more *evolved* as a finite → infinite self by receiving the legacy from his infinite, immortal, godly self. I call this state the attainment of the "transcendent position" (Grotstein, 2000a, p. 35).

It is tempting to speculate from the above that the issue of incarnation is central to the hidden order of religion as well as psychoanalysis.

Put succinctly, if the "thoughts without a thinker" (which, I argue, *are* "thought" *a priori* by the godhead) seek incarnation in human experience to achieve *realization*, then might we not speculate derivatively that, from the religious vertex, God is incomplete and needs to incarnate mortals in order to *realize* Him—and might we not speculate that the system *Ucs.* is likewise incomplete and need its more mortal and quotidian twin, consciousness, to complete its mission?

NOTES

1. I should like to take this opportunity to broaden Bion's concept by suggesting that this toxic object may also include Klein's (1928) concept of the dangerous, omnipotent "combined-parent" function as a "symbolic equation" (Freud, 1924d, p. 179; Segal, 1957, 1981)—to render it all the more formidable---*and the desultory release of unbound inherent pre-conceptions, O.* Moreover, this malevolent object may constitute the organizing principle in negative messiahs and charismatic dictators.

2. Bion distinguishes between "pre-conceptions", which are Platonic Ideal Forms, and "preconceptions" which are traditionally held, unmodified categorizations (see chapter 7).

3. See also Godbout (2004).

CHAPTER 10

The "Language of Achievement"

> "I had not a dispute but a disquisition with Dilke on various subjects; several things dove-tailed in my mind, and at once it struck me what quality went to form a Man of Achievement, especially in Literature, and which Shakespeare possessed so enormously—I mean Negative Capability, that is, when a man is capable of being in uncertainties, mysteries, doubts, without any irritable reaching after fact and reason."
>
> John Keats (1817; cited in Bion, 1970, p. 125)[1]

Bion adumbrated the concept of the "Language of Achieve-ment" in *Learning from Experience* (1962b), but he developed it more fully in *Attention and Interpretation* (1970). He borrowed "Achievement" from Keats along with "Negative Capability", which is Achievement's obligatory counterpart. The Language of Achieve-ment (note Bion's capitalizations) was conceived of by Bion in order to rectify problems he encountered—and believed all analysts encoun-tered—in communicating their analytic experiences with analysands to other analysts. He had created the Grid (1963) for the same reason. With the discovery of O, however (Bion, 1965, 1970), he applied the Language of Achievement to the analyst's emotional interaction with the analysand. Ordinary language, being sensuously derived, was unsuitable for conveying the ineffability of the analytic experience to analysands, to colleagues, or to oneself. By "sensuously derived", Bion seems to mean that ordinary language, which he calls the "language of *substitution*", is based upon *representations* of objects: that is, substitutive symbols derived from images that are, in turn, derived from the sense organs. The sense organs are sensitive to external—not internal—stimuli. Sensations produce *impressions* about the object, but the object's aliveness and propensity to be in flux defies any representation to reproduce it. Consciousness alone is the sense organ receptive to psychic qualities, according to Freud (1911b) and Bion (1962b, p. 4). Stated from another perspective (vertex), the Language of Achievement is the language of *emotions* before they become represented as concepts or ideas—and it also is the language of *models*—that is, analogue models and experiences outside the system under investigation.

Put another way, the language we normally speak and write is symbolic. In order to communicate our observations about or address an object, we use a language based on images (internal objects, representations) *about* an object (individual). (I dealt with this matter in chapter 5, where I discussed Bion's rationale for using models as opposed to theories.)

The analyst must consequently become a "Man of Achievement"—one with indomitable patience and equanimity and one who is inured to uncertainty—so as to be qualified to listen to and speak the "Language of Achievement". This means that with *patience* and *security* this person can suspend the distracting din of the language of substitution so as to keep himself open to the unconscious emotions that are spontaneously—meditatively—welling up from within him as he fully experiences himself experiencing the full presence of his analysand: that is, experiencing himself "becoming" the O from within himself that is resonant with the analysand's O (the "psychoanalytic object"). He is Bion's image of the disciplined army officer stationed in a veritable trench behind the couch. I should like to extend Bion's concept of patience ↔ security (P–S ↔ D) from the analyst to the patient. As, according to Bion, P–S operates simultaneously with D, this would mean that: (1) the infant is born into both positions but becomes principally involved with P–S as a defence against the emotional consequences of D. (2) Likewise, the analytic patient generally operates from D to deal with his P–S (O).

Bion states:

By resorting to abstraction and its products, α-function and its factors, I have been able to discuss psychoanalytic unknowns. I continue by concretization [the opposite of abstraction—JSG], that is, by using terms approximating to those used on a level of empirically verifiable data, to speculate on what part of the early psychic apparatus it is that is deflected to the provision of the apparatus needed for thought. Freud, describing thought as providing a method of restraint for motor discharge which had become necessary, simply says it developed from ideation. In his discussion of dream interpretation Freud was impressed by the value of the reflex apparatus as a model for the psychic apparatus involved in dreaming and evolved his theory of primary and secondary systems in the light of this model. *I suggest that thinking is something forced on an apparatus, not suited for the purpose, by the demands of reality, and is contemporary with, as Freud said, the dominance of the reality principle.* A modern analogy is provided by the fact that *the demands of reality not only forced the discovery of psycho-analysis, but have led to the deflection of verbal thought from its original function of providing restraint for motor discharge to the tasks of self knowledge for which it is ill-suited and for the purpose of which it has to undergo drastic changes.* [1962b, pp. 56–57; italics added]

Bion seems to be saying that ordinary (sense-based) language is unsuitable for use in psychoanalysis. He refers to his use of abstraction, linking abstraction to the creation of *ad hoc models* that work analogously and resonantly with the variations in the subject. As one more fully contemplates how Bion conceives of the Language of Achievement, one is tempted to think of Schreber's (1903) "ground language"—a language that is fundamental, mostly unconscious, and syncretistic, like poetic and artistic images. Just as a painting can be worth a thousand words, so certain well-chosen words and word-combinations, as well as well-crafted artistic images, can indicate far more than they express literally. One is reminded of Peirce's (1931) distinction between words that are "iconic" and those that are "indexical", the former conveying a narrower and more immediate range of meaning, the latter a much broader and far-ranging spread of associative meanings, of ever-elaborating metaphors. Bion was searching for a way of expressing psychic qualities in a language that was worthy of them—that is, one that could address complexity and non-linearity. He states:

In his sphere the psycho-analyst's attention is arrested by a particular experience to which he would draw the attention of the analysand. To do this he must employ the Language of Achievement. That is to say, *he must employ methods which have the counterpart of durability or extension in a domain where there is no time or space as those terms are used in the world of sense.* [1970, p. 2; italics added]

Bion's reference here to "counterpart of durability or extension in a domain where there is no time or space as those terms are used in the world of sense" implies that only a language that is free from sense-derived limitations and one that is sensitive to the timelessness and spacelessness (the infinity and absolute symmetry) of psychic reality can be suitable for intercepting the unconscious emotional life operant there.

Bion continues:

> Therefore, the Language of Achievement, if it is to be employed for elucidating the truth, must be recognized as *deriving not only from sensuous experience but also from impulses and dispositions far from those ordinarily associated with scientific discussion.* Freud, like others before him, felt the need to isolate himself—insulate himself?—from the group in order to work. This would mean insulating ourselves against the very material we should study. [1970, p. 3; italics added]

In other words, the Language of Achievement does derive from sensuous experience as well as from non-sensuous experience. With regard to the former, I believe that Bion has the faculty of "observation" in mind. It is my understanding that Bion recommends that when listening to the patient, the analyst should employ "binocular vision": that is, the two perspectives. It also implies that consciousness, the sense organ receptive to psychic qualities, is bimodal in that it is also sensitive to external sensory qualities.

He states further:

> Set over against and *in contrast with the Language of Achievement I consider the language that is a substitute for, and not a prelude to, action.* Language of Achievement includes language that is both prelude to action and itself a kind of action; the meeting of psycho-analyst and analysand is itself an example of this language. [1970, p. 125; italics added]

> The psycho-analyst's *attention must not wander from areas of material characterized either by the Language of Substitution or by the Language of Achievement; he must remain sensitive to both.* I do not claim that sensitivity can be achieved easily: the mental space available to the analysand and the material observed are subject to so many transformations that such a claim suggests inexperience of the practice of psychoanalysis. . . . *Experience leads to an extension of the area over which the Language of Achievement operates and therefore an extension of the area in which its operation can be recognized.* [p. 126; italics added]

Note Bion's use again of "binocular vision"—that is, the recommendation to the analyst to be sensitive to the Language both of Achievement *and* of Substitution. Note also his rationale for the use of the Language of Achievement: the range of the area over which it operates. Bion (1963, p. 103) urges the analyst to employ "sense, myth, and passion" in his search for the "analytic object", O, in the patient's material. The first of these, "sense", can be understood as "observation", which we now realize includes the use of the Languages of Achievement *and* of Substitution. "Myth" implies the whole range of collective and individual myths and phantasies as well as the body of psychoanalytic theories that subtend them—that is, the Oedipal myth. "Passion" implies the analyst's reverie and its receptivity to the analyst's own native emotions, which are evoked by his intimate experience with his patient. This analytic receptivity is yet another aspect of the Language of Achievement.

Christian mystics—Meister Eckhart and others—speak of the metaphatic and apophatic mystical language of unsaying, by which is meant that any spoken word must be followed by its opposite[1] (McGinn, 1994, 1996; Sells, 1994, and personal communication, 1997; Webb & Sells, 1997). This dialectical procedure was deemed necessary so as not to defile the essence of the deity by capturing him in language. This, I believe, is what Bion is getting at. The language of substitution acts like a photographic snapshot to extract a numinous idea or object from the mythic stream and *capture* it forever, thereby arresting its vitality and motion. Bion's Language of Achievement is the language of *paradox*. Perhaps I can reveal this idea more clearly with a quotation from Plato that López-Corvo (2006) cited:

> What is that which always is, and has no becoming;
> and what is that which is always becoming and never is?
> [Timaeus, § 27]

Conclusion: The Language of Achievement is the paradoxical, apophatic language of becoming.

NOTES

1. This is strikingly similar to obsessive–compulsive doing–undoing.

CHAPTER 11

Bion's discovery of O

Following a brief clinical illustration in his third major book, *Transformations*, Bion states:

> I am . . . concerned with theories of psycho-analytic observations, and the theory of transformations, the application of which I am here illustrating, is one of them. Can this theory be applied to bridge the gap between psycho-analytic preconceptions, and the *facts* as they emerge in the session? . . . I shall apply the theory to my own account of the session: something occurred during the session—the *absolute facts of the session. What the absolute facts are cannot ever be known, and these I denote by the sign O.* [1965, pp. 16–17; italics added]

With this statement, Bion crossed the Rubicon of psychoanalytic respectability in London (as described in chapter 9) and launched a metapsychological revolution whose echoes are still reverberating across the psychoanalytic landscape worldwide. Standing veritably on a "peak in Darien", he perforated the flat world of Freud's and Klein's positivism (the instinctual drives as first cause) and introduced inner and outer cosmic uncertainty, infinity, relativism, and numinousness as its successor. *If Bion's theory of O is correct, then it just may be that Freud's and Klein's episteme constitutes an inadvertent manic defence against the primacy (first cause) of uncertainty and the Absolute Truth about Ultimate Reality. In other words, the instinctual drives—particularly the death instinct in*

DOI: 10.4324/9781003348665-12

Kleinian theory—would be relegated to the status of mediators of O. Ferro (2002a, p. 4) goes so far as to suggest that the death instinct is really a way of talking about the intergenerational neurosis in which, when one generation fails to contain its own O, it unconsciously projects the responsibility onto the next to be its messiah–saviour from O.

O is Bion's arbitrary iconic term for a third domain, yet really the first—the original and fundamental domain that is unknown and unknowable to us, one that both subtends and interpenetrates consciousness as well as the unconscious *and* transcends them, one that expresses the Absolute Truth about an Ultimate Reality that is always evolving (always in flux) and is indicative of inner and outer cosmic unknowability, infinity, and ultimate *in*divisibility, *Ananke* (Necessity), chaos, complexity, and, finally, "godhead"[1]—that is, the imagined Presence of the fabled one within us who "knows" all the Ideal Forms and noumena, but who is incomplete and seeks to become incarnated (realized) in the human being by being transformed from an inherent pre-conception to a human conception → concept in the vale of *experience*. O is first cause and marginalizes and replaces Freud's and Klein's libidinal and death instincts as "first cause", the deepest source of mental and biological life, and, in *my* thinking, includes Aristotle's *entelechy*, the actualization of our total teleological potential, and Spinoza's *conatus*.[2]

O is the source of all our anxieties and eternally hovers as the "emotional turbulence" (Bion, 1965, p. 48) that is inescapable when two or more people or objects encounter one another or during any experience of "catastrophic change" (Bion, 1965, p. 11) from one state to another. In psychoanalysis it is the "analytic object" (Bion, 1962, p. 68), to be fathomed by the analyst. The libidinal or life instinct both expresses it and defends against it, as does the death instinct, which attacks the infant's—and analysand's—capacity to think, to contemplate, and to link with objects internally and externally when O is felt to be overwhelming, thus helping the individual stricken by O to "die a little" emotionally, adaptively, in order to remain alive as a self. *O, then—not the death instinct, nor the life instinct—is the instigator of the persecutory anxiety that characterizes the paranoid–schizoid position and ultimately the depressive anxiety of the depressive position: for example, the haunting dread of becoming an "orphan of O".*

O may also be understood as "raw, ever-emerging, ever-intersecting Circumstance". An interesting simile for it is a driving game that can be observed at fairs or penny arcades: a glass booth, on the front surface of which is an automobile steering wheel, and on the viewing screen is a moving road zigzagging in an unpredictable manner towards the person at the controls. The aim is to control the wheel so as to remain on the ever-approaching, unpredictably zigzagging road. This unpredictable road is O; it represents any kind of interaction with an object or objects, within or without. Put another way, life forces itself upon the hapless subject both from inside (entelechy) and from outside (circumstance).

O is the essence of the unconscious as well as of the Unknown, that which lies beyond both consciousness and the unconscious. O, not the drives, constitutes the "seething cauldron", the ultimate "uncontained" of an ineffable, infinite "container", infinity. *From this point of view (vertex) all internal objects can be understood as "radioactive waste-dumps" of unprocessed (uncontained and /or undreamed) β-elements from untransformed O (failures of containment by self and/or by rearing objects) except for those compensatory, putatively good objects that have been internalized in order to counterbalance the former* (Fairbairn, 1943). We must patiently tolerate—suffer—the evolutions of O until they first become ac-knowledged in K, and then we "become" O. In other words, Bion's theory of the transformation of O seems to be a cyclic one in which *impersonal* (indifferent) O becomes transformed ultimately into our *personal* O, which becomes one—and/or which one becomes—as we physically become the food we eat, within the constraints of our self-defining self-organization (conatus). *Knowledge (transformations in K) constitutes, consequently, an intermediary position, an obligatory detour, in the process of the person evolving as an individual in consonance and in parallel with evolving O.*

"'O' is a dark spot that must be illuminated by blindness"[3]

Whereas his conception of container ↔ contained represented a needed extension of Kleinian theory into external reality, his conception of O was a sortie into the surreal. Bion broke the procrustean confines that characterized the time-warped logical positivism of Freud and Klein and thrust psychoanalysis into the "deep and formless infinite", O. To his erstwhile flatlander colleagues he had gone over the edge of the known world. I believe that in fact he had transcended the strictures of our known psychoanalytic *Weltanschauung* and the limitations of the pleasure principle, and he had thrust past the limitations of the death instinct, realizing all the while that they were merely stepping stones, markers—signifiers to or hieroglyphs of an ineffable, O. If I read Bion correctly, the task of each analytic session is for the analyst to discipline himself with the suspension of memory, desire, and understanding (suspension of ego) in such a way that he becomes all the more intuitively responsive to his inner sense receptor that is sensitive to his "waveband" of O, which then resonates with the analysand's *psychoanalytic object*,[4] his own O, which is characterized by his Ultimate Reality, his Absolute[5] Truth. Thus, the analyst's O becomes resonant on that ineffable "waveband" with the O of the analysand, which the former must then transduce or transform for the analysand in K as symbols in the form of interpretation; if accepted, it then becomes retransformed into the analysand's personal O (Grotstein, 1985).

O is either Sodom and Gomorrah or harmony and serenity, depending on the vertex of our ontological disposition. There is a pendulum that inexorably swings between Beauty and Horror. The fulcrum of the pendulum is O. With O in place, we realize, along with Heidegger, that the tongue is the listener to an inner ineffable voice. Words depict but do not encompass Truth. They are a transient reward for the achievement of the depressive position but, like Derrida's erasures, must be barred and erased once we use them so that we can keep our rendezvous with the ineffable, inscrutable, unknowable—that domain where words and their quotidian meanings end and O begins. O—or should I say O-ing, as O is always evolving, in flux?—is paradoxically ineffable but is also immanent and seeks revelation and realization as the psychoanalytic object, as the symptom, or, as I should like to put it, as the phenomenal or immanent subject of psychoanalysis.

O as ultimate reality

O is a hovering, ethereal, placeless landscape that dreamily interpenetrates our reality with its all-too-subtle yet all-too-powerful Ultimate Reality that is beyond our senses, beyond our imagination, and beyond our conception and which belongs to the category of a meta-conceptualization that includes Ultimate Unknowable Truth, chaos, the thing-in-itself, and the so-called "β-elements". It also includes Plato's theory of Eternal Forms and Bion's "thoughts without a thinker",[6] by which he often means "inherent pre-conceptions", those inherent entities that search for confirming realizations in conjured moieties anticipated in their future. To these ideas I would also add yet another relevant idea from the *Kabbalah*, the mystic Hebrew text in which Bion was deeply interested (personal communication, 1976). In the *Kabbalah*, according to Bloom (1983), there once was a unitary Godhead, but, in order for the world to be created, God had to "shrink" (Hebrew: "*zimzum*") from His Godhead ("Keter-Ayn Sof" ["Everything and Nothing]") in order to become immanent. The immanent God has been referred to in Greek texts as the "Demiurge", the creator of the world. When we are in a state of "transformation in 'O'", we *feel* at one with the Godhead itself, the Ultimate Subject. "God", the Demiurge (God as creator of the universe, not the God of essence), is the colloquial way in which we innocently yet sacrilegiously refer to Him (as the Object, which He never can become). In that state we once would have "turned into a pillar of salt" because of our terror of experiencing it. Ultimately, if we can face it, we evolve into a state of *serenity* that is experienced by the mystic. Yet we must also be prepared for the dark face of O—that is, O's reversible perspective, the ineluctable journey to which Bion cryptically refers as "Dawn of Oblivion", and which at the same time constitutes Bion's ultimate theory of eschatology.

O, symmetry, and the death instinct

Thanks to Matte Blanco's (1975, 1981, 1988, 2005) radical mathematics-based revision of our conception of the unconscious, which is isomorphic to O, we are now able to comprehend a graded, stratified layering to O. In other words, by Matte Blanco's reasoning there is a lack of uniformity in the unconscious, which, along with its quality of infinity and properties of infinite sets, presents itself as chaos or, paradoxically, as "asymmetrical symmetry" or infinity. He postulates that the unconscious is characterized by 15 graded layerings or stratifications of varying descending and ascending "bi-logic structures", which consist of differing proportions of symmetrical logic (infinity) and *a*symmetrical logic. Side by side with this binary-oppositional structure there exists "bivalent logic"—that is, classical or Aristotelian logic. According to Matte Blanco, the mind is ultimately dominated by the dialectical interaction of two principal modes, the *homogeneous* (infinity, infinite sets, symmetrical logic) and the *heterogeneous* (divisible, classically logical). In consequence O (the unconscious, the psychoanalytic object) would be characterized as being infinite with varying degrees of asymmetrization of that infinite symmetry, which would characterize an infinite number of sets of infinity itself—thus *chaos*.

Consequently, it is conceivable to postulate, via Matte Blanco's "psycho-mathematical" theorems, that the inchoate infant's proto-experience of O is one of Absolute Chaos. When the infant "experiences"—that is, takes in—the impact of this first confrontation with Prime, Absolute Otherness (other than the breast), its very experiencing of it conveys a sense of *agency* and *personal subjectivity* to it. I suggest that primal transformation causes the infant to believe that it has been attacked by its own death instinct, a tropism that it now assesses as belonging to itself. Subjectivity and agency have then begun (Grotstein, 1996b, 1997a, 1997b, 1997c).

An "imaginative conjecture" on Bion's personal relationship to O

Bion, the intrepid explorer of "the deep and formless infinite", seems to have navigated the passage to O by consulting the "stars of darkness". He arrived at this new concept of transformation *and* evolution in O, first by intuiting the existence (presence) of the absent breast, the "no-thing", in the clinical situation. According to Meg Harris Williams (1985), he may also have arrived at it from having experienced the terrors and traumas of his own life.[8] When we read in his autobiography that he ". . . died on the Amiens–Roye Road on August 8, 1918", we get a haunting piece of subjective archive that informs us with graphic certainty that he had been baptized into and thus had become an "orphan of O", and he had been certified in the experience of "nameless dread" (Bion, 1982). Who could be more qualified to be our guide in that indescribable domain, the very existence of which most of us are privileged never even to have suspected, let alone experienced? With regard to those experiences, one wonders whether, by his few but trenchant critiques of Melanie Klein, his analyst, in his autobiography Bion is not suggesting that Klein effectively analysed the envy, greed, and omnipotence of the putatively surviving Bion (i.e. she helped him to evolve from P–S to D), but she may have neglected the "dead" Bion—the one who was amberized on the holocaustal side of O.

Bion, who had received the DSO (Distinguished Service Order), always maintained that he was a "coward". This paradox is understandable if we think of him as having suffered from what we now prosaically term "post-traumatic stress disorder", in which he may have believed that he had surrendered his soul to the darkness of dread. His autobiography and metapsychology may constitute desperate "radio signals" from an "undead"/"dead" self who is struggling to be heard—from the other side of being. When he spoke of "making the best of a bad job", we perhaps begin to realize that, in his attempted rehabilitation from that ultimate trauma, he was trying to put his agony, surrender, and reconciliation to optimum use: to experience hope under the shadow of intimidating dread and to demonstrate how to use our sublimated agony as an analytic instrument.

NOTES

1. I remind the reader that "godhead" should be read as "godhood" (as I initially stated in chapter 1).

2. Damasio defines "conatus" as follows: "The conatus subsumes both the impetus for self-preservation in the face of danger and opportunities and the myriad actions of self-preservation that hold the parts of the body together. In spite of the transformations the body [and mind—JSG] must undergo as it develops, renews the constituent parts, and ages, the conatus continues to form the same individual and respect the same structural design" (Damasio, 2003, p. 36). Thus, to me conatus and entelechy constitute different sides of the same coin, O, and are the unconscious' seething cauldron.

3. Thus, Bion's idiosyncratic translation of the Freud/Andreas-Salomé Letter and thus the title of this book!

4. I am aware that my earlier statement that O, like the concept of the deity, is the Subject of subjects and can never be the object and Bion's equating O with the "psychoanalytic object" are contradictory. In my opinion Bion is here inconsistent with his own theory of O, the ultimate Subject of Being.

5. Paradoxically, Bion himself was caught up in his own conceptual trap. By daring to *name* Truth "Absolute" and Reality "Ultimate", he reduced them to name-confinable entities, to verbal conventions that now limit them. I said more about this contradiction when I referred to the "apophatic language of unsaying" of the mystics in chapter 10.

6. At times he refers to these inherent pre-conceptions as "memoirs of the future".

7. From the Theurgic Kabbalah of Zohar.

8. See also Meltzer (1978, 1980, 1985) and Joan and Neville Symington (1996) for their readings of Bion's *A Memoir of the Future* (1975, 1977b, 1979, 1981).

CHAPTER 12

The concept of the "transcendent position"

I suggest that Bion's concept of O (see chapter 6) both transcends and *precedes* and *succeeds* Klein's concept of the paranoid–schizoid and depressive positions. I could also have said that it goes *beyond* not only Freud's pleasure and reality principles[1] and his topographic and structural models of the psyche (Systems *Ucs.*, *Pcs.*, and *Cs.*, ego, id, and superego) but also *beyond* Freud's and Klein's notions of the death instinct, each of which my thesis renders as signifying *mediators* of O, thereby making O ultimate, though unknowable. From another perspective one can think of O as analogous to "dark matter"—that amorphous mass hidden in our universe that thoroughly perfuses it (Tucker & Tucker, 1988). It also summons concepts of pure ontology for psychoanalysis, especially the idea of *Ananke*[2] (Greek: "Necessity" or "Fate"; Ricoeur, 1970), Lacan's (1966) concept of the Register of the Real, and Peirce's (1931) concept of "brute reality".

I believe that the concept of O transforms all existing psychoanalytic theories (e.g. the pleasure principle, the death instinct, and the paranoid–schizoid and depressive positions) into veritable psychoanalytic manic defences against the unknown, unknowable, ineffable, inscrutable, ontological experience of ultimate being, what Bion terms "Absolute Truth", "Ultimate Reality". It is beyond words, beyond contemplation, beyond knowing, and always remains "*beyond*" in dimensions forever unreachable by man. Yet at the same time, paradoxically,

DOI: 10.4324/9781003348665-13

even in its beyondness it thoroughly perfuses and interpenetrates our conscious and unconscious existence and the objects with whom we interact.

The cycle of return in O's transformations

Yet, paradoxically, this beyondness is within us as our unconscious, and therefore this numinous transcendence is also *immanent*. Bion believed that we achieve what I am calling transcendence when our immanent godhead—that is, our inherent pre-conceptions (Ideal Forms, noumena)—achieves realization in actual experience. We then become one with our immanent, infinite transcendent self. As I discuss in chapter 19, I believe that Bion's transformational protocol constitutes a cycle of mental and emotional processing on two fronts:

A. On one front—the sensory input aspect—transformation begins with the mentalization of β-elements (O's imprint) and courses through their conversion into α-elements by α-function, followed by their distribution to dream thoughts, memory, contact-barrier, and feelings.

B. On the second front emerge, simultaneously, the inherent pre-conceptions (Ideal Forms, things-in-themselves). Bion also calls them β-elements. Thus the β-element constitutes an amalgam of *sensory stimuli* (from both outside and inside the mind) and *pre-conceptions* (inherent and/or acquired). The infant who can tolerate frustration ("no-breast") long enough, in the faith that the departed breast will return (thereby conceiving of a reassuring cycle of its departure and return), will be able to *realize* the experience and thereby transform the pre-conception into its realization, the conception. Either mother's α-function originally or the infant's α-function subsequently transforms this O (the combination of the sensory stimulus and the pre-conception) from O to K. Once K has been achieved and accepted by the infant, it is *my* hypothesis that the infant does not just acquire K: by acquiring and accepting K, which is impersonal O's (Fate's) derivative symbol and now transformed agent, the infant then *becomes* O, but his personal O, completing the cycle.

The completion of the cycle in which the infant (or the personality in general) becomes O—that is, accepts the personalness of one's Fate without denial—is the achievement of *transcendence*: namely, becoming a more evolved self and entering the transcendent position: that is, becoming a mystic.

O, transcendence, and "Dasein"

I believe that Bion's O interfaces with Heidegger's (1968) concept of *"Being"* or *"Existence"*[3] and Lacan (1966) "Register of the Real". Although Bion never referred to the works of Lacan, Sartre, or Heidegger, I believe that he was attempting to re-position psychoanalytic thinking away from its *ontic* (deterministic, scientific) roots and recast it in an *ontological* perspective. While I shall endeavour to explicate the concept of *transcendence* as it was used by Bion, this very term may be misleading unless one takes into consideration that the intrinsic aim of psychoanalysis is to help the analysand transcend the veils of illusion (sensory images and symbols that *represent* the other) that obtrude between him and the Other and between him and his Being-in-itself—his *"Dasein"*—as well as his *desires*. Thus, the seeming "beyondness" of transcendence signifies being just beyond the veil of illusion on our way to the unknown that is immediately near, both inside and out.

Put another way, what we commonly call reality is itself an illusion that disguises the Real (O). Bion broke through the veil of a constrictive modernism, characterized as it had been by deterministic certainty, and introduced us to relativism, intersubjectivity, and the ineffable. For Bion, O is the question behind the question that embarrasses every answer. Yet at the same time O *is* the unknowable answer. I again remind the reader that when I use the term "transcendence", I am not using it in the religious sense, but to signify immanence. Put another way, our potential transcendence is located with us as O. When as a result of going through emotional experiences we "become" these, our immanence (the godhead) becomes incarnated and realized, and we become self-transcendent—that is, evolved.

Brief clinical vignette
with dream demonstrating transcendence

The following is a brief excerpt from a session with an analytic patient:

> In the beginning of the dream I'm at *schule* [Jewish house of worship—JSG] with my father. I put on a ragged talis. Father tells me

to put on a finer one. I say, "No. I like this one. This is who I am."
The service then begins. I say, "This is not where the real service
is taking place." I then go on a pilgrimage to find the real service.
A woman and a mysterious stranger accompany me. We wander
far and live the way pilgrims do—eating grains, walking through
the fields, sleeping by the road. We then come to some place where
crystals and body oil are available. The woman takes a bubble bath.
Meanwhile, the various grains we have been eating have caused
the woman to develop urinary tract disease. She can no longer
travel with us. I go on alone, enjoying this recognition, *following the
dictates of a consciousness larger than one in my mind* [italics added].

The patient's associations:

> The pilgrimage is only a fraction of our concerns. We all have this
> dailyness to deal with. There is an Oversoul (Emerson) that makes
> a pilgrimage of our lives, but we are not supposed to be aware of
> it. There are so many scenarios going on in our lives. The mind
> transcends the body. The woman left the universal pilgrimage for
> a minor one. I decided to forge ahead despite my anxieties. A car
> is only one symbolic mode of transportation. I travel in a different
> dimension. We've allowed imagination to fall asleep. Now is the
> time for us to allow it to awaken. The novel is the delegate of the
> novelist. We become distracted by a literalization process which we
> mistake for the real. We are not supposed to know this.

O is the numinous Kantian cathedral-and-hell-without-walls that is
intuited from its phenomenal derivatives, the gradual but progressive
contact with which is manifested the experience of approximating and
then becoming alone ("communion") with O. Each of us *is* O, but our
O-ness is normally unrecognizable to ourselves because we are "civilized" and "gentrified" in K. Our O-ness is achievable only through,
by, and for the other. We are O incognito and doomed or tantalizingly
destined to become realized in the disciplined, dedicated intuition of
the other's unfocused gaze. We are O and are terrified of it—thus the
need for inward-directed "sunglasses" that allow diminished illumination and disguise. O *is* the Real. What we believe we experience is a
"virtual reality"—a Reality that has become "virtued" ("laundered")
by the refractions of phantasy, imagination, illusion, and symboliza-
tion, leaving us with a "cooked" "Real" (O) suitable for our timid
digestion.

"Thoughts without a thinker" are O's offspring. They are the "unborns", the "intimations of immortality" that we seemingly experience to be located within our inner cosmos, but they are placeless, unlocatable: they cannot be found because they can never be the object—they are always already the ever-emerging subject. Aesthetics, perhaps the most satisfying of the vertices, constitutes the organic, living, changing/unchanging template of O and of all O's formless forms moving across an (apparently) inner galactic landscape in a dazzling infinitude of discrete patterns that are both implicitly intricate *and* holistic—transiently, seductively revealing themselves for precious half-moments only to disappear once again into their numinous, mystical vapour.

In Bion's conception of O and its association with "thoughts without a thinker" waiting for a mind to think them, we are introduced to the possibility of a conception of mental activity that may perhaps transcend what is ordinarily meant by "thinking". In order to achieve this state, we have to be open—either exploratorily curious or passively unsaturated, but in either case open to and ready for the unexpected. Once we encounter it—perhaps it is better to say that once we are encountered by the unexpected "it"—and are able to allow it entry by our readiness to tolerate it (because we are able to attenuate our fears of its potential awesomeness and are thus indemnified from turning into pillars of salt by its confrontation), we process it. In effect we unconsciously stamp it with the imprimatur of our personalness (autochthony): that is, we allow ourselves to "create" it imaginatively before "discovering" it and then allow it to be internalized and enter into the digestive alchemy of transformation. It must be noted that "thinking" for Bion is not necessarily a conscious, intentional act.

By allowing familiarity with the unfamiliar, we are allowing thoughts without a thinker to be thought about by a receptive mind that realizes the presence of its lost yet nevertheless remembered echomoiety from its future, which now has a home-mind in which it can play and be played with—thoughtfully—in the pre-conscious. Thus, August von Kekulé could discover the yet unknown and unsuspected hexagonal ring of the carbon molecules that defined the aromatic series of chemicals—but not through conscious thought. He could only unconsciously intuitively anticipate and thereby summon this thought without a thinker. It was in a dream that this realization was able to make its dramatic and historic epiphany.

The Gnostic within me presupposes a concept here that Bion all but stated: that there seems to exist a numinous "thinker" of the "thoughts without a ('recognized') thinker", and this "thinker"—

actually "creator" of "imaginative conjectures"—is the *"ineffable subject of the unconscious"*, O, who is the author of the narrative enacted by its counterpart O, the *"immanent"* or *"phenomenal subject of psychoanalysis"*, what Bion terms the "psychoanalytic object" (Grotstein, 2000a). From this perspective, consequently, O forever seeks its rendezvous with O through the channel of human K—that is, O's trajectory is cyclical. Professor Chaim Tadmor of the University of Jerusalem, perhaps the world's foremost authority on ancient Assyria in the days of Assurbanipal and Tiglath Pileser, informed me that the ancient Assyrians believed that dreams constituted the sacred god-language—that gods communicated with each other through the channel of humans while they dreamed. Humans had to consider dreams sacred and had to resist the temptation to understand them. The "thinker who thinks the thoughts" is akin to the "dreamer who dreams the dream" and the "dreamer who understands the dream" (Grotstein, 1981d, 2000a). The "thinker who understands the thoughts" is the constantly expectant internal playmate of this unsaturated, disciplined unconscious thinker. Together, they patiently await the entry from the future of their long-exiled, unknown but always suspected "thought without a thinker", which is borne by "memoirs of the future".

The point is that thoughts, from the point of view of associationism, seem to think themselves if we are optimally able to allow them their intercourse in our receptive containers. At the same time but from another perspective, they are pre-thought and thought by an ineffable thinker-subject, one that we arrogantly claim as being ourselves and with which we seek to identify but who really is Other to us while it is within us. Perhaps what we call thinking, consequently, constitutes the afterthoughts and "bare-bones" derivates of a numinous thinking couple.

Bion's endeavour

The question that Bion confronted was *how do we format (anticipate) the events we face in order to render (transduce) them first into personal and then into objective experiences?* He was aware that the rationalistic enterprise required *transcendental*[4] (*a priori*) considerations beyond the drives that could account for the uniqueness of how we format our experiences—that is, prepare a suitable *container* that can anticipate its future contents. In considering these *a priori* categories, he borrowed the concept of the Ideal Forms from Plato and termed them "inherent pre-conceptions" (or "memoirs of the future"), which, along with the sensory apparatus (as "common sense"), container ↔ contained, L, H, and K linkages, and intuition, became the instruments of apprehending the "psychoanalytic object" and resonating with O (Absolute Truth, Ultimate Reality).

In his epistemological pilgrimage Bion retraced the philosophical contributions of leading thinkers of the past, including Plato, Aristotle, Meister Eckhart, Hume, and Kant in particular. He also consulted mathematicians like Poincaré and Georg Cantor. The point of resorting to mathematics was to arrive at tools for understanding that were unsaturated with preconceived meanings. His endeavour was to find out what inheres within us that allows us to grasp, process, and internalize our experiences so that we can grow from them—by *becoming* them, much the way we physically become what we eat. Ultimately, he was to come upon O and *intuition*, the former being, in the Kantian sense, a *transcendent* entity and the latter a *transcendental* (*a priori*) entity that allows us to divine the beyond from the beyond within us (Bion, 1965, 1970, 1992).

These achievements are difficult to overestimate. They constitute an epistemic and ontological metapsychological metatheory that elegantly extends and graces Klein's enterprise and transcends that of Freud. This metatheory, especially with the Truth[5] of emotional experience as its centrepiece, Faith as its guardian and hovering presence,[6] and O as its initiator *and* realization, introduces not only epistemic and ontological theory into psychoanalysis but also teleology and especially transcendence, as I hope to demonstrate. The focus here is on the capacity to experience[7] O, the Subject of Subjects that, like the conception of God, can never be the object of the senses or of contemplation. The capacity to experience O is the privilege of the ineffable subject of psychoanalysis (Grotstein, 1997a, 2000a), the "Man of Achievement". It is my belief that the ineffable subject of psychoanalysis, the unconscious aspect of ourselves that experiences *being O*, is presented to the patient as what Bion (1963) terms the "psychoanalytic object", as symptoms, dreams, and free associations, especially with regard to its being the locale of significant "*constant conjunctions*" of elements that, when united, signify unique meaning. It is my belief that that aspect of the analysand that experiences O and awaits realization or incarnation with the analyst's interpretation is the ineffable subject of the unconscious, a numinous entity who may also be known as the "once-and-forever-infant-of-the-unconscious" (Grotstein, in press-a).

Through self-abnegation (abandonment of ego), we *become* O,[8] according to Bion. In so doing, becoming O represents the achievement, albeit transitory, of what I propose is the *"transcendent position"*—the individual's gradually developing capacity, from infancy (or perhaps even fetaldom) onward, to tolerate (suffer) and therefore to resonate with O, the ultimate reality of anything and everything. This capacity, therefore, exists before, during, and after, hovers over, surrounds, embraces, and is beyond (in every dimension and perspective) the paranoid–schizoid and depressive positions, both of which constitute, I believe, an emotional and epistemic "ozone layer" or protective lens or filter against the blinding illumination of the Absolute,[9] O's nom de plume. As mentioned earlier, O is but another name for "Being or Existence-in-itself" (*Dasein*)—without disguise and what Being purely and meaningfully experiences. It is *"aletheia"* ["without concealment"] (Heidegger, 1927).

Caveats

Some caveats are in order before I proceed. First, I use the term "transcendent" or "transcending" as a way of approximating Bion's quintessential episteme, and while it may seem to have religious/spiritual/ "mystical" overtones as well as a parallel usage in analytic psychology (Jung, 1916), my usage is confined to the psychoanalytic and epistemological vertices even when applied to mysticism itself. The concept of a transcendent position does not constitute a whimsical journey into lofty, ethereal abandon, nor does it necessarily validate religion, spirituality, or belief in God, except as the need in response to which humans attempt to close the maw of the ineffable with an all-encompassing name. It is not in the oeuvre of W. Somerset Maugham's Larry Darrell, who sought "enlightenment" atop the Himalayas in *The Razor's Edge* (1945). In other words, it is not a blissful "autistic enclave". O is one's reality, without pretence or distortion. This reality can be a symptom, the pain of viewing beautiful autumn leaves, gazing upon the mystique of the Mona Lisa de la Gioconda, contemplating the horror of Ypres (for Bion), trying to remember Hiroshima, Nagasaki, Auschwitz, Viet Nam, or Iraq, or resting comfortably beside one's mate trying to contemplate the exquisiteness and ineffability of the moment.

Transcendence is the mute "Other" that lies "just beyond, within, and around" where we are. It is the core of our very Being-in-itself. The mystic[10] or genius is that aspect of us which is potentially able to be at one with transcendence as O—but only after we have "cleared" with P–S and D. *The mystic, according to Bion, is one who sees things as they really are—through the deception or camouflage of words and symbols.* It is fascinating how the term "mysticism" has acquired such prejudice. The generally feared connotation of "mysticism" has occurred through the projective identification of "mystique" onto it by those who are, according to Bion, afraid of truth and so mystify its clarity.

Transcendence carries in its sweep an epistemological tradition that began among the pre-Socratic philosophers, flourished with Plato, continued in other forms in the so-called mysteries (Orphic, Eleusinian, and others), traversed the ancient Hebrew and early Christian mystics, became prominent in the Gnostic Gospels and in Zoroastrianism and later with so-called apophatic mystical writers such as Meister Eckhart, Ibn'Arabi, John Scotus Eriugena, Marguerite Porete, Plotinus, surfaced again in the Zohar Kabbalah, became bleached out by the glare of the Enlightenment and further dismissed by the proud certainty and determinism of logical positivism, surfaced briefly with the transcendentalistic movement of Carlyle and Emerson in the nineteenth century, and resurfaced in yet another form in the mystical works of Kierkegaard. Elsewhere it arose as a Zoroastrian revival in the works of Nietzsche and played a prominent position in Schreber's (1903) *Denkwürdigkeiten*.

The mystic seed then took root in metaphysics. It appeared as such in Hegel and especially in Kant's *Critique of Pure Reason* as the epistemological quest for the transcendent—a concept that was to find its consummate expression in the existential literature, such as Sartre and particularly the works of Heidegger, the latter of whom left us the legacy of his obsession with the nuances implicit in the subjectivity of Being—in contrast to Hegel's legacy of the object. Jung was the first psychoanalyst to appreciate its importance.

Mysticism has long been claimed both by religion and by epistemology. Spiritualism overarches both areas. Lacan had the profoundest respect for mysticism, and the totality of his works can be read as an appreciation of its importance in mental life. Bion had profound respect for the presence in man of what he termed the "moral or religious instinct". Not formally religious himself, he was one of the profoundest secular mystics of our or any time—certainly within psychoanalysis—as well as its foremost epistemologist generally—and this includes Freud. Briefly put, Bion's works represent a consummate distillation of the collective wisdom of Western and Eastern civilization and are focused on the episteme of how man seeks and hides from the ineffable. Reality had become so saturated that it shrunk into a positivistic enclave. The realness of the other is in contrast to the mystery, the Otherness of the other.

A reconsideration of Klein's positions in light of the transcendent position

The paranoid–schizoid position, according to this formulation, constitutes a primitive digitalizing mode that reduces the chaotic, infinite, non-linear complexity of O to linear, Manichean good and bad mythic objects, phantasmal chimerae with which we can live in our ever so limited waveband of perceptual and apperceptual tolerance until we are ready for the depressive position, in which mode we can further process these elements of thought into *realizations* within the waveband of objectivity. The Kleinian concept of the depressive position has been moored to its provenance in the death instinct, and both P–S and D remain constitutive of Klein's theory of the *infantile neurosis* (actually, as "psychotic" positions because of the *omnipotence* that characterizes their operations and worldview). With O as the centrepiece of this new metapsychology, P–S and D can then be understood as adaptive (normal) paranoid, manic, and/or depressive defences against the inexorable emergence of O. Furthermore, atavistic prey–predator anxiety becomes sexualized and aggressivized and therefore personalized as categories of autochthonous subjectivity and agency.

The long and the short of the above reassessment of the positions is as follows: With O as a new consideration, we can now distinguish between *terror* (*dread*) and *persecution* and *guilt* or, put another way, between *infantile catastrophe* and the *infantile neurosis* (*psychosis*). Put yet another way, ultimate terror or dread predicates the experience of the impersonal meaninglessness of O, whereas persecution is our attempt to personalize O for mastery.

P–S mediates O by primary subjectivization (personalization) whereby nameless O becomes "baptized" with a *personalized* subjective stamp of "persecutor" and is no longer "dread" namelessly and pervasively adrift. The hope that unconsciously subtends both P–S and D is that chaos (O) *is* organized by a "fact selector" ("strange attractor") that gives it a coherence unto itself before our own α-function can bestow personal and objective meaning to it. As I have already adumbrated, I believe—and I think that Bion hinted—that the paranoid–schizoid position is not primary; rather, it has been set up as an operational filter to contain and process (triage) the chaos, infinity, randomness, *Ananke* of O, which may also be associated with Fate. The other filter is the depressive position. This concept of "filter" requires more development, and I shall take up that idea later. Theoretical questions and clinical experience tell me that even though mourning, the quintessential capacity that is achieved in the depressive position, is thought never to end, in fact it does and should, notwithstanding the probability that reparations and restorative attempts may normally continue throughout one's lifetime. Wounds heal, and the need to continue mourning past its proper time becomes pathological, as the *Talmud* advises us. Put another way, while the *capacity* for mourning becomes the legacy, as a *personality trait*, of having *achieved* the depressive position, the continuation of "mourning" as a *clinical state* would be an indication of the *presence* and *continuation* of as yet unresolved *clinical depressive illness* (melancholia).

This contribution concerns a transcendence that exists before, beyond, during, and following both the paranoid–schizoid *and* the depressive positions. I am merely suggesting that there is a *"beyond" the depressive position*. The same principle applies to the *paranoid–schizoid position*. A position—shall I say a *"position*ing*"?—of non-linearity hovers over the microcosm of our limited linear *Weltanschauung*. Furthermore, in consideration of P–S, is it not true that the very name explicates two major defensive functions, "paranoid" (projective identification) and "schizoid" (splitting), which together help the infant reestablish the "purified pleasure ego" (Freud, 1911b, p. 222)? By using the concept of transcend-ent(-*ing*) position, one is able to interpose a positioning that exists with, before, during, and after the other positions, one that interpenetrates them and conveys the supraordinate theme of transcending impersonal O to get to P–S, transcending P–S to get to D, transcending D to get to personal O. Put another way, it is as if we human individuals must, from the very beginning and with the benignly collusive help of our objects, establish an ongoing and ever-varying covenant with the Absolute Truth about Ultimate Reality—so as gradually to come to peace with it finally as *our* O. Its primal name is "emotional turbulence" (Bion, 1962b, 1963), the state that inescapably evolves when two individuals meet.

Towards the concept of the transcendent position: transcendence (evolution of self)

With regard to transcendence Bion states:

> My object is to show that certain elements in the development of psycho-analysis are not new or peculiar to analysis, but have in fact

a history that suggests that they *transcend* barriers of race, time, and discipline, and are inherent in the relationship of the mystic to the group. [1970, p. 75]

and:

One result of separation [from the Establishment] is no direct access of the individual to the god with whom he used formerly to be on familiar terms [as in the Homeric concept of man's relationship to his gods]. But the god has undergone a change as a part of the process of discrimination. The god with whom he was familiar was finite; the god from whom he is now separated is *transcendent* and infinite. [1970, pp. 75–76]

As mentioned above, I understand Bion to employ both *transcendence* and *transcendentalism* (*a priori*) in his episteme. The former includes his concept of O, whereas the latter includes his concepts of intuition, L, H, and K linkages, container ↔ contained, and inherent pre-conceptions. His theory of transformations in and from K and O represent the epitome of the phenomenon of *transcendence*, perhaps what I might now also call "transcend*ingness*.

Kant's theory of transcendence and transcendentalism

My re-reading of Kant's (1787) *Critique of Pure Reason* suggests to me that Kant's concept of "*a priori*", including the categories of reasoning, along with the noumenon or the thing-in-itself, constituted what he meant by "transcendental", the *deep structures* of the mind. To them I would extend O (the "Real"). Here is how I believe it is configured: O has two arms: *one arm* is the transcendental analytic, the deep structures within our unrepressed (inherent) unconscious. The *other arm* is raw inner and/or outer sensory experience itself. The individual is sandwiched between the two arms of O and must *become* the experience of raw indifferent O by personalizing it into personal O via transforming it through dreaming—that is, α-function—from the first arm.

Thus, the fundamental nature of the psychoanalytic concept of psychic reality is basically "*transcendental*" in so far as it depends on *a priori* assumptions.[11] In contrast, however, infantile developmental progression—say, from orality to anality or from the paranoid–schizoid position to the depressive position—can be considered "*transcendent*" (my view, as well as that of Jung, 1916). Kant himself differentiates between "*transcendental*" and "*transcendent*" by assigning the notion of *a priori* to the former and speculative expansion beyond reason to the latter—that is, speculations that are as yet unwarranted by logical reasoning. It is at this juncture that my own views—and, by association, Bion's—differ somewhat from Kant's. In his *Prolegomena* (Kant, 1783) he archly responds to a critic of the first edition of his *Critique of Pure Reason* (Kant, 1787). After first quoting an unnamed critic's evaluation that his work, "is a system of transcendent (or, as he translates it, of higher) Idealism", Kant then states in a footnote:

> By no means *"higher."* High towers, and metaphysically-great men resembling them, round both of which there is commonly much wind, are not for me. My place is the fruitful *bathos*, the bottom-land of experience; and the word transcendental, the meaning of which is so often explained by me but not once grasped by my reviewer . . . does not signify something passing beyond all experience, but something that indeed precedes it *a priori*, but that is intended simply to make cognition of experience possible. If these conceptions overstep experience, their employment is termed transcendent, a word which must be distinguished from transcendental, the later being limited to immanent use, that is, experience. [Kant, 1787, p. 150–151]

My reconciliation between my views and those I believe to be Bion's and Kant's with regard to "transcendent" as "something passing beyond all experience" is that O is not "experienced" *per se*—that is, as an *object* of experience. O, like the God of Moses in *Exodus* ("I am that I am") is the *subject*, something with which one can only subjectively resonate—that is, "become". Put another way, one does not really *experience* O; one experiences *being* O.

In *Cogitations* Bion (1992) entitled a chapter "Reverence and Awe". As soon as I read it, I could not help wondering whether he had me in mind when he discussed the patient who experienced the propensity of reverence and awe towards an object that could not be apprehended (by the senses). I believe that reverence, awe, and the aesthetic vertex are yet other manifestations of O. In that regard it should be mentioned that Neil Maizels, an Australian analyst, has, simultaneously with me, found inadequacies with the Kleinian formulation of the depressive position (the issue between "attaining" and "transcending") and independently conceived of the *"spiritual position"* (Neil Maizels, personal communication, 1990). Because of our common interest in the theme we have decided to embark on a reassessment of the conception of the depressive position.

NOTES

1. Britton (2006) proffers the concept of the "uncertainty principle".

2. I am indebted to O. H. D. Blomfield (personal communication, 1995) for this idea and its source in Ricoeur (1970).

3. Heidegger states: "Every philosophical—that is, thoughtful—doctrine of man's essential nature is *in itself alone* a doctrine of the Being of beings [i.e. what it means for a being to be]. Every doctrine of Being is *in itself alone* a doctrine of man's essential nature" (1968, p. 79).

4. At the end of this chapter I cite the distinction between *transcendental* and *transcendent* drawn by Kant in his *Prolegomena* (1783).

5. I am indebted to Elizabeth de Bianchedi (1993, 1997) for her deep understanding of Bion's ideas on truth, lies, and falsities.

6. By "presence" I mean my concept of the background presence of primary identification (Grotstein, 1978).

7. At the point where K is transformed to O, the verb "experience" changes from a transitive verb into a linking verb. My reading of Bion's conception of O is that it is the consummate Subject and never the object.

8. Though it seems that I have earlier introduced a contradiction when I said that Bion hints that O is the Subject and now I cite him as stating that O is the psychoanalytic "object", I must, with the greatest of humility, disagree with Bion on this point. To me, O is never an object. It eludes all verbs except for the linking verb "*becoming*". Beta-element is the object.

9. Here again, the idea of the Absolute might be "traded in" for something like "*Absoluting*", but this gerund is awkward.

10. While writing these lines, I could not help wondering what the relationship was between the mystic *qua* mystic and his α-function: how did it affect him?

11. In this regard Freud (1915e) states: "Just as Kant warned us not to overlook the fact that our perceptions are subjectively conditioned and must not be regarded as identical with what is perceived though unknowable, so psycho-analysis warns us not to equate perceptions by means of consciousness with the unconscious mental processes which are their object. Like the physical, the psychic is not necessarily in reality what it appears to us to be" (p. 171). In other words, the internal world is *transcendental*, if not also *transcendent*.

CHAPTER 13

The quest for the truth, Part A: the "truth drive" as the hidden order of Bion's metatheory for psychoanalysis

Freud (1915e) conceived of the unconscious as a "seething caul-dron" because of the constant irruption of the instinctual drives that he posited, principally the libidinal drive, to which Klein (1935) added the prime importance of the death drive. To Bion the unconscious constituted a seething cauldron because it was the quin-tessential seat of infinite, ineffable uncertainty, which he designated as O, his arbitrary, unsaturated sign for the *Absolute Truth* about *Ultimate Reality*. Quite recently I attempted to amplify, extend, and synthesize Bion's ideas about the endangering aspects of truth by positing that he hinted at but never came out and said what I now say for him and in his name: that there exists a relentless truth drive in the psyche, which Freud mistook for the libidinal drive and Klein for the death drive (Grotstein, 2004b).

Bion the polymath and erstwhile Oxford student went a step fur-ther than Freud and Klein in yet another way. Freud briefly alluded to the ideas of Immanuel Kant but never explicated his ideas, or, for that matter, those of Plato or Hegel, with regard to their proper provenance for psychoanalysis. Bion did. Plato's Eternal Forms (inherent pre-con-ceptions, archetypes, "memoirs of the future") and Kant's primary and secondary categories and noumena (things-in-themselves) found an enthusiastic reception in Bion's thinking.

DOI: 10.4324/9781003348665-14

Put succinctly, first cause and its sequelae are for Bion as follows: Evolving O, which not only constitutes the Absolute Truth about Ultimate Reality[1] but is also the denotation of life's (inner and outer) constant impingement upon us as a sensory stimulus, impacts on our emotional frontier and becomes registered as a β-element. The individual's α-function then intercepts it[2] and transforms it into an α-element[3] that is capable of mentalization to become dream thoughts, memory, and/or reinforcements for the contact-barrier that separates consciousness from unconsciousness[4] so as to guarantee our capacity to sleep, to be awake, and to think.

Before these phenomenological stimuli (β-elements) undergo transformation by α-function, however, they instantly recruit and become conjoined with elements from the unrepressed unconscious—that is, inherent pre-conceptions, archetypes, noumena. This is a significant but little-noticed contribution by Bion. Consequently, unconscious never-thought thoughts—what Bion whimsically terms "thoughts without a thinker"—awaiting a thinker (mind) to think them—comprise the results of the impingement of raw circumstance (O), which becomes registered as a β-element and in the next instance becomes conjoined by the infinite sets of categories of inherent pre-conceptions and noumena, which amount to all the conceivable and inconceivable symmetrical possibilities that can link up with the new stimulus (β-element) in order to anticipate it and to format the mind to prepare for it.

The problem is that this format emerges from infinity and is experienced as chaos. It requires α-function to transduce it to finite integers and dreaming for ultimate comprehension. That is where the containing mother comes in for the infant and where ultimately the mind comes in, for which the mother may be considered either as the forerunner or as the facilitator and developer of the infant's own inchoate mind. Part of the maternal or analytic sorting-out process consists of a transduction from the infinity and infinite sets of the Absolute Truth about Ultimate Reality downwards to finite, tolerable, personal—and, later, objective—meaning. Another, according to Bion, is learning what is *not* the meaningful truth implicit in the communication, thereby engendering relief from what had been initially anxiously anticipated as a fateful premonition (use of Column 2 of the Grid).

Bion thus subtly revised the psychoanalytic concepts of first cause (emotional stimulus as opposed to libidinal or death drive), hinted at but did not specify a truth drive, and relegated the libidinal (L) drive and the aggressive (H) drive, in a new conjunction with the epistemophilic (K) drive, to the status of emotional links between self and objects: in other words, one knows (K) an object by how one feels (L and/or H) about it. Consequently, L, H, and K linkages join α-function in assigning categories (emotionally encoding) to β-elements as they become α-elements.

The immanent "godhead" ("godhood" or "godliness") in man

It would take some time before psychoanalysts and psychotherapists would be able to comprehend the profound significance of Bion's paradigm change. That time has not arrived even now, but hints of it are beginning to emerge (Grotstein, 2004a, 2004b). In the meantime resistances to his ideas have begun to develop around what is commonly thought to be his religious, spiritual, and mystical leanings. Bion himself was not religious, but he keenly observed the religious nature of mankind. He often mentioned to me that Freud seemed to have neglected the power of religion and how important the religious instinct was for mankind. He was interested not only in theology generally, because of its many parallels with psychoanalysis, but especially in the spirituality of the mystics, Christian, Hebrew, and Islamic alike. In fact, he did something very daring. Having read the mystical work of Meister Eckhart, he borrowed Eckhart's heretical distinction between the idea of an immanent "god" and a transcendent "godhead"[5] as the God of Essence and placed the transcendent "godhead" within man as immanent and as a cognate of O. It is my belief that another reading of the meaning of "godhead" for Bion was the Gnostic one, where godhead is equated with pure thought—that is, pure intelligence, in the Neoplatonic sense of the Ideal Forms. This godhead is a pure essence and is not to be confused with God, the Creator.

Bion (personal communication, 1977) believed that man has an instinct to worship and must create a god to justify it, and that theology and psychoanalysis ran parallel courses, so that, roughly speaking, whenever a theologian speaks of "God", a psychoanalyst could substitute the unconscious or O. If Bion were ever to have subscribed to a religion at all, I should think it would have been "agnostic Gnosticism". As for Bion, the mystic, as I have stated earlier, the mystic does not need K to experience O. He is one who sees the obvious in complexity and complexity in the obvious.

The deeper significance of Bion's "experiment perilous" with the deity is, as mentioned earlier, in the spirit of Prometheus: to allow man to be introduced to—be incarnated by—his "godhood", the composite

archetypal term that embraces O and which act designates man's becoming O, which means transforming indifferent, impersonal O into
personal O in the transcendent position (Grotstein, 1993a, 2004b). One
can now begin to see that Bion was introducing a very different view
both of the unconscious and of the human struggle, to say nothing
of a very different view of psychoanalysis that miraculously remains
within the classical boundaries and just barely avoids being heretical,
except in the minds of some.

NOTES

1. Bion (1965, 1970) assigns separate status to "Absolute Truth" and "Ultimate
Reality", dividing them with a comma; I unite them causally with the premise that
truth always predicates the acceptance of reality.

2. When the adult was an infant, his mother's α-function in her action of containment initiated this transformation, translation, conversion function.

3. One must remember that "α-function, "α-elements", and "β-elements" are
Bion's *models* for explicating a putative function in the mind. They do not exist in
their own right; they are constructed analogue models.

4. Bion initially deals with a presence of consciousness and the unconscious;
soon he will replace this dialectic with that of infinity versus finiteness.

5. It seems odd that Bion neglected to cite the one who is, in my view, his
Doppelgänger—Spinoza, who also conceived of the immanent, as opposed to the
transcendent, godhead.

CHAPTER 14

The quest for the truth, Part B: curiosity about the truth as the "seventh servant"

After numerous readings of the entirety of Bion's published works, I was finally struck by what, for me, became a "selected fact": that the Ariadne's thread that seems to run through all of his works and ultimately to define them is his conception of the "quest for the truth" (curiosity) (Bion, 1970, p. 46), which I have reinterpreted as the "truth instinct or drive" (Grotstein, 2004a, 2004b). This quest for truth (or truth as an instinctual drive) underlies his whole notion of transformations and the theory of O. In other words, the function of transformation is to transform the Absolute Truth about an indifferent and impersonal Ultimate Reality into personal, subjective truth about reality. Bion lists "Absolute Truth" alongside "Ultimate Reality" as comprising O, together with "noumena", "godhead", and "β-elements".

Transformations operate on the Absolute Truth about Ultimate Reality and the latter's infinite sets and infinite container to transduce them via α-function from their indifferent, impersonal, and infinite status to personal, subjective meaning, initially in the form of binary oppositions in what Klein terms the "paranoid–schizoid position", where they are encoded as unconscious phantasies consisting of internal objects as "symbolic equations" (Freud, 1924d, p. 179[1]; Segal, 1957, 1981) in the form of opposites, such as good versus bad, inside versus outside, and so on, and then sent along to the depressive position (P–S ↔ D) as symbols for whole objects for more objectification.

I postulate that the truth drive can be assigned to what Freud (1911b) called "consciousness", which constitutes "the sense organ for the perception of psychical qualities" (Freud, 1900a, p. 615, cited in Bion, 1962, p. 4) (". . . Of things invisible to mortal sight"). I think of "consciousness"—and especially "curiosity" within consciousness—as Bion's (1977) *"seventh servant"*:

> The Seven Pillars of Wisdom are:
>> "I keep six honest serving men
>> (They taught me all I knew);
>> Their names are What and Why and When
>> And How and Where and Who.
>> I send them over land and sea,
>> I send them east and west;
>> But after they have worked for me,
>> *I* give them all a rest."
>
> *The missing one completes the seven.* [Bion, 1977, *Seven Servants*, Introduction (poem from Rudyard Kipling's *Just So Stories*); italics added]

It is my impression that the "seventh servant", the consciousness that is responsive to psychic qualities (internal world), functions complementarily to the other consciousness, the one that represents the sense organs that are responsive to external qualities ("what", "why", "when", "how", "where", and "who"). Furthermore, I posit that it is linked with Bion's "quest for the truth". Together, they comprise *curiosity.*

> "Like one that on a lonesome road
> Doth walk in fear and dread;
> And having once turned round walks on,
> And turns no more his head;
> Because he knows a frightful fiend
> Doth close behind him tread."
>
> The "frightful fiend" represents indifferently the *quest for truth* or the active defences against it. [Bion, 1970, p. 46; italics added]

I consider Bion's use of this passage from Coleridge's "The Rhyme of the Ancient Mariner" as supporting the notion of a truth drive (Grotstein, 2004a, 2004b) as a relentless, hounding *"quest for truth"*. Bion continues:

Assuming that there is some standard by which one could distinguish what is true and what is not, namely, that there is some sort of *truth function*, it is difficult to believe that I, as the object of investigation, am likely to give you a correct (truthful) answer as to what it is that I am or contain. [1973, p. 59; italics added]

Thus, Bion seems to equate "seventh servant", "truth function", "quest for truth", and the "regard for truth" with curiosity and its dangers (Bion, 1992, p. 126). I should like collectively to nominate them as a *"truth principle"*, which accompanies the reality, pleasure, and uncertainty (Britton, 2006) principles and predominates in relation to them.

Bion speaks often about truth throughout his works. Some examples can be found in *Learning from Experience* (1962b, e.g. pp. 11, 56, 100–101); in *Transformations* (1965, e.g. pp. 37, 38, 147); in *Attention and Interpretation* (1970, e.g. pp. 29–31, 59, 97, 99, 102–104, 117–118); and in *Cogitations* (1992, e.g. pp. 99, 114, 117–118), among many others. Truth was a very important concept for Bion, one that is pre-eminent in his thinking. It also should be emphasized that for Bion truth meant *emotional truth* both about oneself and about one's relationships with one's objects. He seems to think of truth as something that goes beyond moral integrity, something that is "scientific", a respect for the undeniable. His concept of *faith* is closely related to it. One might say that faith is a function of truth.

Curiosity and its dangers

Bion frequently speaks about the putative dangers of curiosity. He encountered proscriptions against it even as child, from his parents and from "Arf Arfer" ("Our Father Who Art in Heaven") (Bion, 1982). He also lists the Garden of Eden myth, the myth of the Tower of Babel, and the Oedipus myth as myths in which curiosity is forbidden by the deity. Furthermore, he suggests that Oedipus was guilty of hubris or arrogance in being determined to learn the truth about the tragedy in which he unknowingly participated.

Having considered Bion's formulation with regard to a constant conjunction normally between curiosity and arrogance and pathologically between these two and stupidity (1967c), the following speculative thoughts emerged:

A. The "deity" represents O, and the curious investigator must reckon with the danger of *actively*—that is, *sacrilegiously and invasively*—

penetrating the contact-barrier between infinite O, which is associated with the godhead (godhood), and consciousness. In other words, man—that is, man's curiosity—must not selfishly (like Faust, or what Bion attributed to Oedipus and I attribute to Prometheus) invade the holy of holies (the unconscious, mother's body, godhead). Man must develop patience—that is, negative capability—so that godhood (the Eternal Forms, inherent pre-conceptions, the things-in-themselves, noumena) can spontaneously enter man when properly summoned by circumstance, O. It is as if the unconscious works like a Hollywood producer who might characteristically say to an actor auditioning for a part: "Don't call us! We'll call you!" This is how the Eternal Forms, O, godhead become realized in human experience as a conception. Curiosity must learn humility! The rewards are enormous. Put another way, when Bion speaks of the deity's proscription against curiosity, he is linking the myth of the sentinel pagan deities of yore who served as threshold gods to protect that which was sacred—the Hebrew mezuzah, the Greek Hermes, the Norse Troll Dahl, and so on. Ultimately the proscription against curiosity is to become the contact-barrier that guards and guarantees the integrity of System *Ucs.* with regard to System *Cs.*—and the reverse.

B. The other interdiction against curiosity is due to the consequences of its being fulfilled. Curiosity is a function of a developing self who has become epistemologically ambitious. Each fulfilment of curiosity imposes a growing sense of ever-expanding responsibility for the evolving self. In other words, it creates greater and greater developmental asymmetry, separation, and a greater sense of vulnerability in terms of responsibility. Thus, *curiosity* is constantly conjoined with *catastrophic anxiety*.

Bion frequently alludes to Oedipus' arrogance in seeking the truth. This requires discussion. Oedipus, the appointed tyrant of Thebes, owed it to the populace of Thebes to get to the bottom of the matter of the pollution that had affected the city. His curiosity was therefore a responsible one, not necessarily an omnipotent one, in my opinion. On the other hand, it could be said that it may have been a sign of illusions of omnipotence for Oedipus to believe that he could tolerate the ultimate truths his curiosity revealed. But another source of hubris may be laid at Oedipus' feet. Dodds (1965) points out that Sophocles' three Oedipal plays, *Oedipus Rex* (Tyrannus), *Oedipus at Colonnus*, and *Antigone,* seem to have been moralistic plays. Greenberg (2005), in his study of the Ancient Greek "middle voice", asserts that Oedipus' hubris lay in his answering the riddle of the sphinx with his own wisdom—without acknowledging the wisdom of the gods who had helped him. To support this idea he acknowledges his sources in the works of such Greek scholars as Dimock (1989), Vernant (1990), Fagles (1991), and Lebow (2003).

Bion writes frequently about curiosity and its interdiction by the deity. He then cites the following myths to support his thesis: The Garden of Eden, the Tower of Babel, and the Oedipus myths. He might also have cited the myth of Prometheus. The question I propose is: Who is the "deity" that opposes curiosity? Is it the deity, "god" → godhead (O) or is it another dimension of the deity? I suggest that the answer lies in the latent content of the Garden of Eden myth. If one regards God in that myth as a version of the newborn infant who believes, like a god, that he has *created* everything and everyone he opens his eyes to as he *discovers* them, including himself, then the following scenario is conceivable: The god-infant is his own creator and also the creator of his parents, Adam and Eve. Once he learns that it was their intercourse that created him, he is ousted form his Edenic paradise of omnipotence and becomes a normal dependent infant who now envies the parental primal scene from which he is excluded. In his bitterness his curiosity seeks to observe and thus to "know" the primal scene, from which even his curiosity must be excluded in respect of the "law of the father".

The intermediate transformation of Absolute Truth about Ultimate Reality (O) to tolerable truth (K) and its cyclic return to O

Learning from experience

Bion held that each accepted, processed, and transformed emotional experience is accompanied by unconscious realizations of emergent Ideal Forms and/or noumena—that is, inherent pre-conceptions ("thoughts without a thinker")—thereby allowing the recipient to "learn from experience" and to evolve as a self and as a soul. In propounding this line of thought, Bion infused psychoanalysis with ancient and Western Enlightenment epistemology and mysticism to create a psychoanalytic epistemological ontology similar to that of Heidegger and Sartre (C. Williams, 2006).

Clinical vignette

A female analysand was expressing her feelings about my forth-coming departure for my summer vacation. She first expressed consternation about how her out-of-work, now "house"-husband was letting her down by placing the responsibility for making a living on her. I was able to help her see that, by analogy, she was also perceiving me as a soon-to-be out-of work analyst's-partner who was leaving her with the sole burden of caring for herself as well as her family. I first interpreted to her that she believed that she was now being abandoned by a husband-me in retaliation for her having "divorced" (a key element in her history) her childhood family. She wondered about this idea and felt it might be right, but it didn't sufficiently relieve her. She then began—as analysands have done ever since the first days of psychoanalysis—to specu-late on another reason why I was leaving. As is the case with so many analysands, she wondered whether I were leaving at this particular time because she had exhausted and depleted me due to her excessive neediness of late. Although I believed that *she* believed that that phantasy may have had merit, I was struck by its cliché-ness and then replied to her: "Suppose that that wasn't the reason. Suppose that my leaving had nothing to do with you and your neediness." Her reply was instant and animated. "My God! That would be terrible, unthinkable. It has to be my doing, otherwise I'm nothing to you and therefore nothing to myself. At least I have a connection and an identity if I can have driven you away to your vacation!"

I report the above analytic scene as a model to demonstrate what I believe to be the universality of the need for an unconscious phantasy to accompany the analysand's perception and conception of a real event—in this case in the transference. By developing a phantasy—in this case an unconscious one of which she was able to become con-scious (it must be pointed out that on previous occasions I had already interpreted this to her as an unconscious phantasy)—of her own puta-tive sense of agency with regard to an external event, she was able to become the author, for that moment, of her own life scenario with an object (me) and achieve a sense of identity as a moving force: "I caused this to happen, therefore I am." I have elsewhere referred to this phe-nomenon as "autochthony", the unconscious phantasy of self-creation and creation of one's world order ("cosmogony") by the self—that is, self-creation and self-organization (Grotstein, 1997c, 2000a). I also suggested there that trauma can be understood to be the occurrence of a real event before one has had the opportunity to have "created" it beforehand (even by microseconds) in unconscious phantasy.

This phantasy, like all others, emerges from the workings of the primary processes, according to Freud (1911b) and of α-function or dream-work-α, according to Bion (1962b, 1963, 1992), who disagrees with Freud's separation of the primary and secondary processes from one another and unites them as coterminous gradient processes instead, as α-function. Bion thereupon revised Freud's concepts not only of the primary and secondary processes but also about dreams and dreaming and about the psychic apparatus.

I return to the discussion of Bion's radical extension and revision of Freud and Klein further on. For now, let me reveal an idea that Bion implies: *every perception, conception, or act in external reality must be "dreamed" in order to become a part of the unconscious as well as become conscious as a result of initial unconscious processing.* Put another way, *every perception, conception, or act in external or internal reality must be accompanied by the creation of a corresponding unconscious phantasy* (Bion does not seem to distinguish between dreams, phantasies, and myths).

Why (how) do interpretations produce relief?

Freud (1911b) discusses the conflict between the pleasure principle and the reality principle and asserts that the former originates earlier, is predominant in psychic reality, and organizes the primary processes. When an analysand feels relieved by an interpretation, is this because he has achieved enough of a capacity for reality-testing and the pleasure in understanding because the pleasure of wish-fulfilment has become transcended? That is the theory, if I am not mistaken, that informs traditional psychoanalytic thinking.

My own current view, following Bion, is as follows: When the analysand accepts an interpretation (that is presumably correct), several events occur: (1) The analyst's α-function (dreaming) enables, enhances, and fortifies the analysand's own hitherto impaired α-function and dream-work to reconstitute in binding the loose cathexes of imminent primary processes (Freud, 1911b) or in transforming disturbing "β-elements", O (Bion, 1965, 1970), into more reassuringly manipulable symbols, K (knowledge). (2) With a transformation from O to K, there also occurs a simultaneous and pre-emptive transformation of β-elements from O to corresponding "P" (unconscious phantasies)—that is, phantasies (or dreams by day and by night) that match up phantasmatically with their counterpart in symbolic thought. This latter idea, which I shall discuss later, corresponds to one application of Bion's (1965) concept of "binocular vision"—the need to establish and repair the dream-phantasy floor of the psyche to support symbolic reality. (3) But at the same time and on another level, I believe that the very presence of the analyst as well as his courage and the effect of his interpretative activity offer a profound reassurance to the analysand that, at its deepest roots, can be thought of as being close to the operation of the pleasure principle.

I know from all the analyses I have conducted as well as from my own personal analyses that the very act of being with the analyst offers wish-fulfilling feelings such as hope and a relief at being listened to, at the mirage of fairness in the world, and especially at having the opportunity to share one's feelings with an analyst whose role is as a very unique "notary public" (Grotstein, unpublished-b) for one's inner-most life. Thus, one can conceive of a dual track between the operation of the primary and secondary processes or of dream-work in which psychic reality works together as a binary opposition (not necessarily in conflict) with external reality (one could use the analogy of conjoined twins, who are separate and fused at the same time).

Conclusion: The truth drive is the operant agent of curiosity, which constitutes the "seventh servant".

NOTE

1. I am indebted to Thomas Ogden for the Freud reference on the "symbolic equation".

CHAPTER 15

Lies, "lies", and falsehoods

lizabeth Tabak de Bianchedi (1993) and her long-term study group (de Bianchedi et al., 2000) studied "the various faces of lies" in Bion's work and in the work of others over many years. After considerable deliberation they were able to forge a categorical system of untruths along a gradient: falsehoods or falsities → lies → Lies. (Note that the first "lie" is spelled with a lower-case l and the second with an upper-case L to in order to differentiate significantly between the two.) Bion seems to have been the only—or at least the first—analyst since Freud to deal with the theoretical and clinical aspects of prevarications, including the question of whether liars could even be analysed. Bion, unlike Klein, believed that they could be.

De Bianchedi and her colleagues also trace the history of Bion's encounter with the subject of falsehood and lies, as here:

> "What is truth", said jesting Pilate . . . and would not wait for an answer. . . . We probably cannot wait for an answer because we have not the time. Nevertheless, that is what we are concerned with . . . inescapably and unavoidably—even if we have no idea what is true and what is not. Since we are dealing with human characters we are also concerned with lies, deceptions, evasions, fictions, phantasies, visions, hallucinations—indeed, the list can be lengthened almost indefinitely. [Bion, 1977b, pp. 41, 42]

Bion could also have added dreams. Earlier in his work (up to *Transformations*, 1965), Bion sets truth against its counterpart, falsity, according to de Bianchedi (1993), who then goes on to show how he significantly altered this distinction once Bion had uncovered O, the Absolute Truth about an Ultimate Reality, a domain that must forever remain ineffable to and unreachable by human knowing. In uncovering this concept of Absolute Truth and Ultimate Reality, Bion transcended the positivistic notion of reality for its ultimate, unknowable forebear by the invocation of unknowable Truth, that which was needed to face this Reality. Bion then postulated the operation in human beings of transforming/transducing operations: α-function and later dreaming, which convert the Absolute—indifferent, impersonal—Truth into personal emotional, subjective truth, an entity that allows us to think, to feel, to grow mentally: in other words, to be enabled to "learn from experience" by being able to convert Absolute Experience into personal experience that can be felt and thought about (reflected upon). In the meantime Bion's older polarization between truth and falsehood had to be altered in favour of a gradient, Truth → truth → falsehood → lie, to which gradient de Bianchedi and her group add lie → Lie. They distinguish lie from Lie as follows:

> [W]e ... differentiate the "lie" (with a small letter), related to defence mechanisms, from the "Lie" (with a capital letter), specifically related to conscious and denuding lying". [de Bianchedi et al., 2000, p. 224]

In *Attention and Interpretation* Bion discusses truth and lies:

> For satisfaction, the liar needs an audience; this makes him vulnerable, since his audience must set a value on his fabrications. It is therefore *necessary that the analyst-victim should attach importance to the patient's statements as formulations of a truth*. It must be possible to observe incoherent elements and to detect a pattern that brings together the disparate elements, showing a coherence and a meaning that they had not without it. . . . The Ps ↔ D reaction reveals a whole situation which seems to belong to a reality that pre-exists the individual who has discovered it. *The lying discovery lacks the spontaneous bleakness of the genuine Ps ↔ D. The lie requires a thinker to think. The truth, or true thought, does not require a thinker—he is not logically necessary.* . . . Provisionally, we may consider that the difference between a true thought and a lie consists in the fact that a thinker is logically necessary for the lie but not for the true thought. *Nobody need think the true thought: it awaits the advent of the thinker who achieves significance through the true thought. The lie and its thinker*

are inseparable. The thinker is of no consequence to the truth, but the truth is logically necessary to the thinker. . . . The only thoughts to which a thinker is absolutely essential are lies. . . . *The paranoid–schizoid state may then be seen as peculiar to the thinker who is in a state of persecution by thoughts that belong to a non-human system, the O domain.* [1970, pp. 102–103; italics added]

To elucidate the above italicized comments:

- *"It is therefore necessary that the analyst-victim should attach importance to the patient's statements as formulations of a truth"*: I take this to mean that the analyst should regard the liar as inadvertently employing the equivalent of dream-work, if not actually using dream-work to disguise the truth (Truth) that he fears. Put another way, the liar's lie predicates the truth in disguise—like dreams.

- *"The lying discovery lacks the spontaneous bleakness of the genuine Ps ↔ D"*: My understanding of this citation is that the analyst can detect an emotional difference between the way one tells the truth and the lie.

- *"The lie requires a thinker to think. The truth, or true thought, does not require a thinker—he is not logically necessary"*: I take this to mean that the liar must think—defensively—to protect the "truth (consistency) of the lie", all the while knowing it is untrue.

- *"Nobody need think the true thought: it awaits the advent of the thinker who achieves significance through the true thought. The lie and its thinker are inseparable. The thinker is of no consequence to the truth, but the truth is logically necessary to the thinker"*: Truth just is and awaits its thinker but does not depend on the latter to think it. The "true thinker" (as opposed to the thinking liar) must seek the truth, though in vain, only being able to approach it obliquely or tangentially because of its "blinding glare".

- *"The paranoid–schizoid state may then be seen as peculiar to the thinker who is in a state of persecution by thoughts that belong to a non-human system, the O domain"*: I find this last statement to be unusually profound and explanatory for all the preceding statements. From the positivistic Kleinian stance, P–S constitutes the reaction of the infant to the experience of its drives, both from within and then from without via projective and then introjective identification. In other words, the drives constitute first cause. In Bion's radical revision of psychoanalytic metatheory, P–S is our first defence against the indifference, impersonality, and absoluteness of a non-human cosmic system yet to become "humanized and personalized by α-function and dreaming, the infinite, ineffable, and numinous domain of O, Bion's nomination for first cause.

I have also come to believe that one of the significant differences between the "liar" and the "Liar" is in character. Weak characters (liars) may be prone to lying when difficult situations arise, whereas Liars (those who are called "pathological liars") seem to lie characterologically—even when it is not necessary. They seem unable to help themselves. It is my belief that these characterological Liars are dominated by a pathological organization or psychic retreat (Grotstein, in press-c; Steiner, 1993).

On the other hand, I believe that it is important to consider the obverse of the situation: we analysts are so imbued with respect for the truth, both the analysand's and our own, that we tend to moralize against lies, Lies, and falsehoods and the liars who propound them. The very terms seem pejorative. Lies reveal the hapless analysand's passion and anguish in reverse—as truth in the negative as it is transmitted by a spokesman for a putatively protective psychic retreat. Lies are but an alternative mode of revealing the truth: "To tell you the truth, I cannot tolerate the truth except through the filter or lens of a lie!" (Grotstein, unpublished-b).

CHAPTER 16

The container and the contained

Early origins of the concept

Of Bion's numerous contributions, certainly his development of the concept of *container* ↔ *contained* ranks as the best-known and most widely used, both in theory and in technique (see chapters 4 and 5). It seems to have been incubating for some time in the observations Bion had made on psychotic patients. We find the first adumbration of the concept in "Development of Schizophrenic Thought":

> In the patient's phantasy the expelled particles of ego lead to an independent and uncontrolled existence outside the personality, but either *containing* or *contained* by external objects where they exercise their functions as if the ordeal to which they have been subjected has served only to increase their number and provoke their hostility to the psyche that ejected them. [1956, p. 39; italics added]

The "negative container"

We can deduce from this and other passages that Bion seems to have come across the idea of a pathological or "negative container" prior to his later formulation of a "positive container". In a subsequent paper, "On Arrogance", he states:

> [I]t appears that overwhelming emotions are associated with the assumption by the patient or analyst of the qualities required to pursue the truth, and in particular a capacity to tolerate the stresses associated with the introduction of another person's projective identifications. Put into other terms, the implicit aim of psycho-analysis to pursue the truth at no matter what cost is felt to be synonymous with a claim to a capacity for *containing* the discarded, split-off aspects of other personalities while retaining a balanced outlook. [1957a, pp. 88–89; italics added]

A few pages later Bion observed that the patient believed (1) that Bion could not bear his communications, and (2) that by insisting on verbal communication between the patient and himself, he was attacking the patient's form of communication—that is, projective identification:

> In this phase my employment of verbal communication was felt by the patient to be a mutilating attack on *his* methods of communication. From this point onwards, it was only a matter of time to demonstrate that *the patient's link with me was his ability to employ projective identification.* . . . On this depended a variety of procedures which were felt to ensure emotionally rewarding experiences such as . . . *the ability to put bad feelings in me and leave them there long enough for them to be modified by their sojourn in my psyche,* and the ability to put good parts of himself into me, thereby feeling that he was dealing with an ideal object as a result. *Associated with these experiences was a sense of being in contact with me, which I am inclined to believe is a primitive form of communication that provides a foundation on which, ultimately, verbal communication depends.* From his feelings about me when *I was identified with the obstructive object,* I was able to deduce that the *obstructive object* was curious about him, but *could not stand being the receptacle for parts of his personality* and accordingly made destructive and mutilating attacks, largely through stupidity, upon his capacity for projective identification. [1957a, pp. 91–92; italics added]

Here we see Bion, the genius, at work: his unusually keen observation of the patient's interaction with him, and his ability to deconstruct (abstract) the results of his observation into their elements and to reconstruct or reconfigure them into more meaningful entities. In short, Bion subjected his abstractions to dreaming (wakeful thinking) and thereby "stood on a peak in Darien".

The obstructive object
and the "super"ego as a persecutory negative container
(projection-in-reverse)

It is in these early passages—recognized by us retrospectively—that Bion laid the groundwork for his later conception of the container and the contained. He thus first associated the development of containment in its negative or pathological form with a "primitive catastrophe" (Bion, 1967c) having occurred in the infancy or childhood of his psychotic patients; from this he formulated the idea of the positive container in the mother as the critical function that had been lacking. He further deduced that this negative container was characterized, when internalized, by (1) an *obstructive* (internal) *object*, which represents an amalgam of (a) *a real mother* who cannot tolerate her infant's emotional outpourings (projections) in addition to her hatred of the infant for emoting, and who projects in reverse; (b) the infant's hatred of her for her rejection of him, which the infant projects into his image of her; and (2) an infant who can *only* communicate his emotions via projective identification because he does not yet possess the capacity for *verbal* communication.

Bion continued this same theme of the "obstructive object" in his succeeding paper, "Attacks on Linking" (1959) and then, in "A Theory of Thinking" (1962a), as well as in his "Commentaries" (1967a) in *Second Thoughts* (1967c), where he gives it the central position in his first contribution on his radical psychoanalytic metatheory, an ontological and phenomenological epistemology harvested from his experiences while treating psychotic patients.

In *Learning from Experience* Bion refers to this obstructive object as a very (unreasonably) moralistic "super"ego:

> In the first place its predominant characteristic I can only describe as "without-ness". It is an internal object without an exterior. It is an alimentary canal without a body. It is a super-ego that has hardly any of the characteristics of the super-ego as understood in psychoanalysis: it is "super" ego. It is an envious assertion of moral superiority without any morals. In short it is the resultant of an envious stripping or denudation of all good and is itself destined to continue the process of stripping . . ., as existing, in its origin, between two personalities. The process of denudation continues till $-♀ -♂$ represent hardly more than an empty superiority–inferiority that in turn degenerates to nullity.
>
> In so far as its resemblance to the super-ego is concerned – (♀♂) shows itself as a superior object asserting its superiority by finding

fault with everything. The most important characteristic is its hatred of any new development in the personality as if the new development were a rival to be destroyed. The emergence therefore of any tendency to search for the truth, to establish contact with reality and in short to be scientific in no matter how rudimentary a fashion is met by destructive attacks on the tendency and the reassertion of the "moral" superiority. This implies an assertion of what in sophisticated terms would be called a moral law and a moral system as superior to scientific law and a scientific system. [1962b, pp. 97–98]

Perhaps without realizing it, Bion seems to have reconfigured the role of this primitive "super"ego, not merely as the pathological agent that pre-empts the formation of the ego with its harsh, hypocritical moral system, but also as a pathologically "protective" agent for the now demoralized infant who is denied a reasonable container–mother into whom to project. The very severity and harshness of this "super"ego offers, through its omnipotence and hardness,[1] a sadistic security to the now masochistic infant who comes to depend on this default security. Elsewhere, I have referred to this phenomenon as the "Faustian bargain with the devil" (Grotstein, 1979, 2000a). The demoralized infant must then, according to Fairbairn (1943), selectively introject the badness of the intolerable aspects of the needed object, identify with them, and thereby preserve the fiction of a dependable object. It also amounts to an identification with the aggressor (A. Freud, 1936).

It is very interesting to note in retrospect that Bion found this pattern of the negative container in psychotics. I think that were he alive today, he would no doubt see its relevance for traumatic disorders, for which it is highly apposite (Brown, 2005, 2006; Grotstein, in press-c). Today clinicians treat post-traumatic stress disorders resulting from dysfunctional family upbringing. It is also my opinion that the negative container—which, as I have already mentioned, absorbs Bion's earlier concept of the obstructive object and his later idea of the malignant "super" ego—may constitute the bedrock of pathological organizations or psychic retreats (Steiner, 1993), to say nothing of endopsychic structures (Fairbairn, 1940; Grotstein, 2002, 2005). More recently, I have drawn a parallel between the negative container and the psychic retreat (Grotstein, unpublished-b; Steiner, 1993).[2]

Container ↔ contained

The fundamental intersubjective experience of emotional communication between infant and mother, and between analysand and analyst, introduced two new themes to psychoanalysis, particularly to the Kleinian analysis of the time: (1) the importance of the container ↔ contained relationship, and (2) the prime importance of relationships as the *sine qua non* and irreducible factor in the infant's development. It also anticipated subsequent developments in infant development and attachment research (Bowlby, 1969), as well as the rise in intersubjective thinking in other analytic schools—albeit Bion was not alone. Elsewhere I have stated that the container ↔ contained concept, as well as Klein's positions (P–S ↔ D), constitute the unconscious template for attachment phenomena (Grotstein, 2005, 2009):

> An infant endowed with marked capacity for toleration of frustration might survive the ordeal of a mother incapable of reverie and therefore incapable of supplying its mental needs. At the other extreme an infant markedly incapable of tolerating frustration cannot survive without breakdown even the experience of projective identification with a mother capable of reverie. . . . We have thus approached a mental life unmapped by the theories elaborated for the understanding of neurosis. [Bion, 1962b, p. 37]

We can conclude from Bion's container ↔ contained concept, consequently, that *it is the proper counterpart to the concept of attachment and constitutes its unconscious template.* I should further hypothesize that there is a relationship between the container ↔ contained link and a living *covenant* between the partners in the relationship, each of whom owns a portion of the responsibility for its welfare. Furthermore, this covenant becomes the *sine qua non* for the development of the experience of *faith* in one's objects (Bion, 1965, p. 159).

Bion often uses icons—♀♂—to designate the container ↔ contained. He may have had many reasons for this that he never revealed. One possibility that comes to my mind is that Bion believed that the breast, vagina, and penis constituted *linking organs* between objects, and that one of the greatest challenges the infant must confront is the primal scene, which this icon beautifully symbolizes and which represents the original creative act.[3]

The shift from drives to emotions and emotional communication

Bion's shift from the hegemony of the instinctual drives to emotions and emotional communication is notable and would ultimately achieve realization in five successive stages of his theorizations:[4] (1)

the formalization of the *"container ↔ contained"* concept (1962b, p. 99); (2) the model of *"α-function"* as the requisite property of the maternal container; (3) *"transformations"* by the container's α-function of β-elements (unmentalized sensory impressions of emotional experience) into α-elements (mentalized elements suitable for subsequent thinking, memory, dreaming, etc.) (see chapter 7, note 1); (4) the formulation of *"attention"* as a specialized version of "consciousness" as a sense-organ responsive to psychic qualities (unconscious consciousness, intuition, *nous* (for a further development of this concept see Grotstein, 2004a, 2004b; see also chapter 22); and (5) the ultimate apotheosis to his metatheory, *O*, the one that represents the culmination of and the organizing, defining "selected fact" in relation to all his previous conceptualizations. With the last two of these contributions, and particularly with "transformations in O", we find yet a sixth, quintessential conception, one that is still psychoanalytically "heretical" among London Kleinians: (6) the concept of *"truth"* (emotional truth) as it transformatively descends from O, the Absolute (indifferent, impersonal) Truth about Ultimate Reality, to tolerable (acceptable) personal truth.

The component functions of the container

As mentioned earlier, Bion conceptualized first a *negative* container-object as the issue of his original theme of the obstructive internal object that attacks one's thinking and linking with other objects, and then *positive* container-objects, which constitute a necessary element in the act of thinking: the infant projects his raw proto-emotions—β-elements, "thoughts without a thinker"—into his maternal container, who, in a meditative state of reverie, (1) absorbs, (2) sorts out (triages, prioritizes), (3) detoxifies, and (4) transduces the β-elements from infinity to finiteness (good vs bad, etc.), (5) reflects upon these projected emotional communications, and (6) allows them to incubate within her, while, at the same time, she (7) allows them to resonate with her own native, autochthonous emotions and her repertoire of conscious and unconscious experiences (memory). From this incubation and resonant interchange emerges spontaneously a "selected fact" that gives coherence to the entirety of the communication. Meanwhile (8) the infant's original β-elements (proto-emotions) have become transformed into α-elements suitable for *mentalization*. The mother then (9) appropriately responds to or informs her infant (interpretation) what it is feeling. She may also (10) withhold what she has absorbed for a delayed future return (the basis for repression). The analogy to renal dialysis is striking. It is important to realize that the container is not merely the processor of the infant's proto-emotions; it is also the generator of independent thinking in response to the infant's β-elements (co-creation). The act of containment involves the transformative reconfiguration of the infant's/analysand's raw, unprocessed proto-emotions (β-elements) into α-elements (unconscious phantasies, myths, reconstructions, shifting of perspectives) so as to achieve *personal* meaning from the *impersonalness* of O and ultimately to achieve "damage control". From a more simplified point of view, however, the function of the container can be seen generically for an individual (infant, analysand, or whomever) to be able to *share* their emotional experiences with another caring individual whose very act of *caring* acts to *circumscribe* the emotional moment for the disturbed infant/patient.

There is yet another aspect of the container ↔ contained function that needs to be addressed: (11) The container ↔ contained concept has, since its inception, been thought to be, along with communicative projective identification, the basis for intersubjectivity between infant and mother and between analysand and analyst. In this process the infant, like the analysand, is communicating with himself—that is, with his own unconscious—through the intermediary function of the mother (or analyst) as the *channel* between the infant/patient and the mother/analyst. Bion believes that, subsequently, the infant introjects this experience of the successful operation of the container on its contents and is thereafter able to project into his own internalized container, thereby establishing the origin of his own spontaneous, autonomous thinking. In other words, the infant can now begin to mentalize within himself (the beginning of thinking). It is my belief, however—and here I am at variance with Bion—that the infant is born with his own autochthonous α-function as a Kantian primary category, akin to Chomsky's (1957) inborn "transformational generative syntax": in other words, the infant is born ready to communicate with a pre-lexical (sensory) language.

The container functions not only as a *communicative translator*, but also (12) as a *mediator, filter* (detoxifier), and *transducer* of emotional energy states from the uncontainable domains of infinity to the containable dimensions of ordinary reality. Furthermore, the container's act of containment also presupposes that it not only translates emotional communication and transduces emotional volume or valence, but it also *withholds* some of what it contains, sometimes indefinitely. This act constitutes the function of *repression* and is associated with what Freud (1896b, p. 169) called "the return of the repressed" and Klein (1929, p. 222) "persecutory anxiety". The infantile part of the personality begins to experience the return of the repressed persecutory anxiety as it encounters—or is encountered by—the threshold of the depressive position, which signals the homecoming of former projective identifications in their sojourn in objects. Though Bion never stated it outright, he certainly intimated that *internalized objects, including those that have been reprojected in other objects, ultimately constitute unsuccessful containers of β-elements—that is, untransformed O* (Grotstein, 2000a). In psychoanalysis yet another function of the container—that of *stimulation*—manifests itself. The relative silence of the analyst automatically encourages (stimulates) the analysand to associate freely—and thereby to regress. This regression can be seen as the drawing to the surface of deep reservoirs of emotions and memories. Furthermore, the container and the contained can inspire one another to higher functioning.

Clinical and theoretical implications

The clinical, if not the theoretical, implications of these conclusions are vast. Klein—and, early on, Bion—emphasized the clinical importance of the infant's experience, intolerance, and the subsequent projection of its death instinct into its objects, thereby autochthonously creating, first, external objects and then, upon internalization, internal objects that have become transformed by the projection. With the concept of container ↔ contained Bion burst through the one-dimensional envelope of Kleinian solipsism into the third dimension of intersubjectivity, stressing the *prime importance* of the function of the maternal—and the paternal—container. Having stated the above, I hasten to add that, clinically, I adhere to and support—as, in fact, did Bion—the Kleinian focus on autochthony: that is, not what *actually* may have happened to the infant in terms of poor or inadequate containment, but how the infant in unconscious phantasy *accounts* for his role in damaging mother so as to have rendered her a poor container. Having said that, however, Bion's discovery of the intersubjective modification of the results of projective identification constituted a paradigm change for Kleinian psychoanalysis and introduced the clinical fact of intersubjectivity.

Alternating container and contained
♂ ↔ ♀

The relationship between the container and the contained is generally pictured unilaterally—that is, the infant or the analysand/patient as the contained and the mother or analyst as the container. It comes as no surprise, I am sure, that the process proceeds both ways—rapidly, alternately—on different levels: While the analyst is listening to his analysand and trying to understand what he is hearing, he acts as a container. As soon as the analyst presents an interpretation, he becomes the contained who is addressing the analysand, who has, in turn, become the container (for the moment). Ultimately, however, the infant's (analysand's/patient's) content is primary, and that of the mother/analyst becomes a derivative. Ideally, what the content (contained) that the mother/analyst returns to the infant/analysand/patient, now as *ad hoc* container, is a modification of his original contained. Practically, the returned contained may all too often be intermixed with the personality (good and bad) of the original container (mother/analyst), so that the infant/analysand/patient is left with the task of "secondary containment"—that is, sorting out those aspects that have been returned as food for thought or interpretations that conform to or match up with his authentic and recognized needs and separating out and discarding those returned aspects that are, upon contemplation, idiosyncratic to the container–mother–analyst and are not appropriate for the infant/analysand/patient. Hanna Segal (personal communication, 1970) pithily stated that the infant is responsible for obtaining good mothering from a bad mother, and the analysand a good analysis from a bad analyst.

Container ↔ contained, constructivism, and self-organization

The container function of the infant/analysand/patient functions according to the principle of *self-organization* or *autogenesis* (Grotstein, 2000a, p. 50; Schwalbe, 1991), which pre-empts "social constructivism" (Hoffman, 1992, 1994). Put another way, infants/analysands/patients, through their own container function, always bear as "co-construction" the responsibility for what they experience. If they incorporate something that is inappropriate to their basic nature, they traumatically develop a "true-self/false-self" dichotomy (Winnicott, 1960a); if they incorporate something from the other that is agreeable to their true nature, they metaphorically "masticate" it until it is theirs (with their own native "saliva" on it) and it becomes a natural part of them.

Categories of container ↔ contained relationships

Bion defines the categories of the interrelationship between the container and the contained thus:

> The theory is that an object is placed into a container in such a way that either the container or the contained object is destroyed. In pictorial terms the container is represented by a mouth or vagina, the contained by breast or penis. The relationship between these objects, which I shall represent by the male and female signs ♀ and ♂, may be commensal, symbiotic, or parasitic. By "commensal" I mean a relationship in which two objects share a third to the advantage of all three. By "symbiotic" I understand a relationship in which one depends on another to mutual advantage. By "parasitic" I mean to represent a relationship in which one depends on another to produce a third, which is destructive of all three. [1970, p. 95]

By using ♀ and ♂, Bion is conflating the infant–mother relationship at the breast (nurture) with the Oedipus complex (sexual, creative). The commensal relationship has as its model the fetus–womb experience, the symbiotic has the mouth–breast relationship, and the parasitic has the intrusion of pathology into the relationship, either by bad containment by mother and/or by too intense an enfilade of the infant's projective identifications and/or the invocation of envious attacks on mother's residual goodness.

To these we could add other geometrical iconic relationships. First, picture the infant (contained) and mother (container) iconically as conjoined twins—that is, separate heads but one body, as in symbiosis (emotionally united but perceptually separated). Then picture all the possible geometrical configurations that can occur between them: (1) mother in back with infant on her lap, (2) mother in front with infant on her back, (3) infant and mother side by side, and (4) infant and mother together but facing in opposite directions, as in the Janus-face configuration. Next imagine the types of object relations that would derive from each of these configurations. In the first the mother–container is a background presence or holding object, which would include bonding and attachment and all Kohut's mirroring selfobject function. The second typifies Kohut's idealizing selfobject function (of the mother or father by the infant). The third designates Kohut's twinship selfobject function, and the fourth either a complementarity of functions ("You look out for me, and I'll look out for you") or an oppositional selfobject function.

What also stands out in Bion's container ↔ contained formulations is his emphasis on the irreducibility of *relationships* between self and objects and between objects rather than on the self or the object independently. Bion was clearly an intersubjectivist and a relationist, having been profoundly influenced by Einstein's theory of relativity and Heisenberg's theory of uncertainty. Thus, the container ↔ contained theory has come to constitute a pattern or model for all relationships on all levels, normal and/or pathological.

Container ↔ contained and their associations

Bion's thinking, like his writing, was associative rather than algorithmic. He associated the concept of container ↔ contained with α-function, dreaming, the caesura, and the contact-barrier. By so doing, he was creating the analogue of an emotional–epistemophilic *network* of interlocking functions. The container functions optimally when the contact-barrier maintains the protective separation between Systems *Ucs.* and *Cs.* But a cycle or a closed loop is involved. The container, whether within the mother/analyst or the infant/analysand, must produce α-elements from the β-elements in order to reinforce the contact-barrier, which must optimally vouchsafe the functioning of the container. Dreaming allows for the α-elements that are produced by the container to be aesthetically arranged and configured into narrative images. These narrative images become dreams and/or unconscious phantasies that mediate (modify, transform) the original message from evolving O, first as β-elements, then as mentalized α-elements, and now as dreams or phantasies in order to process and further transmit the Truth from O and transform it into "truthful fiction", whereby the indifference and impersonalness of Absolute Truth is translated into a mercifully and personally tolerable and *meaningful* but *fictive truth*—yet, as in all good art, all the more emphasizing the truth by this aesthetic, fictive reconfiguration.

Put succinctly, Bion's picture of human beings is as follows: the individual is born divided between his infinite godhead–self and his limited mortal self, as Freud (1914d) himself had so intuitively adumbrated with regard to the relationship between the ego ideal and the ego. The caesura that *selectively* divides the fetus from the infant evolves into a metaphoric membrane, the contact-barrier, which selectively divides System *Ucs.* (which may correspond to the fetus) from

System *Cs.* (which may correspond to the experienced conscious self). This metaphoric membrane becomes co-extensive with α-function, and all of the preceding become co-extensive with container ↔ contained. One blends seamlessly into the other. The external object whose task it is to become the container can be thought of as a human "co-enzyme" on a transformational cycle beginning with impersonal, indifferent O and ending for a transient moment in personal, human O, only to return to its next cycle. In the meantime we require good-enough—and I mean *really* good-enough—containers to facilitate the homecoming of our projective identifications, behind which act is our reunion with our infinite cosmic self and its incarnation of us as it becomes a realization in us in emotional experience.

Container ↔ contained and the holding environment

Differentiation between "holding" and "containing"

The words "holding" and "containing" are so simple and quotidian that at first blush one would think they cover the same function. In fact, they do not. Winnicott's concept of "holding" implies a background object (Grotstein, 1981a, 2000a) that (who) *facilitates* the infant's maturation without being involved in a direct "I–Thou" interaction. It is as if the holding (environmental) object is perceived more as a "developmental coach", as an important adjunct to the autonomously developing infant, as contrasted with the "object-using" infant, the one who recognizes his instinctual and affect-attunement needs and the object who meets them.

Winnicott's (1960b) concept of the "holding environment" is often used synonymously with Bion's "container ↔ contained" concept. While there may be a good deal of overlap in their respective functions, a careful reading of each author leads, I believe, to the following differentiation. Winnicott (1960b, 1963) developed the concept of two-infant prototypes, whereas Klein adhered only to one. The Kleinian infant is born separate and in need of a nourishing breast–mother from the very beginning. Winnicott acknowledged the "Kleinian infant" as the "active infant" who roots to the breast. The other infant he posited was the "being infant" who was associated with the environmental holding object. While there is communication between the former pair, there is none between the latter pair because no communication is necessary. The holding-object mother is an intuitive mother who reads her infant's needs—but more to the point, she functions as a background object who is preoccupied with facilitating the autonomous development of her infant. My terms for her are: "existential coach" and "background presence of primary identification". Bion's container concept refers initially to a mother who bears and absorbs her infant's emotional states, transforms them, and "interprets" them to her infant. She is, in effect, an emotional instructor to her infant.

The broader significance of container ↔ contained

As mentioned earlier, the container ↔ contained concept immediately transformed psychoanalysis, particularly Kleinian analysis, into irreducible intersubjectivity. Other schools of analysis had also been involved with either the interpersonal or the intersubjective factor, but none was so systematic as Bion's, in my opinion, and they neglected the container's transcendent function whereby the infant subject is enabled to converse through the medium (channel) of the mother/ analyst with his own other self, his unconscious, infinite self.

Bion conceived of other facets of the container function, such as maternal reverie, α-function, dreaming, and phantasying. The last three constitute the transformation ensemble whose functioning the state of maternal reverie facilitates. If one follows the implications of Bion's theory, one inescapably comes to the conclusion that mental health, on the one hand, and psychopathology, on the other, are direct functions of the activity of the container, first external and then internal. O, rather than the drives—except for the truth drive (Grotstein, 2004a, 2004b)—becomes "*first cause*" and everything hinges on the outcome of the interaction between O and the container.

I should now like to revisit Bion's (1967) experience treating psychotic patients and refer to two of his observations. Bion observed that psychotics, as infants, lacked the opportunity to have mothers who could contain their projections. Another observation was that they could not tolerate frustration and, as a consequence, split off and projected, not only their emotional experiences, but also their minds, which experienced them. Thus, unable to tolerate frustration—that is, the experience of what Bion (1965, p. 54) calls the "no-breast" (the presence of the *experience* of the *absent* breast–mother)—the infant who is destined to become psychotic must get rid of his emotions and his mind because he lacks the experience of a good-enough *external* container and subsequently of a good-enough *internal* container (with its associated α-function, dreaming, and phantasying) with which to regulate and mediate his emotions. Without this internal container, consequently, the psychotic lacks transformational equipment and must then declare a state of emotional/mental bankruptcy and jettison what remaining mind he still possesses, along with its thoughts, into his objects, including his body. The mother's failure to be a good-enough container often results in her projecting in reverse back to the infant, as well as being violently projected into by her infant—in default of good containment—and thereby becoming transformed into an obstructive, link-attacking object, a hyper-moralistic "super"ego. This object becomes the nucleus, in my opinion, of the psychic retreat and is the hallmark of trauma (Grotstein, unpublished-b).

Earlier, I spoke of the importance that Bion attributed to the infant's capacity to tolerate frustration and to be able to countenance the experience of "no-breast", an emptiness or nothingness that signifies where the breast once was—with the belief (faith) that the breast will reoccupy this position. The infant—or infantile portion of the personality—that can abide this experience attains the capacity to think and to reflect: that is, it has developed a psychic space in which to accumulate thoughts and to be able to think them (reflect upon them), to experience them thoughtfully and meaningfully, and to learn (evolve) from those experiences. Put another way, the tolerant-enough infant *becomes* his emotional experiences and thus evolves as a self. This ability to tolerate the frustration of the absence of the breast requires the development of *faith* (Bion, 1965, p. 159). The development of faith fundamentally depends on the infant's experience of the pattern of maternal absence becoming constantly conjoined with the mother's return—that is, the trajectory of the circle ("the sun also *rises*"—after it sets).

As the infant, in its role as the contained, becomes emotionally and epistemologically attuned by its container mother, it is not only knowledge that it receives from the maternal container. The infant looks at its external and internal reality through the periscope of its mother's eyes. If mother can tolerate and mediate the infant's β-elements from O, then automatically it means that she can tolerate her own O and thereby herald an atmosphere of equanimity about herself and security about the world for the infant.

A derivative of the container ↔ contained theory is Bion's concept of *dreaming*. Unlike Freud, Bion believed that we dream by night and day and that we dream O, the reality that impinges upon our sensory–emotional frontier. This reality may result from an external stimulus to which we must adjust or accommodate. Dreaming is our way of accommodating—that is, rendering the experience unconscious and allowing selective aspects of the experience back into our conscious awareness through the selectively permeable contact-barrier (Grotstein, 2002). In terms of the analytic situation, the analyst must dream the analytic session, according to Bion (1992, p. 120). The idea that the analyst should "dream" the analytic session—by "abandoning memory and desire"—became an important extension of his intersubjective theory of projective identification and a critical modification of the concept of countertransference as an analytic instrument.

Still another derivative of the container ↔ contained concept was Bion's (1962b, p. 54) concept of *"binocular thinking"*, which he applied in a number of ways. The container ↔ contained relationship was itself an example in so far as it involved the interaction of two individuals. Another example is his idea that consciousness and the unconscious, *Cs.* ↔ *Ucs.*, rather than being in conflict, as Freud suggests, are in binary (cooperative) opposition in triangulating O. Furthermore, he postulates something similar for the relationship between the paranoid–schizoid and depressive positions, "P–S ↔ D", which also cooperatively triangulate O.

Epilogue

The reader will note that my writing of this chapter as well as the other chapters resembles Bion's own work at least in one regard: it is holographic: each chapter in this book, like each subject within the chapter, recapitulates the essence of Bion's works to one degree or another.

I wish to add here some final comments on aspects of the container ↔ contained concept that I have not yet addressed:

A. What does the container ultimately contain? Is it projective identifications, emotions, experiences, or urges? Let us say it is all the preceding—and more. What the container ultimately contains, what α-function ultimately transforms, what dreaming ultimately dreams, what transformation ultimately transforms, what underlies all projective identifications, what inheres in all experiences is—*truth*! I believe that the "godhead", O, *is* Truth that needs inchoately to be *contained* as *emotion* as it enters into the cycle of transformation to personal truth in the process known as "container ↔ contained".

B. When one considers the functions of the container with regard to the contained, one begins to see striking similarities between it and α-function, to say nothing of the contact-barrier, dreaming, and the Grid. I now see all these functions as either identical, overlapping, and/or cognates of one another.

C. Bion believes that the infant projects his β-elements (proto-emotions) into the maternal container, that her α-function transforms them into useful, mentalizable α-elements, and that in time, after many iterations, the infant introjects mother's α-function, then begins to project into it, and starts thereupon to think *within* himself and *for* himself. As I have stated earlier, my own version—which is a modification of Bion's—is as follows: The infant is born with its own inherent α-function capacity, which constitutes a Kantian innate category, similar to Chomsky's (1957, 1968) concept of the inherent "transformational generative syntax". That is, the infant is born with the syntactical capacity to understand and to generate language and only needs to develop the verbal capacity to generate and understand verbal language. However, infant development research tells us that the infant is capable of *communicating*, not just projecting, *meaning* in a pre-lexical language of sensorimotor gesture (Schore, 2003a, 2003b, personal communication, 10 June 2006). Consequently, *I hypothesize that the infant, under normal and felicitous circumstances, possesses a rudimentary α-function of his own and communicates with his mother from the very beginning. It is only when significant disruptions occur in the attachment relationship between them that the infant is reduced (one of Bion's favourite words) to employing projective identification as an urgent alternative.*

D. Containment tempers the anxiety that follows in the wake of unleashed entelechy—the activation of the entirety of one's inborn potential and also of one's premonition of its imminence. The infant's fear of dying is in part the dread of entelechy and of bad demons from inherent pre-conceptions.

E. The container–mother must be in symbolic contact with her husband (father).

F. Emotions are containers of β-elements signifying the Absolute Truth about Ultimate Reality. The dread of emotions is due to one's unconscious sense about the reliability of the container and the Truth it contains.

G. The container does not dream the infant or patient: it dreams the patient's/infant's dream. It completes the dream.

H. One of the most important functions of the container ↔ contained relationship is that of constituting a bridge or channel between the infant and his unconscious (infinite self), which he has projected into his mother as the analytic patient does with the analyst.

NOTES

1. One is reminded here of Tustin's concept of the "hard object" used by autistic patients to plug their holes (metaphorically) (Tustin, 1981, p. 61).

2. Even as I put the finishing touches to this book, a Middle-East war is being waged. I cannot not help contemplating that fanatic members of Hamas and Jihad are victims of and are being driven by a highly omnipotent and super-moral obstructive object—one that has become the superego of fanaticism and evil.

3. For further developments of this concept see Grotstein (2004a, 2004b), and chapter 22 .

4. The concept of the selected fact is complex. Bion borrowed it from the mathematician Henri Poincaré. That it *seems* to emerge unpredictably and spontaneously belies the fact that from the outset it has always belonged to the total communication and has consequently always been a part of it. The observer's grasp of its "arrival" is, however, another matter: that may constitute an independent aspect (pre-conception or even premonition) of the selected fact.

CHAPTER 17

"Projective *trans*identification": an extension of the concept of projective identification

> "It is a very remarkable thing that the *Ucs.* of one human being can react upon that of another, without passing through the *Cs.*"
>
> Freud (1915e)

Projective identification: summary of the nature of the problem and a proposed solution

Of his many contributions to psychoanalysis, Bion's revision and extension of the concept of projective identification was one of the first and was destined, along with container ↔ contained, to become the most famous. In what follows I explore the origins and varying conceptions about projective identification from differing perspectives but ultimately with the task in mind of revealing Bion's ideas as well as my own extension of them about the subject.

Projective identification has become a widely used concept in the mental health field but still suffers from categorical confusion in its usage. The principal confusions are as follows: (1) The question of the differences from, as well as the similarities to, Klein's (1946, 1955) original concept as a strictly intrapsychic, omnipotent, unconscious, defensive phantasy and Bion's (1962b) "realistic", communicative, intersubjective extension of it: are the two respective uses of it continu-

DOI: 10.4324/9781003348665-18

ous or discontinuous and/or both, or might they be complementary to each other? (2) Is there a difference between projection and projective identification? (3) When a patient uses projective identification, does he actually project himself into the object or into his internal *image* of the object, and, if the latter, how can we explain the object's response to the projective identification? Is there some process in addition to projective identification that allows it to become communicative to another person? Put another way, on the *metapsychological* level, as contrasted with the *experiential* level, the subject can only project into an image or representation of the object, not into the external object *per se*. The projecting subject, however, *experiences* the external object as containing the projections, and, furthermore, the latter may also *experience* containing them.

I shall try to explain how this might happen. I suggest that Bion's (1959) concept of normal, communicative (two-person) projective identification is foundational and subsumes Klein's (1946, 1955) one-person model, which presupposes that the intrapsychic, omnipotent, unconscious phantasy is always a component of it.

Put another way, *in the theoretically perfect experience of container ↔ contained there would be no omnipotent intrapsychic phantasy of projective identification.* Moreover, Klein's earlier versions of it dealt with how the object became altered in the subject's mind by virtue of the projective identifications but did not take into consideration, unlike Bion, how the projective identifications into the object became continuously modified by the responses of the object as container (Bion, 1962b). Whereas with Klein one understands projective identification as being evacuative, aggressive, invasive, and possessive, with Bion's version one understands the infant to be communicating—even pleading—his emotions to the object for the latter to contain and mediate.

Yet I also believe that Bion conflated two aspects of projective identification, which I now call projective *trans*identification, in his revised conceptualization of Klein's concept. These two aspects, already alluded to in chapter 13, are (1) *normal*—α-function (infant) to α-function (mother)—*communication*; (2) *abnormal communication*, when normal communication breaks down, in which case the infant is reduced by default to employing projective transidentification into the mother.

One of the problems in moving between Klein's and Bion's versions is that of (1) considering Klein's intrapsychic version to be subsumed by Bion's intersubjective version rather than being orthogonal to it, and yet (2) maintaining a distinction between the two processes, and, in so doing, being able to name them, and/or (3) to add a third possibility, one that would suggest that yet two other functions must be added to either Klein's or Bion's concepts to account for the actualization of the communication, presupposing that projective identification, in either Klein's or Bion's version, still constitutes an intrapsychic unconscious phantasy. As Bion says:

> Melanie Klein's theory is that patients have an omnipotent phantasy . . . the patient feels that he can split off certain unpleasant and unwanted feelings and can put them in the analyst. I am not sure, . . . that it is *only* an omnipotent phantasy. . . . [W]hen the patient appears to be engaged on a projective identification it *can* make me feel persecuted. . . . *If this is correct it is still possible to keep the theory of an omnipotent phantasy, but at the same time we might consider whether there is not some other theory which would explain what the patient does to the analyst which makes the analyst feel like that.* . . . [1973, pp. 105–106; italics added]

I suggest, consequently, that: (1) Bion's bimodal (as alluded to above) communicative version subsumes Klein's intrapsychic version and adds the intersubjective dimension of the object's role in containing and thereby modifying the subject's ultimate experience of what he has projected. (2) Since Klein's intrapsychic model still persists in Bion's model, however, we come to the problematic consideration that the subject can only project into his personal *image* of the object, not the object *per se*. (3) We now follow Bion's notion "whether there is not some other theory which would explain what the patient does to the analyst which makes the analyst feel like that". I believe there is one. My theory of projective *trans*identification includes yet two other processes: (1) a sensorimotor one—that of gesture, prompting, priming on the part of the projecting subject—and (2) spontaneous empathic simulation within the optimally receptive object. I further propose that the projecting subject and the object of its projection constitute *two independent self-activating systems* (Llinàs, 2001) with *shared representations* (Decety & Chaminade, 2003). Also linked with the preceding category is the phenomenon of the "mirror neuron", which constitutes the neurophysiological basis for empathy (Gallese & Goldman, 1998).

Definition of projective identification

In defining projective identification, Klein states:

> The phantasied onslaughts on the mother follow two main lines: one is the predominantly oral impulse to suck dry, bite up, scoop

out and rob the mother's body of its good contents. . . . The other line of attack derives from the anal and urethral impulses and implies expelling dangerous substances (excrements) out of the self and into mother. Together with these harmful excrements, expelled in hatred, split-off parts of the ego, including internal objects and even the superego, are also projected . . . *into* the mother. These excrements and bad parts of the self are meant not only to injure but also to control and to take possession of the object. In so far as the mother comes to contain the bad parts of the self, she is not felt to be a separate individual but is felt to be *the* bad self. . . . This leads to a particular form of identification which establishes the prototype of an aggressive object relation. I suggest for these the term "projective identification". [Klein, 1946, p. 300]

She goes on:

It is, however, not only the bad parts of the self which are expelled and projected, but also good parts of the self. Excrements then have the significance of gifts. . . . [p. 301]

She also says:

From the beginning the destructive impulse is turned against the object and is first expressed in phantasied oral-sadistic attacks on the mother's breast. . . . The persecutory fears arising from the infant's oral-sadistic impulses to rob the mother's body of its good contents, and from the anal-sadistic impulses to put his excrement into her . . . are of great importance for the development of paranoia and schizophrenia. [p. 293]

In this latter citation Klein spells out the connection between the infant's oral- and anal-sadistic phantasied impulses of projecting into the object and its fear of retaliation by the object in the form of persecutory anxiety as a consequence. We are, in effect, hypnotized by what and whom we projectively re-identify in the object. The bad parts of the self that are involved in the projective identification include oral and anal-sadistic impulses in addition to persecutory internal objects. Although the subject thereafter hatefully disavows ownership of these split-off aspects of self, including internal objects, these alienated aspects, now all objects (which still unconsciously maintain their identification with the projecting subject), become personified (Klein, 1929) and in the projecting subject's unconscious phantasy do *not* disown *their* link with the subject. As Klein states it, the transformed object is treated as if it were part of the self. In other words, the defences of splitting and projective identification do not work completely.

Ultimately, the projecting subject and its projected objects cannot totally disown their contact with one another. Splitting and projective identification are associated with a dis-integration of the self, whereas the propensity towards integration enforces a return (a pulling back) of the projections. The unconscious pull between the projecting subject and the contents of what it has projected is the source of what Klein (1946) terms "persecutory anxiety" (p. 296): that is, the fear of retaliation by the object, which now contains projected aspects of the self. Additionally, the projecting subject may, in phantasy, omnipotently acquire control over the object in order to ward off the anxiety of separation.

Also of note in Klein's definition are the following: projective identification constitutes the prototype of an aggressive object relationship, and the infantile portion of the personality which employs it aims to injure, possess, and/or control the object. The projecting subject may also project good aspects of itself into the object, however. In normal or non-defensive projective identification, the projecting subject may extend itself into its image of the object, but without omnipotence or splitting—as in empathy (putting oneself in someone else's shoes), planning ("thinking ahead"), externalization (Novick & Kelly, 1970), and so on (Grotstein, 1981a, p. 213). Another normal aspect of projective identification is its role in the development of sexuality—that is, as an *Anlage* of the ability to contemplate the loving and passionate invasion of another individual, to say nothing of seduction and all other forms of attempts to influence.

Later, Klein expanded the evacuative–manipulative nature of the concept to include fusional aspects. In the first mode, *parts* of the self are split off and projected into the object (Klein, 1946). In the second mode, the self-*qua*-self enters into a state of identification with the object to *become* the object and, through unconscious *imitation*, either passively disappears to one degree or another (Klein, 1955) or (and), at the other extreme, may seek aggressively to take over the identity of the object altogether—as in Julian Green's (1947) novel, *If I Were You*, upon which Klein's second work was largely based. The consequences of this kind of projective identification range from states of confusion and disorientation to grandiosity.

Following Klein, important advances in our understanding of the concept were made by Rosenfeld and Bion. Rosenfeld (1971) separated the evacuative (defensive) from the communicative (non-defensive) functions of projective identification; Meltzer (1992) distinguished between the "claustrum" and the "container ↔ contained", the former designating defensive projective identification and its consequence—incarceration in the object that had been invaded in unconscious phantasy—and the latter, communication (p. 61). Britton (1998) divided projective identification into "acquisitive" ("you are me") and "attributive" ("I am you") types, depending on the putative intention of the projecting subject (p. 5).

Spillius (1988), following Rosenfeld, summarizes the motives for the use of projective identification: communication, empathy, avoiding separation, evacuating unpleasant or dangerous feelings, taking possession of certain aspects of the mind of the other (p. 62). Her way of distinguishing between the exclusively intrapsychic and the communicative forms of projective identification is to call the former "non-evocative" and the latter "evocative" projective identification (pp. 81–86). She also states:

> Thus, unlike Klein, we [modern London Kleinians—JSG] are now explicitly prepared to use our own feelings as a source of information about what the patient is doing, though with an awareness that we may get it wrong, that the process of understanding our response to the patient imposes a constant need for psychic work by the analyst . . . and that confusing one's own feelings with the patient's is always a hazard. . . . The analyst's aim is to allow himself or herself to experience and respond internally to such pressures from the patient enough to become conscious of the pressure and of its content so that he can interpret it, but without being pushed into gross acting out. . . . [Spillius, 1992, pp. 62–63]

Do projection and projective identification differ?
The obligatory role of identification in projection

There has been considerable debate with regard to the role of identification in the process of projective identification. Questions include: Can there be projection without identification? Who does the identifying—the projecting subject or its object? One reason for this confusion may be that projection was originally used as a mechanism that was separate from—although located within the mind of—the subject. Klein seems to have conflated the mechanistic aspect of projection with its status as an unconscious phantasy *and* as an object relationship. Once understood as the latter, the term "projective identification" seemed more appropriate. The very act of projecting implies a change in the state of the identity within the projector—that is, in perception some aspect (identity) of the subject's internal world is being attributed to the perceived image of the object. As a defence mechanism, some aspect is being disidentified from the subject and re-identified in the object (Sodré, 2004, p. 56).

Klein first implied (1946) and then later explicated (Klein, 1955) that projective identification was not *just* a mental mechanism: it fundamentally constituted an unconscious phantasy about internal and external object relationships. We can see here the subtle transition of Klein's conceptualization of projection from the classical Freudian notion of a putatively autonomous defence "mechanism", as had already been formulated by Anna Freud (1936), to one in which projection, like other defence "mechanisms", became transformed into both an *unconscious phantasy* in its own right but also an *object relationship* (internal as well as external). This subtle transition became pivotal, in my opinion, in the transformation of "projection" into "projective identification". Put another way, since the Kleinian concept of defence "mechanisms" always predicates an unconscious phantasy about an object relationship and is always object-dedicated, "identification" *ipso facto* becomes the *sine qua non* for the operation of projection—that is, the transfer of identities.

When the external object *does* seem to identify with the projection, however, "projective *trans*identification" (my term for the intersubjective form of projective identification) is in operation. In my opinion, projective identification *per se* is transacted not between the subject and the external object, but between the subject and its own *internal-object image* (representation) of the object. I came to realize this from reading, in Bion's *Cogitations* (1992), about the limitations imposed on our grasp of reality when we depend on the senses: that is, that we cannot really *know* the object from the verdict of our senses, and thus an internalized object constitutes an image based upon our sensory impressions, including what we projectively assign to it (p. 118).

Similarly, in intersubjective projective identification the object, now a co-subject, also forms its own image of the projecting subject. *Ultimately, a mutually inductive resonance transpires between the two images,* the nature of which I discuss further on. The infantile portion of the personality may, as a result of projective identification, either misperceive the object as the self or project into the suspected or perceived reality of the object, and subtly induce or put pressure on the object to behave in conformity with the projection.

Bion's contribution

Although this had already been intimated by Klein, Bion distinguished even more clearly between normal developmental and pathological (defensive) projective identification *and* between its intrapsychic and intersubjective modes. Extrapolating from his experiences with psychotic patients, Bion (1959, 1962a, 1962b, 1967c) reasoned that, as infants, they lacked the experience of having had a maternal object into whom they could normally project their emotions (1959, p. 104). He proposed, consequently, that the normal infant needed a mother as a "container" into whom intolerable emotions could be projected (1962b, p. 90). Thus he broadened the concept from an exclusively omnipotent, intrapsychic, unconscious phantasy to *in*clude, *seemingly*, very real interpersonal and communicative, as well as epistemological dimensions, but not to *ex*clude the notion of the intrapsychic omnipotent phantasy. He posited that as the infant projects into mother, the latter, in a state of reverie, employs her "α-function". Bion (1962b) designates "α-function" to represent a counterpart to a mathematical variable that operates as an alternative to both Freud's primary *and* secondary processes (1911b, p. 3), collectively, to absorb, detoxify, and refine the projections in preparation for a meaningful, and appropriate response to the infant: that is, supplying the name of the *feeling* (Damasio, 2003) or the gesture that serves as the interpretation of the infant's internal state that corresponds to the *emotion* (Ogden, 1994b).

It must be noted that the container ↔ contained function shifts by reversing itself, so that the mother then becomes the projector and the infant the container, as in normal dialogue.

In ascribing this process to the basic communication between mother and infant, Bion (1970) developed a unique epistemology in which the inchoate process of thinking begins with the projective identification of the infant's "thoughts (emotions) without a thinker" (p. 104) into its mother-as-container, whose reverie and α-function transform them into thinkable thoughts, feelings, dream thoughts, and memories. When the infant's α-function matures in this environment, it begins to think for itself by projecting into its own internal container–object with its own α-function. Bion's formulation not only broadened and extended Klein's version; it also, in my opinion, pre-empted it in a way by postulating the "infant–mother projecting–container team" as an irreducible two-person model, from which Klein's model became a default consequence upon failed containment. Whereas Klein's one-person model predicated a single, static effect upon the object in

projective identification, Bion's two-person model allowed for multiple dynamic shifts in the *relationship* with the object, depending on
how effective the object was as a container for the projective identifications. Bion states: "the patient does something to the analyst and
the analyst does something to the patient; it is not *just* an omnipotent
phantasy" (1980, italics added).

Spillius summarizes the three ways in which modern British Kleinians use projective identification:

> In Britain ... I think there are what one might call three clinical
> "models" of projective identification: Klein's own usage, in which
> the focus is on the patient's use of projective identification to express
> wishes, perceptions, defences; Bion's container/contained formula-
> tion; and Joseph's usage, close to Bion's, in which the analyst expects
> that the patients will constantly bring pressure to bear on the ana-
> lyst, sometimes very subtly, sometimes with great force, to get the
> analyst to act out in manner consistent with the patient's projection.
> [Spillius, 1992, p. 63]

American versions of projection and projective identification

At the time when the concept of projective identification came to
America, I expressed the more traditionally Kleinian view, whereas
Kernberg (1987) and Ogden (1982) distinguished between projection
and projective identification in—different—modifications of Bion's
version (Grotstein, 1981a). Interestingly, it seems that Bion's version
became the better known and more frequently used clinically.

Kernberg (1987) defined projective identification as:

> (a) projecting intolerable aspects of intrapsychic experience onto the
> object, (b) maintaining empathy with what is projected, (c) attempt-
> ing to control the object as a continuation of the defensive efforts
> against intolerable intrapsychic experience, and (d) unconscious in-
> ducing in the object what is projected in the actual interaction with
> the object. [Kernberg, 1987, p. 94]

So far, Kernberg's definition conforms to Klein's (1946) and to my own
(Grotstein, 1981), but then he—unlike Klein and myself—differentiated projection from projective identification:

> Projective identification ... differs from projection, which is a more
> mature type of defense mechanism. Projection consists of (a) repres-
> sion of an unacceptable intrapsychic experience, (b) projection of
> that experience onto an object, (c) lack of empathy with what is

projected, and (d) distancing or estrangement from the object. . . .
[Kernberg, 1987, p. 94]

By "lack of empathy", Kernberg means the differentiation between whether or not the subject retains contact with the projection. He fails to recognize that what is projected always maintains contact with the subject unconsciously.

It is readily apparent that—with the exception of his allusion to empathy—both his definitions conform to what Klein and her followers include as projective identification alone. It may be that at the time that Kernberg put these distinctions forward, he was concerned with differentiating the borderline personality and syndrome from neurotic conditions and so shaped his distinctions between projective identification and projection accordingly. In terms of empathy, he considers empathy to be absent in projection, whereas

> Projective identification . . . assures the capacity of empathy under conditions of hatred, in a parallel way to the development of empathy as a concomitant of the differentiation self- and object representations under pleasurable peak affect experiences that lead to introjection. [Kernberg, 1987, p. 100]

Ogden, on the other hand, states:

> A distinction must be drawn between the projective mode of thought involved in projective identification and that in projection as an independent process. In the former, the projector subjectively experiences feelings of oneness with the recipient with regard to the expelled feeling, idea, or self-representation. By contrast, in *projection* the aspect of the self that is in fantasy expelled is disavowed and attributed to the recipient. [Ogden, 1982, p. 34]

Ogden's differentiation between projective identification and projection differs from Kernberg's above and recapitulates the distinction Klein made in her two contributions on the subject. For him "projective identification" corresponds to her second contribution (Klein, 1955) and "projection" to her first (Klein, 1946). Thus, Kernberg and Ogden each differentiate between projective identification and projection but each in his own way—and their differences are all subsumed in Klein's definition of projective identification alone. Ogden (1994a) had also been working on his conception of the "analytic third subject": he emphasized an "intersubjective third subject" (p. 37) and thus reasoned—unlike Kernberg—that projective identification was an intersubjective object relation, whereas projection was a non-intersubjective relationship. In other words, Ogden was trying to distinguish between Klein's (1946) first and second (1955) uses of projective identification. While I personally hold to the Kleinian view that projection and projective identification are identical and that the term subsumes both of Klein's views, I do believe that Ogden's concept of the "intersubjective third subject" is an interesting and valuable way of expressing Bion's intersubjective version of projective identification (Ogden, 1994a)

Other American contributions include those of Schore and Seligman. Schore (2003a) studied projective identification in attachment research and believes that mothers and infants communicate via projective identification between each other's right cerebral hemispheres (p. 77). Seligman (1993) studied projective identification in infant research and attachment research and also attempted to integrate it with infant–mother psychotherapy (Seligman, 1994).

The importance of the internal image (object) in projective identification

Klein stated that projective identification was directed *into* the object by the projecting subject. I hypothesize that one cannot—Freud, Klein, and Bion notwithstanding—project *into* an *external* object. I am of the opinion that one can project only into one's *image* (i.e. phantasy, representation, construction—as an internal object) of the individual. That idea is implicit in Klein's description of the process *as an unconscious phantasy*. Bion, while formulating the realistic communicative aspects, never considered *projective identification* as actually taking place in the object—only that the object was *affected*.

The concept of transference presupposes that we form internal, subjectively modified images of real objects and that we confuse the latter with the former. In projective identification, the projecting subject creates within his mind an image of the object to re-present. In manipulative projective identification the subject, in unconscious phantasy, magically (omnipotently) manipulates the *image* of the object (which is identified with the external object) in order to control the latter (action at a distance, sympathetic magic).

Subjects who use defensive projective identification have an omnipotent unconscious phantasy in which they believe that they no longer possess those particularly painful aspects of themselves and feel that the object—whether internal or external—now possesses them. These comprise: (1) either good or bad aspects of themselves, which include good and/or bad emotions, such as love and/or hate, impulses, and internal objects, including superego; (2) modes of relationships, such as sadism, masochism, hatred, aggression, voyeurism, exhibitionism, and so on; (3) omnipotent expectations or obligations of role-responsiveness imposed upon the object to meet the infant's needs (J. Sandler, 1976), with concomitant concordant and/or complementary role assignments (Racker, 1968); (4) omnipotence (as a transformation of the infant's sense of infinite urgency); and (5) attributions of animism and/or personification (Klein, 1929) to the object so that it assumes a preternatural life force. Additionally, the image of the object is invested with the quality of (6) intentionality (will, agency, purpose, or determination). The qualities of expectation, omnipotence, intentionality, animism, and personification prefigure the object's future role upon internalization by the subject as (7) an omnipotent and determined (wilful) primitive superego. Having exported his omnipotence and intentionality to the (image of the) object, the projecting subject is left in desolate emptiness and impoverishment.

The subject may then re-project a demanding superego *and/or* a mutilated object-self (in the ego) into—the image of—the same or another external object, leading to the appearance of *claustrophobic anxiety* (being trapped within the object). The external object is then felt to be very demanding and yet devalued (by the double projection), and the subject needs space in order to resist being suffocated by the projectively compromised object. In the phantasied act of attempting to control the object by entering it via projective identification, the subject feels trapped within the object. Projective identification is involved clinically in distinguishing between *enemies* and *persecutors*—the former being independent of the subject and the latter constituting projective identifications originating in the subject.

Proposed postulates

A. Intersubjective projective identification constitutes the operation not only of Klein's theory of projective identification as an unconscious, omnipotent, intrapsychic phantasy (occurring only within the unconscious of the projecting subject) but, in addition, with regard to Bion's version, two other processes: (1) conscious and/or preconscious modes of sensorimotor induction and/or evocation or prompting techniques (mental, body, speech, posturing or priming, "nudging") on the part of the projecting subject, followed by

(2) spontaneous empathic simulation in the receptive object of the experience of the subject who is already inherently equipped (programmed) to empathize with it. So far I am discussing projective identification in metapsychological *theory*. From the perspective of *experience*, however, the projecting subject feels that he has rid himself of bad (or good) emotional contents and now believes that the object *is* the self or is indistinguishable from it with regard to the projected parts—and, experientially, the object may concur that it has become affected.

B. The projecting subject *and* the object of projection constitute *two separate self-activating systems,* and the interpersonal process should consequently be renamed *"projective* trans*identification"* to designate its unique transpersonal mode so as to contrast it with the unconscious phantasy of intrapsychic projective identification proper.

C. A corollary of the preceding view is that one can never project into another individual *per se*, only into one's *image* (internal-object representation) of them—and then attempt to manipulate that image in unconscious phantasy as if it *were* the external object that was being manipulated. This idea is but another way of stating that the objects we encounter in our daily lives are fraught with personal transferences from our unconscious.

D. Consequently, projective transidentification would function by establishing an inductive resonance between the internal-object images formed by the projecting subject, on the one hand, and those counterpart images formed by the external object of the subject, on the other.

E. Projective identification into the object-image is followed by an introjection by the projecting subject of the now projectively transformed image of the object, which, upon introjection, ultimately lands in the subject's superego and ego. If hatred were projected, the subject experiences a hateful superego and a hated ego, respectively.

F. Projection from the Kleinian/Bionian points of view is inseparable from and identical to projective identification, but in the mainstream American view they differ from one another in various ways.

G. In thinking of communicative (intersubjective) projective (trans)identification, one should distinguish between normal pre-lexical communication and urgent, default projective (trans)-identification.

H. I believe that projective identification (Kleinian version) has yet another function: that of a *"homing instinct"*, an instinctual urge to retrace one's roots.

I. The ideas above appeared in my 2005 publication. I now see fit to modify them in light of attachment studies. I now believe that *the infant normally communicates with its mother, and the analysand with his analyst, with α-function and α-elements from the start—they only resort to using projective transidentification when there is a disruption between mother and infant and between analysand and analyst.*

The operations of projective transidentification: an explication of Bion's model

I wish to explicate Bion's intersubjective model in two ways: (1) from an experiential (phenomenological) perspective, and from (2) a meta-psychological perspective.

Experientially, the projecting subject *seems* to project into the object. If the object responds, it is experientially due to (1) the counter-formation in the object of a receptor site for the projection, which consists of the object's image of the projecting subject; (2) the object receiving a form of projection that Money-Kyrle (1956) suggests is "introjective countertransference" (counteridentification), to which may be added projective aspects of the object's own infantile neurosis, thus constituting what Grinberg (1979) calls "projective counteridentification". In this experiential model the projecting subject's image of the object and the object's image of the subject are in active, communicative *resonance*.

Metapsychologically, however, the subject can only project into his image of the object. The analysand and analyst are conceived of as *two separate self-activating systems* (Llinàs, 2001). If that is the case, then how does the object become affected? My explanation is that *two additional factors or functions must be added to the concept of projective identification in order to render it projective transidentification*: (1) In the case of the projecting subject, we must add the capacity for a hypnotic-like power to induce transformation in the object—one that owes its origin to "body rhetoric": that is, prompting, gesturing, priming, "nudging", prosody, and other similar modes, all being sensorimotor-originating modes of inducing responses on or influencing the object by the projecting subject (Bråten, 1998, Damasio, 2003; Greatrex, 2002; Helm, 2004; Kristeva, 1989; Modell, 1980; Stern, 2004). (2) In the case of the actively responsive object, we must add his capacity for an inherent sensitivity—a capacity to be empathic and to be attuned to the emotional state of the subject—a sensitivity that Stern (2004), after Bråten (1998), calls "altero-centred participation". "Damasio (1999) believes that we are 'wired' to respond to the other's emotions in a preorganized fashion when we receive certain stimuli in the world or in our bodies . . ." (Greatrex, 2002, p. 191).

In other words, a system of bilateral self-activation exists in which *the projecting subject evokes something already extant and dormant within the external object* whose latent capacity for empathic resonance with the subject's intrapsychic projective identifications can be elicited. Under the rubric of the metapsychological perspective I include the distinction, which I addressed earlier, between infant-to-mother communication and infant-to-mother projective (trans)identification. The analyst's unconscious is already inherently formatted ("hard-wired") to anticipate and resonate with the analysand's "body-rhetoric"—that is, sensorimotor induction (Bråten, 1998; Greatrex, 2002; Stern, 2004). To cite Daniel Stern's view of Stein Bråten's concept of "altero-centred participation":

> *Altero-centred participation* . . . is the innate capacity to experience, usually out of awareness, what another is experiencing. It is a nonvoluntary act of experiencing as if your center of orientation and perspective were centered in the other. It is not a form of knowledge about the other, but rather a participation in the other's experience. It is the basic intersubjective capacity that makes imitation, empathy, sympathy, emotional contagion, and identification possible. Although innate, the capacity enlarges and becomes refined with development. [Stern, 2004, pp. 241–242]

Joseph (1989) suggests that the analysand "nudges" the analyst into acting in a manner consistent with the analysand's projections (in Spillius, 1992, p. 63). I suggest that this "nudging" is related to sensorimotor-originating induction, which can include priming, evoking, speaking, hinting, or posturing, all of which belong to either observable or subliminal stimuli from the analysand. These phenomena might include tone of voice or atmospherics, which compound the analysand's initial projective identification and transform it into projective *trans*identification. The two processes together constitute an influencing process whose ultimate effect lies in the vulnerability and the now activated and already constituted empathic capacity of the recipient.

In postulating that a subject cannot project directly into an object, I have already alluded to another problem. My induction hypothesis (which includes resonance, evocation, provocation, priming, prompting, and/or gesture from the subject and spontaneous empathy from within the object) is fully compatible with Bion's conceptualizations, and I suggest that he adumbrated it in his "transformations in O" (1965, p. 160). Briefly, the analyst, upon receiving the analysand's projections—which are equated initially with unprocessed β-elements, emotional imprints of O (Bion, 1962b, p. 7), the unknown and unknowable—is able to contain: that is, undergo a transformation in O, and transform them into K (knowledge about his emotions). The source of the analyst's transformation is from within his own repertoire of experiences and emotions, which he seeks to match (simulate) with those of the analysand and "*become*" the O (the unknown and unknowable truth) of the session (Bion, 1965, p. 146). My understanding of what Bion means by this is that the analyst must recruit his own self-activated simulation of the analysand's experience and "*become*" it as thoroughly as possible. Thus, the source of the analyst's information is largely from within himself, but it is my opinion that it also emerges from the mystery of the projective–introjective transmission process detailed earlier. The concept "become" is an example of the ancient Greek "middle voice" (Greenberg, 2005), in which the passive and active voices coincide.

In support of this latter idea I cite Damasio:

The neural patterns and the corresponding mental images of the objects and events outside the brain are creations of the brain related to the reality that prompts their creation rather than passive mirror images reflecting that reality. [Damasio, 2003, pp. 198–199]

Thus, according to Damasio, we inherit the capacity to create empathically within us virtually the same feelings and emotions experienced by the patient (also personal communication, 6 February 2004). Thus, Damasio and Llinàs lead us to believe that there may exist a mechanism other than introjection to account for how the object becomes sentient about the subject, and this theory is supported by Bion's (1961) statement that a herd instinct or group psychology does not exist, only individual psychologies in a group (p. 169).

Induction by gesture and voice

I should like to develop further the subject of hypnotic-like induction. The analysand, like the infant, may employ overt or subtle levels of language including that of *gesture* and/or *voice* (prosody) or subtle bodily-evoked interpersonal communications ("*le sémiotique*" [preverbal semiology]—Kristeva, 1989, p. 62), or priming (Helm, 2004, Modell, 1980; Ogden, 1994b), in which infant and mother, as well as analysand and analyst, read each other's *gestures*. Priming, according to Helm, includes all the subliminal transactions of information that enter the implicit memory system and, with regard to the psychoanalytic situation, unconsciously affect the analyst and analysand. Modell (1980) believes that priming constitutes a manipulative mode of communicating affects (p. 260). The act of pointing represents an early developmental milestone for the infant. By pointing, the infant is both gesturing to indicate his interest in an object—with, conceivably, a wish to share the moment with his mother—*and* wishing, also conceivably, in unconscious phantasy, magically to acquire the object towards which he is pointing.

If what I have stated above is indeed so, the language of voice and gesture, which I associate with hypnotic-like induction, evocation, provocation, prompting, and priming, differs significantly from projective identification proper but is included within the process of projective *trans*identification and may constitute yet another communicative factor in inchoate mental life. Frazer (1922) long ago spoke of this process as "sympathetic magic".

My modified version of this process, as alluded to above, is that the infant or infantile portion of the personality, under the strain of accumulating emotional distress, *induces* a symmetrical state in the vulnerable-because-willing mother (or analyst) so that the mother/analyst unconsciously surveys (self-activates) her own inventory of past actual or possible experiences within her conscious and unconscious self, selectively recruits the most pertinent of them for conscious consideration, and then *generates* thoughts and/or actions (interpretations) to address the distress in the infant or analysand.

What the mother or analyst contains, consequently, is not really the infant's or analysand's projections but, rather, the emotional results of their corresponding unconscious recruitment of the mother's own experiences, which constitute her own subsequent reconstruction of the infant's experience to which they resonantly correspond. They remain self-contained in the presence of the emotional induction by the infant/analysand. In other words, the mother/analyst and the infant/analysand each contain "*shared representations*" (Decety & Chaminade, 2003). I hypothesize that this process corresponds more closely to what Bion (1965) really meant by the analyst's need to "become the analysand" (p. 146). *The analyst must even more deeply "become" those aspects of himself that most relevantly correspond to (simulate) those of the analysand.*

Projective identification, transference, and countertransference

To my mind projective identification is the underlying common denominator in all transferences, whether displacement of past object cathexes or the projective identifications of current mental representations. Analysands may attempt to project into (the image of) the analyst as an appeal or in order to influence, manipulate, seduce, corrupt, imitate, or fuse with the analyst. When they do so, they unconsciously manipulate the *image* of the analyst within themselves and *try to force the analyst by induction or priming (gesture) to conform to this image.*

I take the position that *countertransference* is the obligatory counterpart to transference and includes the whole range of the analyst's repertoire of feelings and emotions in the analytic situation, whereas *reverie* (Bion, 1962b, p. 36) strictly designates the purposefully directed and induced state of mind of the analyst who "abandons memory and desire" (Bion, 1967a, p. 143) in order to be optimally intuitive and receptive to his own unconscious *vis-à-vis* the analysand. When the analyst does seem to identify with the image created by the analysand, that identification may be a *trial* or *partial identification* (Fliess, 1942, p. 213) functioning as an intuitive analytic instrument. I would think that total identification would correspond to countertransference, and partial identification to reverie.

Mason terms the phenomenon of the analyst being afflicted with contagion from the analysand "mutual hypnosis", or "*folie à deux*" (Mason, 1994; personal communication, 2003). Mason's reasoning is as follows: In order for the object (i.e. the analyst) to be affected by the analysand's projected unconscious phantasy, the analyst must already unconsciously harbour the same omnipotent unconscious phantasy himself and must unconsciously seek to preserve its fiction, thereby entering into collusion with the analysand to preserve their mutual belief—that is, *folie à deux*. I not only agree with Mason's view but suggest that *folie à deux* has a normal function and constitutes the basis for intuition and empathy. The object's own unconscious is inherently structured to match the mindedness of the subject (Stern, 2004, p. 85).

In projective transidentification the analyst, upon experiencing the evocative or provocative induction (sensory, ultra-sensory, or even extra-sensory) stimulus from the analysand, summons within himself those corresponding symmetrical phantasies that match the analysand's experience. This is how a mother functions in maternal reverie when she is attending to her infant. Thus, when the analyst *seems* to act as a container for the analysand's reported experiences, I postulate that the analysand unconsciously *projectively identifies* his emotional state with his *image* of the analyst in the hope of ridding himself of the pain and of *inducing* this state in the analyst by manipulating his image of the latter. The analyst, who is willing to be a helpful co-participant in this joint venture, becomes open and receptive to the analysand's input *via a state of empathic resonance*. This resonance eventuates in the analyst's counter-creation of his own image of the analysand's projections (β-elements). Stern (2004) describes other-mindedness thus: "[I]nfants are born with minds that are especially attuned to other minds as manifested through their behaviour" (p. 85).

In clinical practice we allow ourselves the liberty of using the short-hand expression, "you are projecting your feelings into me" because it is practical to do so and concretely depicts the actual *experience*. My point is that, while this *seems* to work, it oversimplifies the intermediate processes that, when considered, suggest a paradigm shift in our understanding of the overall process *theoretically*. I refer to Bion's (1965) revolutionary conception of "becoming" (p. 146) and dreaming on the part of the analyst. When Bion used the term "become", he did *not* mean "identify with", which would designate a loss of the self—that is, a loss of ego boundaries—with the other. "Become" can occur only when the analyst's contact-barrier (boundary) is intact (Bion, 1962b, p. 17), so that the analyst may become that unconscious aspect of himself that is always already dormant within him resonantly and which always *potentially* corresponds to the analysand's projected emotions. (I refer the reader to my review of Bion's theories on dreaming and becoming—Grotstein, 2002, 2003; see also chapter 25.)

The subjugating third subject of analysis

Klein (1946) posited that in projective identification the infant or the infantile portion of the personality may project its urine and faeces, in unconscious phantasy, into the object in order to control it (p. 300). While she never really explained how the "faeces" and "urine" exert their control, Meltzer (1966) did. I understand him to mean that the infant first equates its faeces and urine with the milk *and* the breast that has just been swallowed, in part because the gastro-colic reflex occurs rapidly after feeding. When the infant squeezes the faeces in its rectum or performs anal masturbation, it is vicariously exerting its control over the maternal object within. In the course of these ma-noeuvres, the infant may, in unconscious phantasy, project its faeces or urine into (the image of) the external object at the latter's rear (anus) as it is departing and seek to enter it in order to control it from within (colonization). This phantasied act of projective identification presup-poses that the object's and the infant's anuses are now fused and/or connected—that is, mutually identified. Thus, the infant *and its* faeces, now equated with the internal breast–object by sympathetic magic (Frazer, 1922, p. 43), are able to control the object.

Ogden's (1994a) explanation for this process is different. He pro-poses that the analytic relationship between analysand and analyst itself constitutes a third subject, one aspect of which can be understood as the "subjugating third subject" (p. 101), which unconsciously directs the subjectivities of the analysand and the analyst. The formation of the subjugating third results from the intersubjective compaction or coalescence of the subjectivities of the analyst *and* analysand. It is a distinctive subject that acts independently of the subjectivities of either participant and directs each of them in the analytic drama.

On the other hand, the engagement may be derailed by the analy-sand's need to undermine the analysis. A collusion, a *folie à deux*, may then take place, though it can be rendered therapeutic if the analyst, who has been in a *partial identification* with the analysand, is able to step back and reflect upon what has transpired so as to render the drama into a mutative interpretation. Ogden's version is *experiential*. My own *metapsychological* version is that a *"dramaturge"* (the creator–architect and director of the drama)—the preternatural unconscious presence or demon that is located only in the unconscious of the analysand—co-opts the subjectivities of the analysand and analyst to create a play in which the relevant unconscious theme is able to be enacted and thus known (Grotstein, 2000a). The other name of the "dramaturge" is the *"ineffable subject of the unconscious"* (Grotstein, 2000a, p. 19). The dramaturge directs and orchestrates the subjectivities of the analysand and analyst to play roles suggested by Sandler (1976) but within the constraints of the analytic frame and the container/contained (Bion, 1962b) safeguard. When the analyst's own dramaturge becomes activated, a countertransference enactment replaces reverie. Furthermore, just as Bion (1961, p. 168) believes that the herd instinct does not exist—there is only the accumulated psychology of individuals in a group—so, metapsychologically, there may be no third intersubjectivity (except in mutual phantasy).

Concluding thoughts

While projective identification, as Klein understood it, helps us to understand the infant's fate in being confronted by objects that are suffused with his projections, Bion's version helps us to comprehend the nature of the pre-lexical emotional communication between infant and mother, the complexity of which warrants a new designation: "projective *trans*identification". I suggest that the latter includes prompting, tracking, or signalling (Couzin & Krause, 2003) to the object in addition to projective identification. I also consider the nature of this intersubjective communication to lie on a continuum in which the object's reverie and intuition range from ultra- or even extra-sensory perception through primary maternal preoccupation and transformations in O, to projective transidentification.

I have thus far portrayed the operation of projective identification as originating in the infantile portion of the projecting subject's personality and complexly resonating within the personality of the object. It must be stressed, however, that during the process of analysis, as in infant–mother transactions, and in daily life generally, the vectors of the transactions of projective transidentification operate bilaterally: the object instantly becomes a sender, and the originating projective sender thereupon becomes a receiver—that is, a dialogue is taking place. Moreover, newer studies on projective identification (what I now call "projective *trans*identification") emphasize the effects, for instance, of the mother's projections on the long-term outcome of the infant's personality development and behaviour. In an extended outcome study of mothers and infants, Apprey (1987) collected unconscious maternal phantasies about their infants from the fetal stage until the third year of the child's life and found significant positive correlations between the unconscious phantasies and the outcome with regard to the child's personality and behaviour.

One final note

I cannot leave the subject of projective identification and projective transidentification without suggesting that perhaps the prime motive for the former is "homing" or returning to the first home, the womb, as the infant is not yet able fully to accept birth and separation. The function of the latter may be an advanced step in which it wishes to communicate its distress about leaving its home. I also believe that projective *trans*identification occurs as a default when normal communicative discourse has broken down, and that no one can ever project into another individual, only into one's internal *image* of that person, and then seek to treat that image as if it were the real person (transference).

CHAPTER 18

Bion's work with groups

My plan in this chapter is first to present an overall general review of Bion's seminal ideas on groups. I think of his contributions as, on the surface, an archipelago of seemingly disparate, disconnected ideas that ultimately reveal to the patient eye a hidden land mass underneath, which connects them. This land mass is the consummate value he accords to *emotional truth* counterposed to the enormity and consistency of the *Unknown, O,* within and about us.

Experiences in groups

Bion began his investigative career with the study of groups. There he made a number of significant observations. He formulated the notion that a group consists of individuals each of whom, though an individual in his own right, also contains a group self. There is no such thing as group psychology in its own right.[1] The psychology that appears in groups expresses the composite psychological grouping of the group aspect of individuals within the group, in which that of the individual tends to submerge. Bion (1992) was later to express this dialectic as that of "socialism against narcissism" (p. 103). The other way of expressing this idea is that each person can be thought of as a group of subpersonalities, and the group can be thought of as an individual

 DOI: 10.4324/9781003348665-19

as well as a group. He later dealt with these putative subpersonalities in "The Imaginary Twin" (1950) and "Differentiation of the Psychotic and Non-Psychotic Personalities" (1957b).

Groups are formed to perform a unified task. Such a group, unified in this purpose, is called a "work group". As time passes, disruption or resistance to maintaining the unity of the group effort develops. These subgroup resistances form clusters known as "basic assumption" subgroups because each respective subgroup is characterized by a specific basic assumption that differs from the assumption of the work group. Group resistance bears some interesting resemblances to those in the treatment of individuals. Resistant subgroups have certain characteristics. One is that of "fight/flight"—either open or passive–aggressive rebellion against the progress of the work group. A second form of resistance is that of "dependency", by which is meant pathological dependency: this subgroup abrogates its sense of cooperative responsibility for working on the common task and projects it back onto the work group or especially onto the group leader. A third form of resistance is that of "pairing", whereby two or more individuals develop phantasies of sexual liaison. Another subsequent aspect of that phantasy is the more mystical idea that the two of the members of this pairing group will get together and produce a messiah or a messianic idea. This last idea—that the pairing group seeks to breed a messiah–child to bring hope to the group—was a brilliant "reach" for Bion. It is certainly not readily apparent to most observers of groups, but once Bion had observed it and formulated it, it became confirmed over and over again. That is an example of the genius in Bion.

The first form of group resistance, fight/flight, corresponds to its aggressive counterpart in individual therapy, whether the aggression is active or passive. The second, the dependency-subgroup resistance, corresponds to the individual patient who dissociates his own sense of responsibility for the treatment and unconsciously attributes (projects) it into the therapist, resulting in an omnipotent narcissistic form of dependency. The case of the third, the pairing group, is more complicated. The first aspect of it corresponds to the individual patient's sexualization of the transference to his analyst—as a defence against experiencing the pain and humiliation of dependency feelings. The subsequent phantasy that the pair will produce a messiah who will ultimately deliver the group from its travail is also more complicated. It may begin in individual psychology as one of the phantasied results of incest, in which the incestuous pair will produce a superior child[2] who will surpass the limitations of one's real family. It also suggests postponed magical deliverance in the future. Bion (1961, p. 164) gives the barest of hints about this idea when he states that group processes and their resistances can ultimately be traced back to Klein's concept of the archaic Oedipus complex. In other words, the incestuous male toddler may believe that *he* can produce a superior *"Wunderkind"* in mother's body—superior, that is, to a child that father can produce, which includes himself, thus its perpetual futurity.

The group leader becomes the magnet for the projection of omnipotent expectations from the individuals in the group. The group makes progress in reunifying and re-owning their projections and returning to their original mission after the group leader is able first to experience, then intuit, and finally interpret the subgroup anxieties that underlie their basic assumption deviations. The action of the group leader prefigured Bion's later work on maternal reverie and containment and that of the psychoanalyst. The fundamental anxieties that underlie the basic assumption group resistances were originally thought of as "proto-mental phenomena" (Bion, 1961, p. 101). These would be the forerunners of Bion's later concept of β-elements and O. These phenomena arise when one personality encounters another, and "emotional turbulence" is produced (Bion, 1976). Why? As is his wont, Bion does not explain this, but I would hypothesize that when two individuals get together for analysis or otherwise, various proto-emotions—rivalry, expectations of persecution or disapproval, fear of shame, love, hate, dependency, and many others—are probably experienced consciously or unconsciously by each.

Thus, we can see the first beginnings of Bion's later contributions here in his early group studies. He emphasized the primitive nature of group phenomena and was able to apply Klein's concepts of projective identification and the archaic aspects of the Oedipus complex, as I have just suggested, to which he added the notion of the paranoid–schizoid and depressive positions. He would continue and extend his group findings when he next undertook the psychoanalysis of psychotics and uncovered the "mystic".

A few citations from specific works show how representative group therapists have integrated Bion's later metapsychological work with his group concepts. I shall not comment on them because they speak for themselves.

Gordon's (1994) paper, "Bion's post-*Experience in Groups* thinking on groups" integrates Bion's original seminal work on groups with his later ideas developed from his individual work with psychotic patients and emphasizes the contrast between K and –K in group situations:

In short, for Bion the struggle to know and to understand (K) or the opposite, mindless evasion and anti-understanding (–K) are as essential for mental life as love and hate. Consequently, attempts to know; anxieties about and defences against that which is known; perversion and obliteration of the truth can be as salient *in any group session* or series of sessions as efforts to express love and hate and the related anxieties, defences, and perversions. [Gordon, 1994, p. 112; italics added]

Gordon goes on to describe a clinical example of a –K object in a group situation constituting a group conflict. He then discusses the application of Bion's later thinking about interpersonal projective identification and how apposite it is for group psychology and goes on to say:

Bion clearly expressed his view in *Learning from Experience* (Bion, 1962b, p. 99) that the clinical theories developed in his post-*Experience in Groups* work with psychotics and other seriously disturbed patients were applicable to groups. He discussed this in *Attention and Interpretation* as container–contained relationships. However, aside from some general examples of commensal (creative: "two objects share a third to the advantage of all three"); symbiotic (mutually satisfactory: "one depends on another to mutual advantage"); and parasitic (mutually destructive; "one depends on another to produce a third which is destructive of all three)" (Bion, 1970, p. 95), encounters between the mystic and the establishment. Bion did not offer clinical material from psychotherapy groups to illustrate the application. . . . I think that the intense feelings of alienation, emptiness and meaninglessness which accompany an "experience of a gap" reflect and express the unconscious effects on the personality of the psychic catastrophe that Bion symbolizes by –K object relationship. [Gordon, 1994, p. 124]

V. Schermer (2003) states:

There is a particular denial of Eros in Bion's group psychology, as he portrays the group forever enmeshed in returns to the ba [basic assumption—JSG] states, *à la* the repetition compulsion and the death instinct. This despair is not so dominant in his later writings, where he seems to have found life in thought itself and where he sets as his task the elaboration of what he calls "transformations in O", "O" being the "thing in itself" or the elusive object of scientific scrutiny. . . . Essentially, Bion's later works challenge the group psychologist to question at the most fundamental level the function of groups in human existence and the goals of therapy and training groups. [V. Schermer, 2003, p. 144]

Sutherland (1994) says the following:

> Bion likened the problem of the individual coming to terms with the emotional life of the group as akin to that of the infant in its first relationship, viz., with the breast/mother. In his later analytic work he spelled out the nature of the infant's task in overcoming frustration, i.e. when instead of the expected breast there was a "no breast" situation. For this achievement he took the mother's role as a "container" to be crucial. . . . It could readily be said that, for the group therapist, Bion advocates a role of considerable withholding. [Sutherland, 1994, p. 1179]

Finally, I should like to cite two passages from Bion's *Experiences in Groups* (1961), both because they are insightful if not recondite but also because they clearly demonstrate a cerebral juggler at work who can balance many ideas simultaneously, each of which seems far afield from the nature of the enterprise, group psychology, until he puts them all together.

> On the emotional plane, where basic assumptions are dominant, Oedipal figures . . . can be discerned in the material just as they are in psycho-analysis. But they include one component of the Oedipus myth of which little has been said, and that is the sphinx. In so far as I am leader of the work group function, and recognition of that fact is seldom absent, I, and the work group function with which I am identified, am invested with feelings that would be quite appropriate to the enigmatic, brooding, and questioning sphinx from whom disaster emanates. . . . . For the group, as being the object of inquiry, itself arouses fears of an extremely primitive kind. My impression is that the group approximates too closely, in the minds of the individuals composing it, to very primitive phantasies about the contents of mother's body. The attempt to make a rational investigation of the dynamics of the group is therefore perturbed by fears, and mechanisms of dealing with them, that are characteristic of the paranoid–schizoid position. [1961, p. 162]

Bion is essentially saying here, I believe, that primitive group anxieties—those that can be categorized as paranoid–schizoid—involve not only anxieties reminiscent of the relationship of the infant's mouth and the mother's breast, but also those reminiscent of the archaic oedipal struggles of the infant when it experiences being left out of the insides of mother's body. Is the sphinx, then, the combined mother–father object who, like an all-knowing sentinel, "knows" that the infant wishes to invade and explore the insides of mother's body? In other words, the infant's newly arrived sadistic and epistemophilic impulses to invade mother's body become projectively identified with the analyst or group leader, who thereupon becomes a frightening and all-knowing sphinx. It is the sphinx as sentinel, like the minotaur (Grotstein, 2000a), who keeps the analysand and/or the group from entering the mother's body and toppling the "aristocracy" (the paternal phallus and the "unborn babies") who reside there.

Later in the same text he states:

> In psychoanalysis, regarded as part of the pairing group, the Messiah, or the Messiah idea, occupies a central position, and the bond between the individuals is libidinous. The Messiah idea betrays itself in the supposition that the individual patient is worth the analyst's very considerable devotion; as also in the view, sometimes openly expressed, that as a result of psycho-analytic work a technique will be perfected that will, ultimately, save mankind. In short, I regard Freud's use of the term libido [for group identification—JSG] as correct only for one phase, though an important one, and feel the need for some more neutral term that will describe the tie on all basic-assumption levels. The tie in the work group, which I regard as being a sophisticated nature, is more aptly described by the word *co-operation*. [1961, pp. 176–177; italics added]

This portion was of some personal interest to me since I clearly recall feelings like this when I was in analysis with Bion. Although Bion does not specifically say as much, I believe that he is hinting that the pairing group constitutes the phantasy, vicariously for the group, but for the individual analysand of an archaic–oedipal victory. The omnipotent infant has killed off the internal penis–father and now has become a privileged "privy councillor" to an idealized mother, or perhaps even to a combined-parent object, thereby sparing him the need to undergo rivalry and castration anxiety with either mother or father.

Bion studied groups only because of the vagaries of a fortuitous military assignment during the Second World War, and then only for a short time. Yet in that short time he rose to the head of his class, so to speak, and broke new ground in getting to the roots of group psychology as well as applying psychoanalytic understanding, first to the psychoanalytic principles of Freud and then to those of Klein. His genius there was due to his own powers of keen observation and his capacity for "wild thoughts" in addition to a gift for integration, especially between Freud and Klein.

Another interesting point comes to mind. Bion cites more references in his bibliography in *Experiences in Groups* than he does in any of his later works. He never dropped the concept of group psychology from his thinking. He thought of the group as an individual and the individual as a group. This is exemplified in his idea of the dialectic (binary opposition) between "narcissism and socialism" (Bion, 1992, p. 103). It is due to Bion in no small measure that Kleinian and contemporary post-Kleinian analysts deal with the internal world of their analysands as if it contained cooperative (work group) as well as dissident (basic assumption groups) internal objects.

NOTES

1. Bion's disavowal of "group psychology" has vast ramifications for the current trend in psychoanalytic thinking that espouses "co-construction" or "constructivism". To put it succinctly, *the subject who becomes influenced by another is individually responsible for being influenced. Put yet another way, self-organization always transcends co-construction.*

2. The child will be superior because it is the product of two omnipotent incestuous individuals.

CHAPTER 19

Bion's studies in psychosis

In *Second Thoughts* (1967c), Bion brought together eight papers that represented an ongoing chronicle of his psychoanalytic work with psychotic patients, which he had either presented or published between 1950 and 1962. At the end of the work there is a "Commentary" that represents a significant caesura in his thinking about his work with those patients and the conclusions he had derived from it. The "Commentary" must have been written between 1962 and 1967, and in that time Bion apparently went from being a "Kleinian" to a *"Bionian* post-post-Kleinian. He moved from the logical positivism and certainty of modern Freudian and Kleinian thinking, which was ultimately based on the drives as first cause, to a position of uncertainty, O. He had already formulated the tools of his new metatheory, which included such concepts as the container and the contained, α-function, α-elements, β-elements, the theory of transformations, the reassignment of the drives to L, H, and K emotional linkages between objects, the notion that a coeval, dialectical, rather than a hierarchical and chronological relationship existed between the paranoid–schizoid and depressive positions, P–S ↔ D, not P–S → D, and the transformations in and from (and to) O.

By the time of the publication in 1967 of *Second Thoughts,* he had already published *Learning from Experience* (1962b), *Elements of Psycho-Analysis* (1963), and *Transformations* (1965), which included his new ideas. Because of Bion's refusal to re-edit the original papers, the reader is compelled to read them, knowing that they are already obsolete, and it is not until the Commentary that they are updated with his radical new views. Yet by reading in this way, one has the unique advantage of being in Bion's shoes, first going through the experience and then, later, reflecting on it.

Summary of the themes in Second Thoughts

"The Imaginary Twin"

In "The Imaginary Twin" (1950) we see a very Kleinian Bion, who is an unusually keen observer of a labyrinthine analysand who uses an imaginary twin to comfort himself but also to substitute for the analyst. With consummate versatility Bion unmasks the many personas that comprise the imaginary-twin ensemble, including the "unborn twin", the one the analysand kept from being born in his unconscious phantasy. It also represents the breast as a twin under his control.

There seemed to be a stalemate early on in the analysis, until Bion became intuitively aware that a rhythm of responses was going on between them. I shall cite the climactic analytic moment.

After a discussion concerning the analysand's feelings of futility about the analysis and his questioning of Bion about whether he should leave, Bion considers this from many different angles and then states:

> Let us now return to the patient whom we left silent after my summary of the issues . . .: I asked him what he was thinking about. He replied that he was thinking about a woman with rheumatic pain "She's always complaining about something or other and I thought", he said, "that she's very neurotic. I just advised her to buy some Amytal and packed her off."
>
> This, I said, was probably a compact description of the treatment he was having from me, treatment of which he doubted the efficacy. My interpretations were felt by him to be vague complaints to which he paid scant attention; his associations were many of them stale associations employed more for the soporific effect they shared with Amytal than for their informative value and designed to keep employed without bothering him. But, I added, we should also consider how this situation was rendered tolerable for himself and I drew his attention to peculiarities in his behaviour, notably *the rhythm of "association—interpretation—association"* that indicated that I was a twin

of himself who supported him in a jocular evasion of my complaints and thus softened his resentment. He could identify himself with any one of the three roles.

His response was striking. His voice changed and he said, in a depressed tone, that he felt tired and unclean. It was as if, in a moment, I had in front of me, unchanged in every respect the patient as I had seen him at the first interview. The change was so sudden as to be disconcerting. [1950, pp. 7–8; italics added]

Bion concludes:

In each case [he had alluded to other similar cases—JSG] the newly achieved powers were used to solve an already existing problem but were found to reveal still other problems that demanded solution. . . . All three patient seemed to feel that the problem had been there all the time but its revelation depended on increased capacity for awareness.

The regression in each case could be stated as being away from (1) the increase in capacity produced by psychological development (2) the phenomena brought into awareness by the increased capacity (3) the physiological development associated with the psychological development which revealed the relationship between the parents.

In each case I had the impression that the patient felt that sight produced problems of mastery of a new sense organ. This had its counterpart in a feeling that development of the psyche, like development of visual capacity, involved the emergence of the oedipus situation. With "A", the change . . . was extremely striking. [1950, p. 21; italics added]

What I think Bion is saying is that his lengthy, condensed, loaded interpretation had a dramatic effect. Why? Presumably because in one fell swoop he identified the internal-object components of the veritable hydra that constituted the imaginary twin as well as the anxiety from which it sprang: damage to the unborn twin as a consequence of a phantasied attack on the parents' intercourse and on each of the parents. By being able to give the interpretation, Bion became a trustworthy container of the patient's destructiveness as well as a reconstituted parent (father) who could lay down "the law of the father". The patient was afraid of the deadly cost of normal development—that is, castration anxiety.

First we see Bion, the clinician in action, and an adumbration of what he is later to call the "*analytic object*", O, the anxiety of the moment in the patient. We see how he detects this via the triad of "*sense*" (observing the rhythm of speech interaction), "*myth*" (the archaic oral as well as phallic–oedipal myth), and *"passion"* (his own passion—that is, suffering what the patient was suffering).

We also see his first acquaintance with the idea of a phantasied twin. Later in this same volume he will apply this concept to the "differentiation of the psychotic from the non-psychotic personalities", and it may also possibly be the origin of his concepts of "binocular vision" and the "reversible perspective".

Another interesting notion is the pathological autonomy he detected in the patient's use of vision. Later in this volume, in "On Hallucination" (1958), he will demonstrate how the psychotic, unlike the neurotic, uses the sense organs, principally vision, as a projective act rather than as an introjective one. Bion shows himself to be a hypervigilant observer and a relentless defender of the analytic frame. He interprets strictly and explicitly in the transference and implicitly from the countertransference (actually, reverie). Although later he will renounce "memory and desire", for the moment one can clearly see his keen and determined motivation to encourage—albeit through interpretations—his patient to separate and individuate, to evolve from the paranoid–schizoid to the depressive position. I experienced a C4 image of him as a determined sheep-herder and football-coach while reading this paper. In later papers in this book we will witness the emergence of another Bion, the one who burst through the bubble of Freudian/Kleinian positivism to discover the container and the contained, which, to my mind, is the first major contribution to the understanding of analytic *resistance*. We are going to see that Bion is about to "cross the Rubicon" and bring us into a new psychoanalytic worldview, the outlines of which we are only now beginning to grasp.

"Notes on the Theory of Schizophrenia"

Although "Notes on the Theory of Schizophrenia" (1954) could just as well have been called "Notes on the *Psychoanalytic Treatment* of Schizophrenia" because of Bion's rich display of interpretative skill, he seems already to be gearing up for establishing the theoretical foundations for an ontological and phenomenological epistemology sometime in the future, and analysing schizophrenics is his research laboratory.

In this paper, delivered to the International Psychoanalytical Association Congress in London in 1953, he delineates many formal and phenomenological defects of the schizophrenic, emphasizing the peculiarities of their object relationships, their derailed thinking, and their difficulty with the use of language.

At one point in a session his patient states (summarized by Bion) that he has a problem he is trying to work out, that as a child he never had phantasies, that he knew they weren't facts so he stopped them, and, finally, that he doesn't dream nowadays. Bion's interpretation is startling and prophetic as a theme for his future metatheory. He states:

> It must mean that without phantasies and without dreams you have not the means with which to think out your problem. [1954, p. 25]

The patient agreed with Bion and proceeded more freely.

In the denouement of the case Bion emphasizes the importance of splitting and splintering of objects and of the ego in the development of the thought and language disorder in schizophrenia and then discusses the destructive negative therapeutic reaction when the analysis became successful. When the schizophrenic reaches the threshold of the depressive position, he is caught in a tightening vice between two terrors. If he proceeds, he is entering the domain of responsibility, regret (of what he has irreparably done to himself and his objects), and challenge (castration anxiety). If he falls back, he will have become a traitor to his former state, which now seeks to persecute him with special ferocity:

> What takes place, if the analyst has been reasonably successful, is a realization by the patient of psychic reality; he realizes that he has hallucinations and delusions, may feel unable to take food, and have difficulty with sleep. The patient will direct powerful feelings of hatred towards the analyst. He will state categorically that he is insane and will express with intense conviction and hatred that it is the analyst who has driven him to this pass.
>
> . . . I did not depart from the psycho-analytic procedure I usually employ with neurotics, being careful to always to take up both positive and negative aspects of the transference. [1954, p. 23]
>
> . . . Evidence for interpretations has to be sought in the countertransference[1] and in the actions and free associations of the patient. [1954, p. 24]

Finally, Bion summarizes:

> The experiences I have described to you compel me to conclude that at the onset of the infantile depressive position elements of verbal thought increase in intensity and depth. In consequence the pains of psychic reality are exacerbated by it and the patient who regresses to the paranoid–schizoid position will, as he does so, turn destructively

on his embryonic capacity for verbal thought as one of the elements which have led to his pain. [1954, p. 35]

We see here a preview of his later theories about the function of dreaming and phantasy in thinking and in defining the boundary between sleep and wakefulness—and between sanity an insanity. We also see a prefiguring of his most famous concept, that of container ↔ contained ("evidence sought in the countertransference"). Bion's keen clinical observations allowed him to sense that the patient believed that he had felt progressively worse with the advent of verbalization—that is, as he approached the depressive position where he felt more separate from the object, more individuated, and more aware of the significance of his being insane. In other words, the increasing strength of the non-psychotic personality allowed that aspect of the patient to be all the more horrified by the presence of the psychotic personality. It is interesting to note that Bion states that his technique for analysing psychotics does not differ from his treatment of neurotic patients.

Summary: Here Bion is boldly showing how he successfully analysed a schizophrenic. Of note is not only the technique he so steadfastly used with such versatility, but also his mapping out of the landscape of the schizophrenic's internal world with such perspicacity.

"Development of Schizophrenic Thought"

In "Development of Schizophrenic Thought" (1956), Bion states:

Schizophrenic disturbance springs from an interaction between (i) the environment, and (ii) the personality. In this paper *I ignore the environment* and focus attention on four essential features of schizophrenic personality. First is a preponderance of destructive impulses so great that that even the impulses to love are suffused by them and turned to sadism. Second is a hatred of reality which . . . is extended to all aspects of the psyche that make for awareness of it. I add hatred of internal reality and all that makes for awareness of it. Third, derived from these two, is an unremitting dread of imminent annihilation. Fourth is a precipitate and premature formation of object relations, foremost amongst which is the transference, whose thinness is in marked contrast to the tenacity with which it is maintained. [1956, p. 37; italics added]

It is interesting here that Bion is adumbrating his later contributions on psychotic thinking, particularly the differentiation between the normal and psychotic personalities, not only in psychotics but also in neurotics and all patients generally. It is also of interest that he purposely excludes the environmental factor. We now know that he is going to take up this factor in a big way beginning with his work "On Arrogance" (1957a) and continuing with "Attacks on Linking" (1959), when the concepts of communicative projective identification, container ↔ contained, and α-function emerge. Bion emphasizes the importance of hostility, sadism, and destructiveness, all properties of the death instinct, which are turned against internal as well as external reality and against the objects that remind him of those realities. His observation about the tenacity of the patient's transference which contrasted with its thinness is an especially acute observation. I have found it to apply to all the patients I have treated who fall into the category of primitive mental disorders.

"Differentiation of the Psychotic from the Non-Psychotic Personalities"

In "Differentiation of the Psychotic from the Non-Psychotic Personalities" (1957b) Bion, with his characteristic keen ability to view things from different vertices or angles, approaches the problem of a psychotic patient, a schizophrenic, and shows us that the psychotic, like the neurotic, has at least two personalities. In the case of the neurotic, the patient's neurotic personality will screen a subterranean or cryptic psychotic personality. In a psychotic patient, however, the psychotic personality is dominant and screens the neurotic personality. In each case the subordinated personality putatively constitutes a danger or threat to the dominant personality. The psychotic fears the problems that the neurotic has to think about: problems in object relations contingent upon separation and the need for individuation—that is, ever-evolving tiers of responsibility. The neurotic, on the other hand, is afraid of the psychotic personality's proclivity for breaking through its repressive barrier and taking over the whole personality. The neurotic personality utilizes repression, whereas the psychotic personality utilizes massive splitting and evacuative projective identification; therefore the latter becomes denuded and mentally helpless. Bion believes that the schizophrenic personality develops its pathology at the very beginning of life, at the inchoation of the paranoid–schizoid position where preverbal sense impressions, the ancestors of later verbal thought, are attacked because for the psychotic to feel them or even to feel time passing is to experience unbearable frustration.

Because of the psychotic personality's hatred of reality, it undergoes minute splitting of its ego and violent projective identification of its proto-emotions *and* the now fragmented mind (ego) that could have felt the proto-emotions as emotions. Bion, who had already begun to think of proto-emotions as β-elements and emotions as α-elements, would soon (1962b) formulate his conception of "container ↔ contained" to explain how the patient, unable to tolerate frustration, foregoes having a mind that can think. Bion would also formulate "α-function in reverse"—a state of psychotic reconstruction of a negative universe based on –K. Eventually, Bion would realize that the psychotic personality attacks, not so much the objects, but the *links between objects* (primal scene) and the links between the self and the object. Thus they cannot form symbols that can articulate (p. 48).

Parenthetically, Bion often refers to material in previous sessions. His injunction to abandon memory and desire applies *only during the session*:

> In the last interpretation I was making use of a session, many months earlier, in which the patient complained that analysis was torture, memory, torture. [1957b, p. 56]

But this is what Bion did with it:

> I showed him then that when he felt pain, as evidenced in this session by the convulsive jerks, he achieved anaesthesia by getting rid of his memory and anything that could make him realize pain. [p. 56]
>
> Patient: "My head is splitting; maybe my dark glasses." Now some five months previously I had worn dark glasses. . . .
>
> I have explained that the psychotic personality seems to have to await the occurrence of an apt event before he feels he is in possession of an ideograph suitable for use in communication with itself or with others. . . . [pp. 56–57]
>
> Assuming then that the dark glasses here are a verbal communication of an *ideograph*, it becomes necessary to determine the interpretation of the ideograph. I shall have to compress, almost to the point of risking incomprehensibility, the evidence in my possession. The glasses contained a hint of the baby's bottle. They were two glasses, or bottles, thus resembling the breast. They were dark because frowning and angry. They were of glass to pay him out for trying to see through them when they were breasts. They were dark because he needs darkness to spy on his parents in intercourse. They were dark because he had taken the bottle not to get milk but to see what the parents did. They were dark because he had swallowed them, and not simply the milk they had contained. And they were dark because the clear good objects had been made black and smelly

inside them. All these attributes must have been achieved through the operation of the non-psychotic part of the personality. Added to these characteristics were those I have described as appertaining to them as part of the ego that has been expelled by projective identification, namely their hatred of him as part of himself he had rejected. [pp. 58; italics added]

I cite this passage at length because it truly exemplifies the way Bion then worked and continued to work in his later years. This is the Bion I knew as an analyst. His left and right cerebral hemispheric functioning are working in elegant, mysterious synchrony. His intuition, his having "become" his patient's psychosis, can only be inferred. This is what I get out of this last interchange: Bion interprets to the patient that he is seeking anaesthesia from his emotional torment by evacuating his unprocessed proto-emotions into muscular action. The patient responds with an ideographic signifier that connotes blindness—to replace the anaesthesia dismantled by Bion's interpretation. Bion then weaves a fascinating tapestry containing a chain of signifiers that extend from "glass" as in "dark glasses" to "glass" as in a "baby bottle" and, finally, "glass" as voyeuristically observing the parental primal scene. Anal references then follow, the contamination of the needed milk. Bion's ability to spot and then to reconfigure these symbolic signifiers attests not only to his clinical genius but, more importantly, to the intactness of the patient's non-psychotic personality to *dream* his psychotic personalities' fragmentation and present it to Bion. Thus, the patient's "dreaming" capacity, which originates in his non-psychotic personality, was able to produce "dreamed" associations that allowed Bion to dream them even further into interpretations.

"On Hallucination"

In "On Hallucination" (1958) Bion reports on his studies of his experience of treating psychotic patients from the vertex of hallucinations. Once again, his unusually keen capacity to detect patterns and nuances in his patients' behaviour is remarkable. Having discovered that hallucination is used by the psychotic patient's sense organs to evacuate mental content and even the patient's mind itself rather than incorporate it into themselves, he correlates their proclivity to evacuate with their exclusive use of the pleasure principle to get instant relief, obtained through sensorimotor actions via projective identification, disregarding the reality principle because of the frustration that it entails—that is, introjecting it by taking the time to alter the frustrating situation:

> The lack of any impulse to alter the environment, together with the wish for speed that is associated with the inability to tolerate frustration, contributes to forcing a resort to muscular action of the kind characteristic of the phase of dominance by the pleasure principle. . . . The unburdening of the psyche by hallucination, that is by the use of the sensory apparatus in reverse, is reinforced by muscular action which may be best understood as being an extremely complex analogue of a scowl; the musculature does not simply change the expression to one of murderous hate but gives effect to an actual murderous assault. The resultant act must, therefore, be understood as an ideo-motor activity and is felt by the patient to appertain to that class of phenomena that I have described as creating bizarre objects. [1958, p. 83]

Bion shows us that psychotics may have two kinds of hallucinations: (1) the frankly psychotic ones, characterized exclusively by the presence of part-objects, and (2) hysterical hallucinations, which are healthier, which may emerge later in the analysis, after the patient has made some progress, and which are characterized by the presence of whole objects (real persons) in addition to part-objects. The ability for the psychotic patient to develop the latter depends on his ability to tolerate depression. We see here especially Bion's proposed invariants for the development of psychosis: intolerance of frustration (later to become a function of negative containment and α-function in reverse) and the use of evacuative projective identification from the sense organs.

"On Arrogance"

Earlier, I alluded to Bion's fateful "crossing of the Rubicon". He begins this crossing in "On Arrogance" (1957a). He has uncovered a syndrome in a group of psychotic patients in which he found a constant relationship—a pattern—between curiosity, arrogance, and stupidity. Arrogance seems to be the most salient one. He then states that arrogance is to the death instinct what pride is for the life instinct. If these three elements are to be found scattered in a patient's material, even scattered over time, it is evidence that an *infantile catastrophe* has occurred. Bion describes a clinical situation:

> I remained at a loss until one day, in a lucid moment, the patient wondered that I can stand it. This gave me a clue: at least I knew that

there was something I was able to stand which he apparently could not. He realized already that he felt he was being *obstructed* in his aim to establish a creative contact with me, and this obstructive force was sometimes in him, sometimes in me, and sometimes occupied an unknown location. . . . The patient had already made it clear that the *obstructing forces* or *object* was out of his control. . . .

What it was that the object could not stand became clearer in some sessions where it appeared that in so far as I, as analyst, was insisting on verbal communication as a method of making the patient's problems explicit, I was felt to be directly attacking the patient's methods of communication. From this it became clear that when I was identified with the obstructive force, what I could not stand was the patient's methods of communication. In this phase my employment of verbal communication was felt by the patient to be a mutilating attack on *his* methods of communication. [1957a, p. 91]

Here Bion found an obstructive object, whose origin lay in the infant's interaction with a rejecting mother (one incapable of *self*-containment and therefore incapable of containing her infant's terrors, O). This combination of circumstances inexorably leads to a *primitive catastrophe*. At this pivotal point in his thinking and his career, Bion is breaking with Kleinian tradition by metapsychologically validating the importance of the environment in mental health and illness. The obstructive object thus formed oscillated between being located in the patient and in Bion. He thus deciphered the deepest message embedded in the interaction. The patient was conveying to him, in the inchoate, unconscious language of projective identification, that he had experienced a primitive infantile catastrophe in which he had become reduced to employing arrogance (defensive omnipotence) and had to abandon his curiosity instinct.

"A Theory of Thinking"

"A Theory of Thinking" (1962a) represents a major turning point in Bion's psychoanalytic episteme. It is the culmination of his work of treating psychotics and clearly adumbrates his future work on emotional epistemology. He introduces the subject of thinking as being dependent, first of all, on the theory that *thoughts* must be distinguished from *thinking*, originate before thinking, and require a mind to think them. By emphasizing the distinction between thoughts and thinking, Bion makes a unique contribution to epistemology generally and to a psychoanalytic epistemology specifically. Psychopathology may originate in either of the two. He devises an epigenetic course of thought development and classifies them as "pre-conceptions", "conceptions" (thoughts proper), and "concepts". Pre-conceptions are analogous to "empty thoughts", which are required for being available for experiences to join up with them for the registration of new thoughts. Conceptions must be constantly conjoined—permanently associated with or linked—to an emotional experience of satisfaction to achieve the status of a realization. He defines "thought" as the mating of a pre-conception with a frustration. Put another way, frustration accompanies the act of maintaining the absent space in one's mind while awaiting the emergent thought, which he will later call a "β-element" seeking to become "α-betized" by α-function.

The infant, and his grown-up adult descendant, must be able to tolerate the frustration of not-knowing (e.g. when mother is returning) in order to preserve his "empty thought" long enough for a conception to fill it as a realization. This empty thought is a "no-breast: that is, the ability to conceive of the absence of the breast rather than because of an inability to tolerate frustration, prematurely filling the empty thought with a concrete "no-breast", which becomes a malevolent internal object. In the former case in which the infant *can* tolerate frustration, the thought is born by emerging from within because the empty space is dedicated for its emergence: that is, the way is prepared for the apparatus of thinking to think the emergent thought. Bion states furthermore that the evacuation of a bad breast (by the infant who cannot tolerate frustration) becomes inseparable from the infant's belief that he has introjected a good breast.

In the case of the infant who can tolerate frustration, a capacity for two-ness, of separation between the infant–subject and its object, can develop. Otherwise toxic bad objects are projected via projective identification—that is, projectively identified into (the image of) the object—thereby producing confusion with the object and thus no separation. Yet, he states:

> If mother and child are adjusted to each other projective identification plays a role in the management through the operation of a rudimentary and fragile reality sense; usually an omnipotent phantasy, it functions realistically. [1962a, p. 114]

This statement marks a change in Bion's conception of projective identification from an evacuatory intrapsychic mechanism to the origins of communication between infant and mother. He then discusses the importance of the mother's "containment" of her infant's proto-emotions. They must be able to arouse in the mother the emotions the infant wishes to be rid of. This act of maternal containment becomes the ancestor of *repression*. Bion subsequently first introduces the concept of "α-function"—a mental function that converts sense impressions into α-elements, which are suitable for sleep, waking, dreaming, and thinking. Then he states formally:

> [T]he failure to establish between infant and mother, a relationship in which normal projective identification is possible precludes the development of an α-function and therefore of a differentiation of elements into conscious and unconscious. [1962a, p. 115; italics added]

Later, Bion adds that maternal failure to receive her infant's projections causes the infant to feel that his "fear of dying" is stripped of meaning. I believe that Bion is presuming here the irruption of the death instinct with unsuccessful containment by the mother for modification. It is my belief that Bion might also have thought of the infant's inchoate dread of uncontainably being alive and not being able to tolerate his frighteningly burgeoning *entelechy* (actualization of one's inherent potential)—that is, the fear of the cost of being alive!

When Bion assigns the function of "translation" of the infant's "fear of dying" to the mother–container, he is implying a hitherto unexplored aspect of the relationship between container and translation. This relationship transcends those of (1) *affect regulation* and (2) interpersonal or intersubjective *communication*.

There is yet another aspect: that of the container–mother (analyst) serving as a *channel* between the suffering infant/patient and his infinite self, his godhood. Container ↔ contained, in other words, constitutes an exercise in a *transcendent evolution* of the self. In being able to suffer rather than endure his emotional pain, the infant/patient is able to transcend himself in the act of suffering due in no small measure to his availability to becoming incarnated by his godhead. Bion's (1962b) concept of the pre-conception (p. 91) (either inherited or acquired) is a bimodal one. One aspect, *psi* (ψ) is saturated. The other, xi (ξ), is the unsaturated aspect, the part that is available to accept experiences. This concept is the equivalent of Bion's earlier formulation in which a pre-conception—that is, the *idea* of the breast—searches for its *realization* of (incarnation in) the actual breast. This act constitutes a *positive* realization. In other words a pre-conception becomes transformed into a conception (positive realization). If and when the infant expects the real breast—that is, hunger—and one does not immediately appear, a *negative* realization takes place in which a pre-conception remains empty but with the idea of a "no-breast" as an ideogram (image); or, if the infant cannot tolerate frustration, the negative realization aspect becomes transformed into a concrete "no-breast", leaving no room available for thinking.

In other words, the inherent as well as acquired pre-conceptions, which include the Ideal or Eternal Forms and/or the things-in-them-selves, become released and fill an unsaturated (empty and available) aspect of the pre-conception—now conception or realization. The infant/patient evolves from this self-transcendence. I am aware that the transaction I have just described bears some resemblance to Lacan's (1966) formulation that the patient projects his unconscious into the analyst and then believes that the analyst is "the one who knows". It is also similar, I believe, to Jung's (1967) concept of "alchemy".

The translation into action of the transformative results of α-function involves *publication* (letting oneself know), *communication* (letting others know), and *common sense* (the result of the verdict about an internal or external perception either by consulting different senses within oneself and/or other objects). Common sense is associated with *correlation*:

> [T]he counterpart of the commonsense view in private knowledge is the common emotional view; a sense of truth is experienced if the view of an object which is hated can be conjoined to a view of the same object when it is loved and the conjunction confirms that the object experienced by different emotions is the same object. A correlation is established. [1962a, p. 119]

Here Bion seems to be alluding to the epistemology that transpires between the paranoid–schizoid and depressive positions (P–S ↔ D) and to the evolution of the splitting of objects into a sustained *ambivalence*.

"Commentary"

"Commentary" (1967a) contains some of Bion's reflections on his earlier work (1962b, 1963, 1965, 1970) from the vantage point of his new emotional epistemology—either brief applications of his contemporaneous ideas or adumbrations of his future work, as mentioned previously. One sees references to his exhortation for the analyst to abandon memory and desire, his concept of the Grid, and, above all, his concern for the accuracy—or, really, the lack of *sense*-obtained accuracy—in the clinical situation. Psychoanalysis is ineffable, he exhorts, not reducible to external sense data. As one reads the chapter, one senses that Bion is beginning to lay the foundation for a new kind of science, a mystical science that can encompass the ineffable, the incomprehensible, and uncertainty. He is also adumbrating the inspired, intuitive language that spontaneously emerges from the unconscious, which he will later call the "Language of Achievement", as contrasted with the "language of substitution"—spoken and written language, which uses icons and symbols (substitutes) for the thing-in-itself. An interesting derivative of these ideas is Bion's proscription against note-taking, notes being conceived of and written in the language of substitution.

He alludes to the idea of *evolution* (p. 127), which he will later take up as O's evolution (flux). He prefigures his later concept of the "selected fact", a concept he borrowed from the mathematician, Henri Poincaré (1963), which resembles the "strange attractor" of chaos theory in that it represents the appearance of an observable or conceivable pattern in a sea of incoherence and uncertainty. This pattern becomes a realization.

Later in "Commentary", Bion states:

> The more experienced and sensitive the psychoanalyst is the more readily he experiences the non-sensuous phenomena unfolding before him. [1967a, p. 132]

Here Bion is retrospectively applying the concept of the analyst's state of *reverie* with regard to the patient. He later follows the concept of reverie with the concept of *intuition*—non-sensuous knowing. Bion's quest for epistemic precision is shown when he carefully discriminates between the actual event reported in an analysis and the verbal representations of visual images, which constitute transformations of the events. The concept of transformations had appeared almost simultaneously (Bion, 1965).

Bion also introduces the notion of "God", whom no mortal imbued inextricably with memory and desire can ever "know" (sensualism). Then he states that for harmonious mental growth to take place man must achieve *atonement* with O (Ultimate Reality) and also says that man needs to worship a god because he is born with a religious instinct, one that matures to become the capacity for *awe* (1967a, pp. 145–146; personal communication, 1978). He also refers to the necessity for mathematical formulations and models in order to achieve precision in studying the mind. He states: "the 'originals' are beyond inquiry without the aid of a model. ... The model is an attempt to bring it [the problem—JSG] into reach" (p. 147). The rest of the "Commentary" is devoted to "cameos", as it were, of aspects of his new emotional epistemology, including container ↔ contained, transformations, and so on.

NOTE

1. Bion would later differentiate between "countertransference" and "reverie", the latter being an analytic instrument whereas the former represents the analyst's own infantile neurosis, which, according to Bion, is always unconscious to the analyst.

CHAPTER 20

Transformations

> Suppose a painter sees a path through a field sown with poppies and paints it: at one end of the chain of events is the field of poppies, at the other a canvas with pigment disposed on its surface. We can recognize that the latter represents the former, so I shall suppose that despite the differences between a field of poppies and a piece of canvas, despite the transformation that the artist has effected in what he saw to make it take the form of a picture, something has remained unaltered and on this something recognition depends. The elements that go to make up the unaltered aspect of the transformation I shall call invariants. [Bion, 1965, p. 1]

So begins Bion's third major book on psychoanalytic metatheory. Bion invoked the concept of transformations to move psychoanalytic thinking from stasis to flux—that is, the constancy of movement and change—and to help us to understand the intermediate processes by which we "learn from experience": how we "digest" experiences and "metabolize" them into emotional meaning *and* objective significance. He frequently alluded to Heraclitus' statement that one could never step into the same river twice. "Transformations", as we shall see, has differing meanings for Bion, but above all it must be considered in context with *evolution*—specifically the evolutions of O, which can be understood as the inexorable flux of circumstance, life, from both the internal and external vertices. It may have been from

DOI: 10.4324/9781003348665-21

Plato's *Theaetetus* that Bion drew the idea that life's happenings—and the objects constituting those happenings—were always in flux, were always evolving, and that the human being who observes this flux constitutes a semiotic receptor who must experience transformations of the ever-evolving experience to be able to countenance his experiences of O.

The act of transformation involves two combined processes: (1) the subject being transformed undergoes an alteration in *form* (thus, "trans"form), and (2) some aspect of the subject shall remain unaltered (the invariant). The concept of transformation follows from Freud's idea of *"Nachträglichkeit"* ["secondary revision"]. In recommending that the analyst "abandon memory and desire", Bion added that he should also, when in the session, forget the previous analytic session because what transpired in that session had already undergone a transformation and the invariant would be represented differently in the present session. Consequently, transformations constitute the ultimate moving backdrop of psychoanalysis!

What is the object upon which transformations operate? We shall soon see that Bion suggests O—but what is O? O seems to be a collective term for noumena, Ideal Forms, Absolute Truth, and Ultimate Reality, at least from the inner world: that is, from the unrepressed unconscious. However, he adds another source of O:

> I suggest that somebody . . . should, instead of writing a book called "The Interpretation of Dreams", write a book called "The Interpretation of Facts", translating them into dream language—not just as a perverse exercise, but in order to get a two-way traffic. [Bion, 1980, p. 31]

The other aspects of O, consequently, are the sensory stimuli of our emotional responses to our interaction with external (as well as internal) objects. Bion believes that external stimuli must be dreamed (transformed by α-function) so as to become unconscious prior to our becoming conscious of them as they are carefully delivered back to our consciousness through the selectively permeable membrane of the contact-barrier.

Self-organization, co-construction, and transformations

A particular aspect of the concept of transformation deserves discussion. In today's psychoanalytic literature we read a good deal about intersubjectivity and social constructivism (Hoffman, 1994). Transformation is certainly involved in intersubjective interactions, but the concept of constructivism is another matter. Yes, we are influenced by others and ultimately *become* the outcome of those influences—that is, we become "co-constructed"—but this co-construction is first mediated by a more fundamental ground plan, that of "self-organization" ("autogenesis") (Schwalbe, 1991) or "autopoiesis" (Maturana & Varela, 1972). Spinoza anticipated the concept of self-organization with his *"conatus"* (Damasio, 2003, p. 36). Put another way, transformation, along with α-function and dreaming, is the principal process whereby the individual *personalizes* (makes personal with regard to himself) the sensory data of O (the impact of other objects upon him), which in the first instance is foreign to the individual and may be *im*personal. Ultimately, self-organization determines how we are to be influenced and supraordinates co-construction. We unconsciously *decide*—through transformations—to impart our metaphoric "saliva" of personalness onto each input from the other and *then* claim it as our own. The default alternative we call *trauma*.

The "alimentary canal" versus the "synapse" as models for transformation

The concept of "transformations" would ultimately attain almost the same prominence as the "container ↔ contained" theory but would fatefully suffer in esteem, at least among contemporary London Kleinians, from Bion's final extension of its reach to embrace O. He uses two major models to conceive of transformations: the *alimentary-canal* model and the model of the neuronal *synapse* or the *contact-barrier*.

The alimentary model

In the alimentary model thoughts are likened to food and the mind to the gastrointestinal tract, which conducts transformative "digestions" or "metabolizations" of the food so as to change (transform) it from raw food to ultimate breakdown derivatives (glucose, fructose, fatty acids, and amino acids) that enter the cells of the body as nutrients. When food enters us and we do not digest it, we experience indigestion. The analogy to "food for thought" is obvious. Bion states, with regard to indigestion:

> The emotional experience must now be considered generally and not only as it occurs in sleep. I shall emphasize what I have said so far

by re-writing a popular theory of the nightmare. It used once to be said that a man had a nightmare because he had indigestion and that is why he woke up in a panic. My version is: The sleeping patient is panicked; because he cannot have a nightmare he cannot wake up or go to sleep; he has had mental indigestion ever since. [1962b, p. 8]

In other words, mental indigestion, as exemplified here as a nightmare, is the result of the failure of "food-for-thought" ("thoughts without a thinker") to be "thoughtfully" processed—that is, "transformed—and the patient consequently suffers from "indigestion" of β-elements while becoming "truth-starved".

The synaptic model

Let me now present yet another perspective on transformations. The synaptic model is first referred to in *Learning from Experience* (Bion, 1962b, p. 17). Briefly, Bion associates the synapse to the contact-barrier and/or the caesura. He replaces Freud's repressive barrier between the Systems *Ucs.* and *Cs.* with a contact-barrier that functions in both directions and is selectively permeable to the passage of elements from either System to the other. More to the point for our purposes, however, is the property and mode of functioning of the synapse. The nerve impulse courses down the neuron and ends at the synapse, which it stimulates. The pre-synaptic membrane induces a potentiation in the neurotransmitters within the synapse, which, in their turn, stimulate and potentiate the post-synaptic membrane. Now here is the major paradigm difference: the post-synaptic membrane always already contains the neural pre-conceptions that anticipate the message carried by the initial and initiating nerve impulse. This mode differs from the alimentary mode because of the break in its continuity. As an analogue this mode applies to signal induction in the projective transidentification process between two individuals (Grotstein, 2005, chapter 14).

Other models

To Bion's two models I should like to add two more of my own: (1) α-function (and dreaming) functioning as an *emotional immune system* or *immune frontier* against the invasion of dangerous β-elements, and (2) the concept of the *Möbius strip* (a ribbon that is cut then reunited with a twist, producing a single surface: anything initially travelling on the outer surface of the ribbon will eventually be located on the inner surface). This is a model for the contiguous and coterminous spatial relationship between Systems *Ucs.* and *Cs.*

In Bion's scheme of transformation the operation of α-function and dreaming, and the movement of a pre-conception to becoming realized as a conception, is subtly implied but nowhere specified. I submit that the synaptic model seems to clear some obscurities in Bion's protocol. In the Grid (Bion, 1977a), for instance, he places β-elements at the top of the vertical (genetic) column of thoughts, in row "A" and pre-conceptions in the same column in row "D". The protocol does not account for the union of β-elements with pre-conceptions. The synaptic model does: β-elements travel down the metaphoric neuron to the pre-synaptic membrane, where they induce a response in the post-synaptic membrane, which is always already pre-conceived as to the nature of the β-element on the other side of the synapse.

The two arms of transformation

The two aspects of O and the two parallel aspects of the transformation of β-elements—because of their dual origin—were discussed in chapter 10. Briefly, the two aspects of O are the inherent and/or acquired pre-conceptions from the unrepressed unconscious (β-element) and the sense impressions of emotional experience (also β-element—Bion, 1963, pp. 22–23). Thus the β-element represents a compound entity derived from two disparate sources. Each aspect undergoes transformation. In the former, the sense-derived β-element is escorted, so to speak, through the transformational cycle to α-elements and then assigned to different aspects of the mind. In the case of the latter, the inherent and/or acquired pre-conceptions become transformed into realizations as conceptions → concepts, and so on.

The question of the "invariant"

Thus, transformation includes the processes whereby "food for thought" is *deconstructed* into its elements and then *reconstructed* into more suitable elements so as to be absorbed. In Bion's use of the term, transformation characterizes the processes whereby the human mind *scans* (actively observes) the data (objects) of ongoing experience internally and externally and unconsciously processes them for intake (assimilation, accommodation, ingestion). But what about the "invariant?" Bion clearly believes that the ultimate invariant in the food for thought are *emotions*—ultimately, the *truth about emotional relationships.* In other words, "just as reason is emotion's slave" (Bion, 1965, p. 171), so emotions are slaves to (containers of) truth. Thus, truth is the invariant, and emotion is its vehicle or container.

A prefatory note on the perspectives of transformation: the transformation of emotions (O)

In the citation at the beginning of this chapter Bion uses the metaphor of the painter and the landscape and explains how the painter has to arrange transformations in the appearance of objects on the canvas that correspond to the objects in reality that are being represented. Bion was in fact a landscape painter and thus well understood the comparison. Perhaps we can go a step further with the analogy to say that mind generally, and the unconscious specifically, *is* a portrait and landscape painter, albeit a mystical one, who paradoxically is able, by consulting his inner aesthetic capacities and knowledge of the laws and hidden order of aesthetics (Ehrenzweig, 1967), to *fictionalize* the initial raw, unmentalized, impersonal Truth about an ineffable Ultimate Reality so as to remove its blunt, intimidating, uncompromising coarseness and horror (horror because of its vast, infinite, unending nature) and to reconfigure it in such a way that, miraculously, the truth becomes unintimidatingly highlighted and all the more mercifully tolerable to bear. Our hidden painter paints by day and by night to get the proper angles and perspectives and the ratios and mixtures between fiction and truth off life's existential assembly line. Consequently, everything we see, hear, smell, touch, think, and feel constitutes an "artistic painting".

The transformation and evolution of the self by experiencing O

So far I have viewed the process of transformation from the vertex (point of view) of the emotional message from O → β-element → α-element → dream thought, and so on. But if we see transformation from the vertex (aesthetic angle) of a reversible perspective, we may obtain another view—one that causes us to see that Bion's view of it may constitute an optical illusion. Is it truth—or, for that matter, emotional thought (β-element)—that undergoes transformation, *or is it the mind that is perceiving* (observing) *the truth* (β-elements) *that undergoes a series of transformations* by applying a system of filters to darken the blinding glare of untransformable O? In this sense *reality and truth can never become transformed*; only our receptive, observing mind, our semiotic apparatus, can. From this vertex, *it is the observer himself who transforms—that is, becomes transformed—by being able to experience (feel) the truth of his emotions,* which are themselves invariant, and thereby *evolve* into a higher self. In other words, all we can do is fictional-ize—mythify—our perception, our experience of Truth (O). We call this *dreaming.* I, the subject, alter the transcription of the received ex-perience with my dream ensemble.

A discussion of transformations

> For my purpose it is convenient to regard psycho-analysis as belong-ing to the group of transformations. The original experience, the realization, in the instance of the painter the subject that he paints, and in the instance of the psychoanalyst the experience of analysing his patient, are transformed by painting in the one and analysis in the other into a painting and a psycho-analytic description respec-tively. The psycho-analytic interpretation given in the course of an analysis can be seen to belong to this same group of transformations. An interpretation is a transformation; to display the invariants, an experience, felt and described in one way, is described in another. [Bion, 1965, pp. 3–4]

Thus, psychoanalysis constitutes a series of ongoing transformations in which the analysand's experience is transformed into free associa-tions, dreams, and behaviour (enactments) by the analysand and into interpretations by the analyst, and then the latter is in turn submit-ted to transformations by the analysand—in a continuing transfor-mational cycle. Bion is saying here that psychoanalysis constitutes, by definition, an ongoing series of transformations and progressive movements of invariants from a pre-conception to a realization. In other words, we find once again that Bion emphasizes the importance of psychoanalytic transformations with regard to the movement and realization of the invariant, which is emotional truth. Furthermore, the invariant must be tied to a particular theory—that is, "invariants under the theory of the Oedipus situation".

Transformations through
the pre- and post-catastrophic stages

After offering a series of clinical illustrations, Bion draws a dis-tinction between the pre- and post-catastrophic clinical stages in the course of the patient's analysis. Using these specific clinical examples, he states:

> There are three features to which I wish to draw attention: subversion of the system, invariance, and violence. Analysis in the pre-catastrophic stage is to be distinguished from the post-catastrophic stage by the following superficial characteristics: it is unemotional, theoretical, and devoid of any marked outward change. Hypochondriacal symptoms are prominent. The material lends itself to interpretations based on Kleinian theories of projective identification and internal and external objects. Violence is confined to phenomena experienced by psychoanalytical insight: it is, as it were, theoretical violence. The patient talks as if his behaviour, outwardly amenable, was causing great destruction because of its violence. The analyst gives interpretations, when they appear to be appropriate to the material, drawing attention to the features that are supposed by the patient to be violent.
>
> In the post-catastrophic stage, by contrast, the violence is patent, but the ideational counterpart, previously evident, appears to be lacking. Emotion is obvious and is aroused in the analyst. Hypochondriacal elements are less obtrusive. The emotional experience does not have to be conjectured because it is apparent.
>
> In this situation the analyst must search the material for invariants to the pre- and post-catastrophic stages. These will be found in the domain represented by the theories of projective identification, internal and external objects. Restating this in terms of clinical material, he must see, and demonstrate, that certain apparently external emotionally charged events are in fact the same events as those which appeared in the pre-catastrophic stage under the names, bestowed by the patient, of pains in the knee, legs, abdomen, ears, etc., and, by the analyst, of internal objects. [1965, pp. 8–9]

Bion goes on to say that the analyst must search the pre-and post-catastrophic stages for the invariants—those aspects that remain unaltered. He concludes, for instance, that what had presented itself to the patient and analyst pre-catastrophically as anxious relatives, impending lawsuits, and so forth, appear in the post-catastrophic stage as hypochondria, and so on. The invariant is the anxiety.

Bion then sets forth three kinds of transformation: (1) "T", representing the emotional response to O; (2) Tα (α) for the beginning of the process of transformation; and (3) Tβ (beta) for the end-product of the transformation.[1] These designations apply both to the analysand and to the analyst with regard to the individuality of their differing transformational experiences.

The use of abstract iconic signs

Bion continues here to plead for a mathematical rigour, the use of analogous abstract, iconic signs, to represent mental phenomena because of his belief that verbal language, like science, only adequately addresses inanimate objects. He applies his transformational signs to the Grid. The category fundamentally depends on the clinical phenomena and the analysand's (and analyst's) associations to it. But something else is simultaneously happening here in Bion's discussion about transformations. It is on page 13 that he quietly and unobtrusively "crosses the Rubicon", as I have mentioned earlier, by introducing the abstract iconic sign, O. Things will never be the same for Bion with the London Kleinians. Let Bion (1965) speak for himself:

> Using the facts (of my illustration) to achieve a formulation in terms of a theory of transformations, I arrive at the following: the total analytical experience is being interpreted as belonging to the group of transformations, denoted by the sign T. The experience (thing-in-itself) I denote by sign O. The patient's impression, T (patient) α, is replaced by category C2. The patient's representation, a resultant of the transformation he has effected, T (patient) β, is replaced by category AI. Since we have not yet come to a decision about the nature of the process of transformation it is convenient to employ a sign showing that the abstraction represented by T is unsaturated. [1965, pp. 13–14]

He then goes on to say that his formulation is analogous to a *model*: an observation has been made that certain clinical elements (phenomena) seem to be constantly conjoined—that is, a pattern that unites them has been discerned. The next step is to learn the meaning of the constant conjunction or pattern. He uses another system of signs, T (ξ) (xi)=C2 → A1, in which (ξ) represents an unsaturated element looking to achieve saturation (knowledge) and C2 → A1 corresponds to the specific clinical illustration Bion used, in which the patient hypothetically misconstrued Bion's handshake C as an attack (C2) and thus as a β-element seeking transformation into an α-element, which would be a transformational saturation of ξ: the silent unsaturated twin of the pre-conception.

Then he states that he, the analyst, will only regard as significant those aspects of the patient's behaviour representing the latter's view of O. *O now becomes the centrepiece of psychoanalysis and the object of transformation*. What he is now postulating is of such critical importance that I shall quote him once again:

From the analytic treatment as a whole I hope to discover from the invariants in this material what O is, what he *does* to transform O (that is to say, the nature of T (patient) α) and, consequently, the nature of T (patient). This last point is the set of transformations, in the group of transformations, to which his particular transformation (T (patient)) is to be assigned. As I am concerned with the *nature* (or, in other words, meaning) of these phenomena, my problem is to determine the relationship between three unknowns: T (patient), T (patient) α, and T (patient) β. Only in the last of these have I any *facts* on which to work. [1965, p. 15]

O is what the analysand encounters—that is, the initial clinical experience. That overall experience is T (patient). His feeling of it is Tp α. The completion of his unconscious transformation of it is Tp β. The analyst initially encounters the patient's experience as Ta α. After the experience, O, has become transformed within the analyst, it becomes Ta β. The analyst can only process (transform) Tp β—that is, what the patient has done with O. For the moment O is merely a new iconic term for Bion, an unsaturated sign to represent the "thing-in-itself", the patient's as yet untransformed experience and the analyst's as yet untransformed version of his experience of the patient's O. No one is yet ready for the psychoanalytic revolution that is about to occur in the name of O as it achieves other associative connections—the Absolute Truth, Ultimate Reality, and *"godhead"*! No one yet sensed that Bion was bursting the envelope of Kleinian—and Freudian—positivism (the drives as first cause) and introducing a Renaissance of psychoanalysis.

Types of transformations

Bion next categorizes types or classes of transformations. He divides them into (1) "rigid motion" transformations, (2) "projective transformations", and (3) "transformations in hallucinosis". The terms "rigid motion" and "projective" derive from geometry. The defining example of the rigid motion transformation is the repetition of the patient's infantile neurosis as a transference neurosis in the analysis. This repetition is understood to be an almost unaltered version in the present of what had occurred either in actuality or in unconscious phantasy in the past. "Rigid motion" is a geometric way of designating the movement of a protractor from one fixed base or vertex to another. *The other distinction Bion emphasizes is that between the patient's experience, O, and the analyst's experience, O.*

Bion differentiates between "transference", which he considers to be a rigid motion (neurotic) transformation and projective transformations, which he considers to be a type of psychotic transformation, one in which the patient appears to be parasitic and assigns cosmic responsibility to the analyst (via projective identification) for all that happens to the patient:

> In the group of projective transformations, events far removed from the relationship to the analyst are actually regarded as aspects of the analyst's personality. [1965, p. 30]

Rigid motion transformations
versus projective transformations

Rigid motion transformations involve the displacement of whole entities, such as past memories, from the past into the present—without alteration. Perhaps one way of distilling the difference between rigid motion and projective transformations is to consider that an as-if quality characterizes the former and concreteness the latter. Bion then puts forth the notion of *"publication"*, by which he means helping the patient to transform an unconscious emotional experience into a conscious one, a "public" one to himself. He then states:

> Our model serves psycho-analytic needs better if T β denotes the emotional state stimulated in the recipient and T represents the emotional state, stimulated in the analyst by O, which Ta α is to transform . . . *no one can ever know what happens in the analytic session, the thing -in-itself, O;* we can only speak of what the analyst or patient *feels* happens, his emotional experience, that which I denote by T. . . . *The theory of transformations and its development does not relate to the main body of psycho-analytic theory, but to the practice of psycho-analytic observation.* [1965, pp. 33–34; italics added]

The last statement helps to clarify what precedes it. Transformation relates to how the patient sees (observes) his emotional experiences, and how the analyst observes the way in which the patient observes his experiences. In sum, thus far Bion suggests that rigid motion transformations are characteristic of patients who can tolerate frustration and can withhold action in order to think, and projective transformations are characteristic of patients who use their muscles as a mind—and that transformations constitute an observational (perceptual) act.

Bion believes that

> What psycho-analytic thinking requires is a method of notation and rules for its employment that will enable work to be done in the

absence of the object, to facilitate further work in the *presence* of the object. . . . [1965, p. 44]

I would retain the freedom to speak of "incorporating" a particular theory "in the main body of analytic theory", with the precision necessary for use [Columns 1, 3 and 4] of Melanie Klein's theories of internal objects. This means that there must be psycho-analytic *invariants*, . . . psycho-analytic *variables*, and psycho-analytic *parameters*. These mathematical terms used . . . as models, row C, need transformation to fit them for psycho-analytic use as row F, G and H elements. [p. 44; italics added]

The differentiating factor I wish to introduce is not between *conscious* and *unconscious*, but between *finite* and *infinite*. Nevertheless, I use, as my model for forms of relatedness in an infinite universe, forms of relatedness operative in a finite universe of discourse ands its approximate realization. [p. 46; italics added]

Just as the individual uses names (constant conjunctions) to designate the objects he encounters, so the analyst must use a more sophisticated and emotion-free notation system as an analogue model to apply to the subtle changes that take place with transformations of one's experience with objects absent and present. One can use the example of the sphygmomanometer (blood-pressure cuff) as an analogue model. Its pressure reading is arbitrary as an analogue of what the real but ultimately unknowable blood pressure really is. The invariant not only represents the truth of one's emotions about the absent and present object. It can also represent an invariant that changes valence if the infant cannot tolerate frustration, in which case the container, ♀, becomes transformed into –♀. The variables may constitute the variability (unpredictability or irregularity) of the adaptive context of the variable environment to which the infant must adapt. Parameters define the universe of discourse in which the invariants and variables operate. Note also that Bion now refers to "finite" and "infinite" rather than to "conscious" and "unconscious" in his mathematical zeal to reduce psychoanalytic elements to unsaturated (conflict-free) integers to facilitate versatile thinking.

The psycho-analyst's domain is that which lies between the point where a man receives sense impressions and the point where he gives expression to the transformation that has taken place. The principles of this investigation must be the same whether the medium is painting, music, mathematics, sculpture, or a relationship between two people, whether expressed verbally or by other means.

These principles must be determined so that they remain constant whether the transformation is effected in a mind which is sane or insane. [1965, p. 46]

I understand Bion here to be reinforcing his notion of the point (of reference) as the invariant ("remain constant").

The L, H, and K emotional linkages (between self and objects) are brought into play by Bion as emotional encoders or "affect catalogues" that assign the emotional properties of personal meaning and subjective importance to the incoming β-elements as they are in the process of being mentally "digested" by α-function into α-elements. O is indifferent and impersonal. L, H, and K impart personalness—that is, personal meaning—to them. Put another way, the very act of accepting the emotion (allowing oneself to feel it) and cataloguing it is tantamount to personally "owning" the experience.

According to Bion, any O not common to both analysand and analyst is not available for analytic discourse.

He then discusses what knowledge the analyst must have at his disposal:

2. Transformation, i.e. Tp α or Ta α, is influenced by L, H and K. The analyst is assumed to allow for or exclude L or H from his link with the patient and Ta α and Ta β are assumed for purposes of this discourse to be from distortion by L, H (i.e. countertransference). Tp α and Tp β, on the contrary, are assumed always to be subject to distortion. . . .

. . . [T]he analyst must have a view of the psycho-analytic theory of the Oedipus situation. His understanding of that theory can be regarded as a transformation of that theory and in that case all his interpretations, verbalized or not, of what is going on in a session may be seen as transformations of an O that is bi-polar. One pole is trained intuitive capacity transformed to effect its juxtaposition with what is going on in the analysis and the other is in the facts of the analytic experience that must be transformed to show what approximation the realization has to the analyst's preconceptions—the preconception here being identical with Ta β as the end-product of Ta α operating on the analyst's psycho-analytic theories. [1965, p. 49]

Many readers who are only casually familiar with Bion's recommendations to use intuition by eliminating "memory and desire" may not be familiar with "left-hemispheric" Bion—the psychoanalytic disciplinarian who also recommends that the analyst should be so well versed in the Oedipus complex (especially the Kleinian part-object version), as well as Klein's concepts of splitting and projective identification and the movement from the paranoid–schizoid to the depressive position, that he can take them for granted. He continues:

> Part of the equipment of observation is pre-conception used as pre-conception—D4 [pre-conception–attention—JSG]. It is in its D4 aspect that I wish to consider the Oedipal theory; that is, as part of the *observational* equipment of the analyst. . . . The analyst's *theoretical* equipment may thus be narrowly described D4, E4 [conception–attention—JSG], F4 [concept–attention—JSG]. [1965, pp. 50–51; italics added]

The theories related to the Oedipus complex that Bion considers necessary to be present in the analyst's mind—projective identification, splitting, intolerance of frustration, envy, greed, part-objects, the theory *that primitive thought springs from the experience of a non-existent object* (*the place where the object is supposed to be but is not*), and the theory of the violence of primitive functions—must be there in a form that allows them to be represented in a wide range of categories (1965, p. 51).

Transformations in hallucinosis

"Transformations in hallucinosis comprise a wide range of phenomena that belong to the psychotic part of the personality" (Grinberg, Sor, & de Bianchedi, 1977). In this type of transformation the patient creates his own external worldview and believes that the analyst's view is rivalrous with his or hers (Symington & Symington, 1996, p. 115). Envy on the part of the patient is consequently quite prominent. "The emotional experience, the result of the session, is transformed into sense impressions, which are then evacuated as hallucinations, yielding pleasure or pain but not meaning" (p. 116).

Bion says:

> This state I do not regard as an exaggeration of a pathological or even natural condition: I consider it rather to be a *state always present*, but overlaid by other phenomena, which screen it. If these other elements can be moderated or suspended hallucinosis becomes demonstrable. [1970, p. 36; italics added]

He is thereby de-pathologizing and reconfiguring hallucinosis: a tendency to it is implicit in all individuals. The psychotic uses hallucinosis as a default technique of survival, and the analyst as intuition (P. Sandler, 2005. p. 321).

Bion says that hallucination

> must be distinguished from an illusion or delusion because both
> these terms are required to represent other phenomena, namely
> those that are associated with pre-conceptions that turn to concep-
> tions because they mate with realizations that do not approximate
> to the pre-conceptions closely enough to saturate the pre-conception,
> but closely enough to give rise to a conception or mis-conception.
> The pre-conception requires saturation by a realization that is *not*
> an evacuation of the senses but has an existence independent of the
> personality. The hallucination arises from a pre-determination and
> requires satisfaction from (a) an evacuation from the personality and
> (b) from conviction that the element *is* its own evacuation. [Bion,
> 1965, p. 137]

Here Bion gives a succinct clarification of the distinction between *illusion* and *delusion*. First of all, illusions and delusions are not necessarily
visual; hallucinations are, except when they use other sense modali-
ties as channels. Furthermore, hallucinations result from a phantasied
evacuation of—and from—the senses and are predetermined. It is not
clear what Bion means by this, but I gather that the psychotic is predetermined *concretely to look away*—that is, evacuate β-elements from his
senses rather than introject—and is gratified to observe the evacuation
outside himself. P. Sandler (2005) notes that *hallucination* "defines perceptions that have no real object to stimulate a sensuous receptor . . . it
is objectless, false perception" (p. 314). In describing hallucination in
a patient, Bion says that

> if the patient says he has seen an object it may mean that an external
> object has been perceived by him or it may mean that he is ejecting
> an object through his eyes. . . . [1958, p. 67]

With regard to *"hallucinosis"*, Bion states:

> Receptiveness [by the analyst—JSG] . . . is essential to the operation
> of psycho-analysis. . . It is essential for experiencing hallucination or
> the state of hallucinosis. [1970, pp. 35–36]

Bion seems to think of hallucination not only in the traditional way
as an indication of serious psychopathology, but also as the patient's
default method of communication with the analyst and, with regard
to hallucinosis, the analyst's way of initiating intuition. As Paulo
Sandler (2005) points out, hallucinosis constitutes the foundation for
the capacity to think in Bion's episteme (p. 321). This concept he
borrowed from Freud (1900a), who stated that the infant attempts
to replace the lost object by a hallucination via the operation of the

pleasure principle. The infant must be able to tolerate frustration long enough to be able to maintain the emptiness of the "no-thing" so that a hallucinatory image of the missing mother can form to incarnate (realize) her as a mental conception. One must also realize that Bion's injunction against memory and desire reflects his distrust of how we normally observe objects—that is, we "hallucinate" them and confuse them with the real object. This dilemma can be expressed by the difference between *sensation* and *perception,* which is subject to dreaming. Winnicott's (1969) concept of the "subjective object" (p. 87) expresses this idea. Bion states:

> Thought consequently [for the psychotic—JSG] is not seen as offering freedom for development, but is felt as a restriction; by contrast, "acting-out" is felt to yield a sense of freedom, *A fortiori* an hallucination is designed through its quality as the-thing-itself (not the thought of a breast but the breast itself) to be indistinguishable from freedom. The patient then may be seen as facing a choice: either he may allow his *intolerance of frustration* to use what might otherwise be a *"no-thing"* to become a thought and so achieve the freedom Freud (1911b) describes, or he may use what might be a "no-thing" to be the foundation for system of hallucinosis. . . .
>
> From this last will spring the set of *transformations in hallucinosis* which it will be necessary to differentiate from transformations in . . . the domain of verbal communication. The importance of making this last distinction is enhanced by the fact that words are used both in the expression of verbal communication and in transformations in hallucinosis. Yet consideration of the nature of differing reaction to the "no-thing" will show that the word representing a thought is not the same as the identical word when it is representing an hallucination. . . . [Bion, 1970, p. 17; italics added]

In the above citation Bion lays the groundwork for our capacity to use and/or misuse our minds. The healthy individual must first have the capacity to bear frustration in order to contemplate and maintain the experience of the absence of the needed object as a "no-thing". This absence becomes the *container for emergent ideas.* The failure to tolerate frustration results in the transformation of the no-thing into a concrete internal object. The difference is one between "unsaturation" leading to ful*fil*ment by spontaneous ideas and "saturation" leading to an inability to think or generate ideas

In the preamble to his exposition on transformations in hallucinosis Bion begins by discussing O and its relationship to Plato's Forms and to the "incarnation of the godhead". Bion's ship has now reached the farther shore of the Rubicon. He has reached the point of no return.

He follows this with a discussion of "hyperbole":

I mean the term to convey an impression of exaggeration of rivalry and, by retention of its original significance, throwing and out-distancing. The appearance of hyperbole in any form must be regarded as significant of a transformation in which rivalry, envy and evacuation are operating. There is a profound difference between "being" O and rivalry with O. The latter is characterized by envy, hate, love, megalomania and the state known to analysts as acting out, which must be sharply differentiated from acting; which is characteristic of "being" O. [1965, p. 141]

Just as exaggeration is helpful in clarifying problems so it can be felt to be important to exaggerate in order to gain the attention necessary to have a problem clarified. Now the "clarification" of a primitive emotion depends on its being contained by a container which will detoxicate it. [pp. 141–142]

In other words, a transformation in hallucinosis results from a state of increasing emotional hyperbole (cry for help) from the patient to a defunct container, which rejects the emotional content. Here we have a revisitation of Bion's (1959) original theory of the "obstructive object" (1957a, p. 91), which later became the hyper-moralistic "super"ego. Bion now adds that the hyperbolic patient becomes rivalrous with and envious of O as well as of the psychoanalyst. The ultimate result is defaulting to evacuate his hyperbolic emotions through the senses as hallucinatory transformations, A6.

Transformations in hallucinosis also seem to account for the phenomenon in which one becomes "a prisoner of the percept" (the hallucinated superimposed image on the object).

"Autistic transformations"

Korbivcher (1999, 2001, 2005a, 2005b), following Bion, conceives of a set of transformations that are categorically linked with, yet separate from, those listed by Bion. Just as Bion generalizes the potential presence of transformations in hallucinosis being undertaken in the "psychotic" personality of the normal individual, Korbivcher likewise generalizes autistic transformations to a similarly separate personality, one that deals with proto-mental phenomena. Korbivcher conjectures that Bion leaves open the possibility that other groups of transformations may be included in this theory. She raises the hypothesis that autistic phenomena could constitute a new group of transformations in addition to those proposed by Bion: the autistic transformations where autistic phenomena prevail. She affirms also that the autistic transformations are characterized by their development within the autistic environment in the absence of the notion of the external and internal object. The relations established are dominated by sensations, and these do not acquire any representation in the mind. Some of the invariables highlighted in them are related to the experience of the "absence of affective life" and of "affective emptiness", and to the presence of "auto-sensuous" activities observed through the relation of the autistic objects and autistic forms (Tustin, 1986, 1990). These manoeuvres protect the individual from terror experiences that would cause a sensation of desegregation and intolerable vulnerability (Korbivcher, 2005a, p. 2).[2]

Korbivcher's unique contribution adds yet a newer dimension to Bion's theory of transformations. In proposing this concept, she is careful to distinguish between actual autistic illness and a primitive level of functioning in normal or neurotic individuals. She states that it "is necessary . . . to stress that the proposal of the autistic transformations applies only to neurotic patients who present autistic nuclei, and not autistic patients (Korbivcher, 2005a, p. 4). She later states that her conception of this archaic level of functioning is one that is characterized by its own unique internal organization and is ruled by its own peculiar rules—rules that differ from those that govern the psychotic *and* neurotic personalities in the same individual.

Transformations in and from O

Transformations (1965) constitutes a watershed for Bion. It marks the high tide of his attempts to render psychoanalytic experience into precise "scientific" mathematical "constant conjunctions" and the beginning of his great paradigm shift to post-"scientific", "intuitionistic mathematics"[3]—namely, the mystical realm of uncertainty, O. I have alluded several times to the fact that Bion "crossed the Rubicon" of credibility with his London Kleinian colleagues with this radical turn in his explorations.[4] He used the term "mystical" in an idiosyncratic way. He meant by it the ability to be in touch with O—to "become O" without having to go through the intermediate transformations enabled by dreaming and α-function. What was most radical was the concept of O itself, which to this very day is never uttered or written about by London Kleinians, although it *is* discussed and written about widely by Kleinians and others throughout the world outside London.

One of the problems with O's acceptability is its esoteric strange-ness. Another is its intimate association with post-modernistic rel-ativism and uncertainty (parallel with the theories of Einstein and Heisenberg). Yet another difficulty lies in Bion's arbitrarily assigning "godhead" as one of the synonyms of O and referring to the need for our "godhead" (our infinite self) to "incarnate" our finite self. Most critics of Bion's postulation of O fault him for what they believe is his religiosity. Nothing could be further from the truth. Bion (1992) him-self refers to "religion as an illusion" (pp. 374, 379).

Having formulated O, Bion refers to the "curtain of illusion" that separates man from reality. That curtain of illusion covers the gap between the noumenon (the thing-in-itself, the Ideal Form) and the phenomenon. Transformation is the set of processes that bridges that gap. I have already discussed rigid motion, projective, and hallucina-tory transformations. The last is transformations in, of, and from O. In psychoanalysis the analyst becomes the container of the analysand's projections. He undergoes first a transformation in O to match the analysand's O (the symptom). He then transforms his own sympathet-ic experience of O into K—knowledge *about* or *from* O—and imparts it to the analysand as an interpretation:

> I propose to extend the significance of O to cover the domain of reality and "becoming." Transformations in O contrast with other transformations in that the former are related to growth in becoming and the latter to growth in "knowing about" growth; they resemble each other in that "growth" is common to both.
>
> Transformation in K has, contrary to the common view, been less adequately expressed by mathematical formulation than by reli-gious formulations. *Both are defective when required to express growth, and therefore transformation, in O.* Even so, *religious formulations come nearer to meeting the requirements of transformations in O than math-ematical formulations.* [1965, p. 156; italics added]

This is the fateful juncture where Bion starts to leave mathematical models and formulations in favour of religious ones. I say "fateful" be-cause, as I have already stated, many critics thought he was deserting sound "psychoanalytic science" for religion. Furthermore, it was in the year 1965, the publication date of *Transformations*, that Bion was begin-ning to plan his exodus to Los Angeles. He continued his explorations into O in *Attention and Interpretation*, which, though published in 1970, had been completed in 1968 while Bion was still in London (Franc-esca Bion, personal communication, 2006). His study of O has been linked by many with his California sojourn as a defamatory "constant conjunction", compounded all the more unfavourably by his publication of *A Memoir of the Future* (1975, 1977b, 1979, 1981), which he wrote in Los Angeles. I personally believe that Bion's use of religious as well as other formulations such as "vertices" of observation was ingenious, as was his formulation of O itself, which may yet qualify as one of the most important contributions to psychoanalysis in the twentieth century and to augur mightily for the twenty-first.

What I believe has had a negative affect on others about his work, however, particularly *Elements of Psycho-Analysis* and *Transformations*, is Bion's Platonic obsession with mathematical formulations that dazzle and confuse many readers who either have not been trained in mathematical thinking or have an aversion towards it and fail to see its connection to emotional life. Psychoanalysts who *are* mathematically sophisticated, however, marvel at Bion's work and are in accord with it. To repeat what I stated earlier, Bion, in the Platonic tradition, was seeking analogue languages with which to address the vicissitudes of emotional experience in psychoanalysis. His progression from arithmetic through plane and solid geometry to algebraic and differential and integral calculus was determined by his zeal to seek a mathematics that, through its capacity for *abstraction*, could be employed in the absence of the object being studied—in complex ramifications. That is, until he came upon infinity, O, which required religious, mystical, and philosophical formulations. Yet his belief in mathematics, a more ethereal and mystical (intuitionistic) mathematics, continued:

> It is said that a discipline cannot be properly regarded as scientific until it has been mathematized and I may have given the impression . . . that I support this view and in doing so risk the proposal of a premature mathematization of a subject which is not sufficiently mature for such a procedure. I shall therefore draw attention to some features of mathematical development which have not hitherto been adequately considered psycho-analytically. As an illustration I shall use the description . . . of the transition from the dark and formless Godhead of Meister Eckhart to the "knowable" Trinity. My suggestion is that an intrinsic feature of the transition from the "unknowability" of infinite Godhead to the "knowable" Trinity is the introduction of the number "three." The Godhead has become, or been, mathematized. The configuration which can be recognized as common to all developmental processes whether religious, aesthetic, scientific or psycho-analytical is a progression from the "void and formless infinite" to a "saturated" formulation which is finite and associated with number, e.g. "three" or geometric, e.g. the triangle, point, line or circle. . . . *The transition from sensibility to awareness . . .*

cannot take place unless the process of change, T α, is mathematical though perhaps in a form that has not been recognized as such. [1965, pp. 170–171; italics added]

From this citation (as well as others) one gathers that Bion *is* religious in so far as he has a deep and abiding faith in mathematics, which I would now term *"the absolute purity of being"* for him. Although consummately human, he ultimately saw individuals and their emotional relationships in terms of integers, circles, lines, angles, and arcs and intersections thereof. All life, human and otherwise, follows mathematical laws as their ultimate template. *That is Bion's Faith!* "Transformations" is the mathematical function of adjusting to being alive. Remaining emotionally human is its incarnation.

Postscript

Before leaving the concept of transformations, I should like to add a postscript. All the while that Bion was focusing on α-function and transformation in his publications, he was quietly dealing with his revised concept of dreaming. In his private, then unpublished notebook, *Cogitations,* Bion (1992) came up with the concept that the "analyst must dream the session" (p. 120). I believe that considerable overlap and/or continuity exists between α-function, transformation, contact-barrier, the Grid, L, H, and K linkages, and dreaming as "editing functions" that mediate, filter, fictionalize, mythify, modulate, transduce, triage, prioritize, detoxify, reconfigure, and recontextualize—O. I believe that all the above models are holographically unified and comprise what I would call the *"dream ensemble"*. (I discuss this in greater detail in chapter 25.)

As I have stated over and over again, Truth (O) cannot be transformed in terms of its own nature. It is—and will always be—what it is. Transformations *to* O is another matter. It is my impression that the ultimate nature of the transformation process constitutes a cycle of mental and emotional alterations of experiences, beginning with the experience of O's intersection with the subject's emotional frontier—as a β-element, according to Bion—through the intermediary mental digestive processes of "α-bet(a)-ization" by α-function ultimately to the finale, in which the subject "becomes" what he has experienced. I call this a transformation *to* O to complete the cycle. Meanwhile impersonal O (Fate) has become personally owned by the subject, and his Grid Column 2 function helps him to discard those aspects of O that do *not* belong to him.

Postscript II

At this point I wish to remind the reader of my Postscript in chapter 6 to the section on "Godhead (Godhood) as the 'Thinker' of the 'Thoughts Without a Thinker'", which applies equally to the theory of transformations.

NOTES

1. Please note how Bion places α before β with regard to the sequence in transformations in contrast to β-element before α-element.

2. I am grateful to Célia Fix Korbivcher for her gracious permission to cite from her paper, which is pending publication.

3. Bion was an ardent follower of the Dutch School of Intuitionistic Mathematics.

4. Certainly, there must have been other factors that caused the alienation between Bion and his colleagues, but they are unknown to me.

CHAPTER 21

Psychoanalytic functions and elements

Caveat

My attempt to do justice to Bion's writings will seem to be un-even. However, I shall write a few words at this time about "functions" as they appear in *Learning from Experience*. I shall not separately discuss *Learning from Experience, Attention and Interpretation, Elements of Psycho-Analysis*, or *Transformations*, because their principal contents have been or will be discussed elsewhere in the text under their own respective headings.

Psychoanalytic functions

In *Learning from Experience* (1962b), Bion states:

"Function" is the name for the mental activity proper to a number of factors operating in concert. "Factor" is the name for a mental activity operating in consort with the other mental activities to constitute a function. . . . The theory of functions makes it easier to match the realization with the deductive system that represents it. . . . The term alpha-function is, intentionally, devoid of meaning [unsaturated and "outside the box" of the object being observed—JSG]. [1962b, pp. 1–3]

He goes on to say that α-function operates on one's sense impressions and emotions to produce α-elements. Failing that, β-elements arise,

DOI: 10.4324/9781003348665-22

which are non-mental and non-phenomenal. Failure of α-function results in the subject's inability to dream and therefore to sleep. In order
to be able to "learn from experience", α-function must be able to mediate the awareness of emotional experience. Attacks on the subject's
α-function capacity may be stimulated by hate or envy (p. 9) but also,
I believe, by the subject's very anxiety about learning and growing
from experience—before he feels ready (Grotstein, unpublished-b). It is α-
function, which processes one's emotional experiences by day and by
night, that allows for the continuing differentiation of consciousness
from unconsciousness. Dreaming, which Bion frequently associates
with α-function, allows for a barrier, the contact-barrier, another function, to maintain the distinction between sleep and wakefulness and
between consciousness and the unconscious—and thereby to facilitate
the generation of a train of thought. The contact-barrier—a term Freud
analogized to the neuronal synapse—is used by Bion to indicate that it
both protects consciousness from the unconscious and the reverse. It is
also characterized by its ability to be *selectively permeable* to data from
within as well as from without.

For me the contact-barrier is a cognate of α-function as well as its
object. It corresponds, I believe, to Column 2 of Bion's Grid in so far as
Column 2 is not only the *lie* column (*denial*) but also the *negation* column,[1] which is necessary for differentiation of one object from another
(secondary process). I see the contact-barrier, in other words, as the
continuation of α-function. Because of the contact-barrier's ability to
differentiate *and* to select, it is of prime importance in the mental function of *abstraction*. Bion reveals his initial puzzlement about a psychotic
who, following the premise of a distinction between the psychotic and
non-psychotic personalities, projected his normal (neurotic) personality as consciousness of psychic qualities into Bion. Bion analogized
this to the projection of maternal emotions into her fetus, where Bion
was the fetus. Bion finally realized that he had been *dreaming* the session—that is, translating sense impressions into α-elements. (Once
again one notes how Bion seems to use dreaming and α-function in-
terchangeably.) He ultimately realized that the patient suffered from a
defective α-function and thus was unable to transform his emotional
experiences.

This awareness explained to Bion that he, Bion, was a "conscious"
(the patient's projective identification) and he (the patient), an "unconscious", was incapable of the functions of unconsciousness. The contact-barrier in this case was one that was formed from the proliferation
not of α-elements but, rather, of β-elements (1962b, p. 22). When the

contact-barrier goes into default, a β-screen takes its place. Bion then observes that the β-screen produces interesting results: it enables the patient to manipulate the response he wants from the analyst and/or that elicits powerful countertransferences in the analyst.

Psychoanalytic elements

> For the purpose for which I want them the *elements of psycho-analysis* must have the following characteristics: 1. They must be capable of *representing a realization* that they were originally used to describe. 2. They must be capable of *articulation* with other similar elements. 3. When so articulated they should form a *scientific deductive system* capable of *representing a realization* suppose one existed. [1963, pp. 2–3; italics added]

Bion lists the following as elements: ♀♂, P–S ↔ D, L, H, and K, R (Reason), I (Idea), α-element, and β-element. I is to represents thought (idea), and R reason, which is to tame the passions of L, H, and K. No sooner has Bion introduced this cast of elements than some of them—R and I—seem to have exited for the remainder of his career.

Bion also states that elements are functions of the personality, and that:

> Psycho-analytic investigation formulates premises that are as distinct from those of ordinary science as are the premises of philosophy or theology. Psycho-analytic elements and the objects derived from them have the following dimensions.
> I. Extension in the domain of *sense*.
> 2. Extension in the domain of *myth*.
> 3. Extension in the domain of *passion*.
> An interpretation cannot be regarded as satisfactory unless it illuminates a *psycho-analytic object* and that object must at the time of interpretation possess these dimensions. [1963, p. 11; italics added]

It now seems apparent that Bion is employing the term "element" because of its scientific cachet, but he seems to be thinking of objects. Sense (attention and perception), myth (unconscious phantasy and its mythic template), and passion (suffering, experiencing O) are the elements of the psychoanalytic session. Later, Bion will espouse abandonment of memory and desire and also exhort the analyst to enter into a state of reverie. It is important to remember that the analyst must, by virtue of the need to attend to sense, myth, and passion, employ his left-hemispheric capacities as well as his right.

Stitzman (2004), following Sor and Senet de Gazzano (1993), proffers two more elements:

Elements are harmonized, conjugated, dispersed, isolated and congealed inside or outside of constant conjunctions, implying conceptually both what is defined inside and also their negative quality. . . . Elements are "elements for thinking". Bion initially proposes two . . . leaving the door open for an extension of the list. These elements are α (the element for transformation into thought) and β (the element for transformation into hallucination). For his part, Dario Sor and Senet de Gazzano (1993) propose including two further elements on the list: gamma (the element of autistic fanatical non-transformations) and delta (the element of at-one-ment or growth transformations). [Stitzman, 2004, p. 1146]

I gather from Stitzman's relaying of Sor and Senet de Gazzano's contribution that they all were seeking to elaborate a spectrum of elements, one of which, gamma, was a more redoubtable element than β, and delta, which is transformationally more facilitating than α.

NOTES

1. As I was using the "Find" function on my word processor, it spontaneously occurred to me that Column 2 of the Grid connoted negation when the reality principle is dominant: the "Find" function was able find what I was looking for by negating everything I was *not* looking for.

CHAPTER 22

Points, lines, and circles

T he process of transformation involves, first, the acceptance by
the infant that the absent breast, the "no-breast", differs from
the breast, and, second, that the "no-breast" can be represented
by the visual image of a point, the place where the breast was. Acceptance of "no-breast" confronts the infant with tolerating the frustration
of the absence of the object. This experience of absence initiates the
experience of time and of space—that is, where the breast used to be:
"The factors that reduce the breast to a point, reduce time to 'now'"
(Bion, 1965, p. 55). He states further that the psychotic patient becomes
concrete in reference to the mentioning of the point and believes that
the point is the "ghost" of the departed object and concretely exists as
a "no-breast" thing. This point is non-representational or non-sym-
bolic—that is, –K, in contrast to K—designating the patient who can
tolerate the concept of "no-breast" as absence.

> O can be replaced by the point or the line or a word such as "breast"
> or "penis" or any other sign representing any constant conjunction.
> . . . I shall suppose the point replaces O as the origin. . . . If "point" is
> to be available for use in K it must be defined to exclude the penum-
> bra of associations with which it is invested. It has to be developed
> so that it reaches the stage represented by D category [pre-concep-
> tion—JSG]. [1965, p. 77]

DOI: 10.4324/9781003348665-23

The clearest presentation I have found on Bion's use of plane (Euclidean) geometry, however, is in the following passage in *The Italian Seminars*:

> Have we any coordinate system which would give us an idea as to where we are, where the pair are—the analyst and the patient? In the narrative story we can get an idea of a person's development by taking any two points, A and B, and the direction would be from A to B. Those two points, A and B, we would call "real and distinct". However, suppose those two points were mobile; then they might travel round the circumference of a circle and become "real and coincident". And if we try to draw in the two points which are real and coincident, we can say that they meet and describe a line which is a tangent. [2005a, p. 31]

Bion's use of plane geometry was, once more, his predilection to find unsaturated, analogue models for precision. For him, points, lines, circles, and tangents seem to constitute a "grid azimuth" (a military term that maps out a terrain). In Bion's usage, it is a moving terrain.

If I can make a pun, the point that is felt to be concrete becomes pointless for thinking. The point that is held to be a representation helps to achieve a transformation of O into K as the constant conjunction; it must shed itself of a penumbra of associations and feelings and must achieve the status of a pre-conception. It is of some note that Bion implicates O in two separate ways (see also de Bianchedi, 2004). One is from the external world and the sense organs that serve stimuli or objects in it, and the other is from the unrepressed unconscious in terms of the inherent pre-conceptions ("memoirs of the future", Plato's Ideal Forms, Kant's noumena). Bion's picture of the human being is of one who seems to be "sandwiched" between the bipolar pincers of O. Psychoanalysts—Kleinians in particular—pay great attention to breaks in treatment, whether holiday, vacation, weekend, or even between ongoing sessions.

The analysand is hard put to hold on to the image of the benevolent analyst (good breast-object), the place of which seems to be usurped by the bad object (Bion's concretized "no-thing"). How does a vacancy of the good object *spontaneously* (at least at the beginning of analysis), inexorably, and ineluctably result in the appearance of the bad object? The traditional Kleinian explanation of this malevolent transformation is thought to be the consequence of the analysand's projective identification of his hatred (death instinct) into a split-off image of the good analyst, who now bears the analysand's hatred for having deserted the analysand and thereby becomes a malevolent object. I believe this formulation is valid, but I wish to add an alternative explanation. When the good mother–analyst departs, the infant or the infantile portion of the analysand's personality is all the more vulnerable to the inescapable irruptions of O, which it tries to self-contain as the concretized "no-thing". I believe that this formulation also helps to explain the origin of Bion's "obstructive object", which he later called the "super"ego.

Bion continues, in *Transformations*:

> The thought, represented by a word or other sign, may, when it is significant as a no-thing, be represented by a point (·). The point may then represent the position where the breast was, or may even *be* the no-breast. The same is true of the line, whether it is represented by the word line or a mark made on the ground or on paper. The circle, useful to some personalities as a visual image of "inside and outside", is to other personalities, notably the psychotic, evidence that no such dividing membrane exists.

> Intolerance of a no-thing, taken together with the conviction that any object capable of a representative function is, by virtue of what the sane personality regards as its representative function, not a representation at all but a no-thing itself, precludes the possibility of words, circles, points and lines being used in the furtherance of learning from experience. They become a provocation to substitute the thing for the no-thing, and the thing itself as an instrument to take the place of representations when representations are a necessity as they are in the realm of thinking. [1965, p. 82]

> The association of the circle with "in and out" contributes to the difficulty of understanding the concepts of the line that cuts a circle in points that are conjugate complex.[1] The difficulty arises from the supposition that the line that does so lies "outside" the circle; as opposed to the line that cuts it in two points, whose roots are real and distinct, and is supposed to lie "inside" the circle. The difficulty is diminished if there is no intolerance of the no-thing to contend with and therefore no opposition to a term of which the meaning is undetermined. [p. 83]

> Two breasts have disappeared. Or perhaps it would be more accurate to say they have shrunk or faded away until only two points remain. The protagonist may feel reconciled to this fact or he may feel quite unable to tolerate these spots (or points or ·) as to him they are either places where the breasts were, or, more poignantly, no-breasts. As he watches they appear to come together until they are coincident with each other and the boundary of his personality. . . . Then they disappear. Where have they gone? If he had an

inside or outside they might have gone inside him or gone the other side. But suppose they are not inside or outside. Worse still, suppose there is no inside or outside, that he himself is only a place-where-he-used-to-be? . . . The elements of the problem are: (I) the no-breast, or point, or (·), (ii) the no-penis, or straight line or (———), and (iii) the no-inside-or-outside, or circle or (O). [p. 84]

I ask the reader at first to forego attempting to understand what Bion is trying to convey and to take a broader look at his use of geometric icons. Bion's zeal to mathematize psychoanalysis has dumbfounded and annoyed many, including Meltzer (1978). Bion gives hints throughout his works and lectures (see *Transformations*, 1965, pp. 73–76) that he is trying to achieve optimum specificity and versatility with minimal penumbra of distracting associations. Mathematics constitutes a pure study with models of the varying kinds of relationships that pure objects have with each other. It is apolitical, impersonal, and optimally expressive. More specifically, points, lines, and circles are the architecture of all the dimensions of space, both external and internal. In their negative forms they constitute the architecture of psychotic spacelessness. Bion thinks of the point and the line as visual images and correlates them with β-elements. They remain invariant under a wide range of conditions.

Bion, having first picked up the idea of the point, the line, and the circle from their use by psychotic patients, then falls back on Euclidean geometry to use them as unsaturated signs to represent object positions. The point represents the *place* once occupied by the breast. The line represents the *position* of where the penis once was—and its future or its past (where it is going or where it has gone). The circle represents *spatial limitation*. Together, these signs define the structure of space for the normal person, but when they become negative entities—that is, –(·), –(———), or –(O), the condition of –K (psychosis) is indicated.

NOTES

1. "'Conjugate complex' . . . is represented by a pair of complex numbers whose imaginary parts are identical but differ only in sign, for example, 6+4i and 6-4i are complex conjugates . . . mirror images of each other, a concept that Bion has used to represent narcissism geometrically. . . . He gives the example of a straight line (representing an object) which cuts a circle (symbolizing the mind) in two different points that could be represented as *point pairs . . . real and distinct, or actual and distinct*: inside the circle, in the internal world, would represent the analyst-analysand relationship working harmonically in search of O and its transformation in K" (López-Corvo, 2003, pp. 62–63).

CHAPTER 23

The Grid

Bion first referred to his concept of the Grid in *Elements of Psycho-Analysis* (1963); he continued to develop his ideas in later works, *Transformations* (1965), *Two Papers: The Grid and Caesura* (1977), and *Taming Wild Thoughts* (1997). The Grid represents that aspect of α-function which mediates elements that are subject to the reality principle and to what Freud (1911b) referred as "secondary process". The Grid is a mathematical device consisting of a plane covered by crossed lines, which creates the image of boxes or squares (containers), or a grating (Bion, 1997, p. 4) that extends both vertically and horizontally. They may be considered "thought bins" to store categories of thoughts and emotions. Every step in the transformational process moves from one bin to another diagonally downward and is constrained by a vertical and a horizontal axis. The vertical axis (the genetic axis) of the Grid designates the progressive transformative sophistication of developing or evolving *thoughts* as it moves downward, whereas the horizontal axis designates the act of *thinking* the thoughts—that is, the use to which the thoughts are being put. It represents the activity of the mind in what Freud termed secondary process. Put another way, the Grid is the *container* for transformed thoughts, the *contained*.

Bion considered the Grid to be apposite for thoughts and emotions that had attained consciousness or were in a state of "emergent consciousness" (the pre-conscious). Although he did not formally consider

THE GRID

	Definitory Hypotheses 1	ψ 2	Notation 3	Attention 4	Inquiry 5	Action 6	...n
A β-elements	A1	A2				A6	
B α-elements	B1	B2	B3	B4	B5	B6	...Bn
C Dream Thoughts Dreams, Myths	C1	C2	C3	C4	C5	C6	...Cn
D Pre-conception	D1	D2	D3	D4	D5	D6	...Dn
E Conception	E1	E2	E3	E4	E5	E6	...En
F Concept	F1	F2	F3	F4	F5	F6	...Fn
G Scientific Deductive System		G2					
H Algebraic Calculus							

that the aspect of α-function that mediates the unconscious β-element impressions from O constitutes a Grid in itself, I do, since α-function acts like a *grating* to sort out raw β-elements (Bion, 1997, p. 4). A Grid is any selective device that receives wholesale input, separates it into its components (triage), and classifies, prioritizes, reorganizes, and reconfigures it for further use. The rows consist of: **A:** β-elements; **B:** α-elements; **C:** Dream Thoughts, Dreams, Myths; **D:** Pre-conception; **E:** Conception; **F:** Concept; **G:** Scientific Deductive System; and **H:** Algebraic Calculus. The columns are headed: **1** Definitory Hypothesis; **2** ψ (lie or falsification); **3** Notation; **4** Attention; **5** Inquiry; **6** Action; and **...n**.

Each of the items listed in the left-hand column (A, B, C, etc.) can be thought of as the Grid's "software" and/or contained, whereas the items listed in the column headings (1, 2, 3, etc.) can be thought of as the container or "hardware". Bion thinks of the left-hand column as the genetic column since it accounts for the genesis (ontogeny, development, maturation, sophistication—in the direction from the concrete to abstraction) of thought, whereas the column headings designate the uses to which the mind puts these thoughts—that is, how the mind thinks them or about them, and then acts upon them.

As one progresses down the axis of thoughts, one moves from the *concrete* to the *abstract*. Ideas or thoughts become more applicable to complex thought-manipulation as they become progressively more abstract—that is, as they become freed from the penumbra of associations that characterize their more concrete form. In other words, they become more like neutral numbers that lend themselves to higher-order thinking and meta-thinking. Bion originally created the Grid in order to find a scientific categorization of mental life that would help analysts from different analytic schools to be able to come to some sort of agreement. He was motivated by the struggles between the Kleinians and the Freudians in the British Institute (Bion, "Lecture on the Grid" to the Los Angeles Psychoanalytic Society in 1975, which I attended).

Frequently in his discussions of the use of the Grid Bion suggests that it should not be used by the analyst during the analytic session, but only afterwards, to get their objective clinical bearings on what might have happened during a session. I have a different view. In laying the foundation for the Grid, Bion borrowed heavily from Freud's (1911b) theory of the two principles of mental functioning, the primary and secondary processes. Here is why I feel that Bion's suggestion may be somewhat misleading: The categories on the horizontal axis constitute Bion's elaborations of Freud's notion of the categories of secondary process (thinking). The elaboration on Freud was Column 2, the ψ (psi) column, representing *falsehood*[1] on the one hand, which I believe represents *negation* on the other. Negation is necessary, after all, to transform primary-process thinking into secondary-process (Aristotelian) thinking.

The vertical categories constitute secondary-process (thoughts to be thought about). Consequently, the Grid constitutes efforts at abstraction, a *model for thinking*, Thus, what the Grid actually represents is *what analysts naturally and habitually do most of the time during the analysis as they ponder and reflect upon what they observe and hear from the analysand*—that is, it constitutes normal reflective thinking. Bion must certainly have been aware that the primary and secondary processes that he united under the concept of "α-function" constitute the analyst's preconscious equipment to be employed during the session. More to the point, the Grid is simply a way of categorizing, of diagramming (parsing), secondary-process thinking—that is, what we do most of the time *during* the analytic session without conscious awareness that we are doing so—in other words, automatically. This preconscious/conscious secondary-process thinking that we do refers to the thoughts–emotions–feelings that are being automatically transformed while we are thinking about them. Moreover, the observing aspect of the analysand also preconsciously employs the Grid as he freely associates.

The Grid represents that aspect of α-function that mediates elements that are subject to the reality principle and to what Freud (1911b) referred to as "secondary process", but what Bion, differing somewhat from Freud, assigns to the collaborative dual functioning of the reality *and* pleasure principles operating as a binary-oppositional structure, now under the hegemony of the reality principle (whereas in the unconscious this binary-oppositional structure, as in dreams and phantasies, would fall under the hegemony of the pleasure principle). Despite all the mystique Bion himself seems to have assigned to the Grid, my own view of it is that it is simply a mathematically schematized model for normal reflective, ratiocinative thinking—*something that analysts routinely do after they have been affected by their own private emotional responses to their analysands.*

The Grid, as just stated, is a mathematical model, an abstraction, consisting, in this case, of a plane covered by crossed lines, creating the image of boxes or squares (containers) that extend vertically and horizontally. They may be considered "thought bins" or gratings[2] (Bion, 1997, p. 4), as mentioned above. Every step in the transformative process moves from one bin to another. The Grid constitutes a functional *matrix* which facilitates the *matriculation* of crude thoughts (definitory hypotheses, "wild thoughts", "thoughts without a thinker") into refined (thought out) thoughts. The vertical axis (the genetic axis) of the Grid, as it moves downward, designates the progressive transformative sophistication of *thoughts*, whereas the horizontal axis designates the act of *thinking* the thoughts. It represents the activity of the mind in what Freud termed secondary process. It also designates the use to which the thoughts are to be put. Put another way, the Grid is the container for and generator of transforming thoughts. In *Elements of Psycho-Analysis* Bion states:

> In this instance the importance of the myth lies in the fact that it represents a feeling and as such its place in a grid category denotes a psycho-analytic *element*. Taken with other similar psycho-analytic elements it and the other elements together form the field of incoherent elements in which it is hoped that the *selected fact*, that gives coherence and relatedness to the hitherto incoherent and unrelated, will emerge. Thus "nominated," "bound," the psycho-analytic object has emerged. It remains to discern its meaning. This verbally same myth may then be a psycho-analytic object which is instrumental in giving meaning to the totality of elements, one of which was the feeling represented by the myth in its category. Correct interpretation therefore will depend on the analyst's being able, by virtue of the grid, to observe that two statements verbally identical are psycho-analytically different. To reiterate, a verbal statement observed to have aspects falling in rows B, C and G represents a psycho-analytic object. A verbally identical statement seen to fall in, say, D2 is a psycho-analytic element. In the example I have taken the myth in category D2 represents a *feeling* of foreboding and is a premonition of a particular kind employed to exclude something else. (*Incidentally the whole of the preceding discussion can be taken as an example of the use of the grid for an exercise designed to develop intuition and the capacity for clinical discrimination.* [italics added]) To conclude: the *elements* of psycho-analysis are ideas and feelings as represented by their setting in a *single*-category; psychoanalytic objects are associations and interpretations with extensions in the domain of sense, myth and passion . . . requiring three categories for their representation. [1963, pp. 103–104]

This citation epitomizes Bion's concept of the use of the Grid in locating, forming, mythifying, and binding the analytic object (O) by the use of the selected fact, after which the analytic object, now bound as a constant conjunction, can be submitted to the Grid for further categorization. Meanwhile, in referring to the Grid, the analyst's capacity for intuition (right-hemisphere processing) and discrimination (left-hemisphere processing) becomes sharpened.

Bion also distinguished between the psychoanalytic element and the psychoanalytic object. The former occupies only one category, whereas the psychoanalytic object, apperceived via the troika of sense, myth, and passion, must occupy the three categories apposite to each member of the troika.

Unmasking the mystery of Column 2 (ψ)

In defining Column 2, Bion, states:

> Column 2 is to categorize the "use" to which a statement—of whatever kind it may be and however untrue in the context—is put *with the intention of preventing a statement, however true in the context, that would involve modification in the personality and its outlook*. I have arbitrarily used the sign ψ to emphasize the close relationship of this "use" to phenomena known to analysts as expressions of *"resistance"*. [1997, p. 9; italics added]

> Column 2 resembles row C in that it requires expansion into a "grid" of its own.[3] My original idea was that it would supply a series of categories for palpably false statements, preferably known both to the analysand and the analyst to be false. . . . [p. 10]

I wonder whether Bion may be confusing or even misleading here. As I have expressed elsewhere in this text, the association between Column 2 and "palpable" falsehood has more to do, in my opinion, with the Aristotelian concept of the law of the excluded middle or, put another way, with deciding what an object *is* and what it *is not*, negation. We must remember that Bion owes the origin of the Grid to Freud's (1911b) concept of the two mental principles, the primary process and secondary process. The Grid is a mathematical model of secondary process. A thought coming from Column 1 (Definitory Hypothesis) to Column 2 becomes categorized by the latter into what it *is* and what it *is not*. I believe that the category "what it is not" is what Bion really means by "falsehood". Yet, in deference to Bion's view, I can conceive of the possibility that Column 2 can be the lie column in the way he suggests—when the subject renounces the reality principle! Then, Column 2 would become the Lie Column—giving the lie to reality in favour of the pleasure principle.

As one carefully follows Bion's journey into the exploration of dreaming on the one hand and α-function on the other, at one time uniting them into one concept, "dream-work-α", and then separating them again, *one begins to realize that α-function is the abstract, unsaturated model that directly corresponds to the actuality of the activity of dreaming—in the flesh!* Moreover, as one carefully re-examines the mystery of Column 2, the ψ (psi) Column on the Grid, a category that Bion assigns to –K (falsification), one begins to experience what was for me a selected fact—that Column 2 paradoxically serves two oppositional functions (binary opposition), to which I then add a third:

A. Column 2, to me, constitutes the *dreaming column—that is*, the α-*function column*—which must aesthetically alter (*quasi-falsify*) the β-elements from Column 1 (Definitory Hypothesis) to make α-elements suitable for subsequent mentalizable portage through the rest of the Grid. In other words, whereas the other horizontal categories of the Grid primarily involve the activity of the reality principle—I say "primarily" because Bion, differing from Freud (1911b), has ingeniously united the primary and secondary processes in his concept of α-function)—Column 2 primarily involves the activity of the pleasure–unpleasure principle—with varying combinations of the reality principle—on a spectrum. At one end of that spectrum one would observe resistance, psychic equilibria, and/or negative therapeutic reactions (all being varying expressions of –K), whereas at the other end normal, "successfully dreamed" α-element derivatives are being sent along their way for further refinement (via Notation, Attention, and Inquiry) to become objective, abstract thoughts. Put another way, β-elements, derived from O's impressions on the emotional frontier, must become altered (transformed, *fictionalized*) to some extent so as to escape total repression. Thus one aspect of the β-element becomes altered, protectively, while the emergent truth about the reality that composes the β-element remains unaltered. A parallel to this idea would be a work of art or of fiction, which skilfully alters the initial *presentation* of the truth about reality so that the truth can survive and be transmitted. Thus, from this perspective, Column 2 reveals the activity of the *pleasure principle*.

B. *Conversely,* however, we recall that Bion borrowed from Freud's (1911b) work on the two mental functions (the primary and secondary processes), and the horizontal axis in Bion's Grid corresponds to Freud's concept of the *secondary process.* What principally distinguishes secondary process from primary process is the function of *negation,* which, I believe, Bion should have assigned to Column 2. Thus, according to this reasoning, Column 2 functions as the introduction of the reality principle to *de*fine and *re*fine the "wild thoughts" (Bion, 1997), which he assigns to Column 1, "Definitory Hypothesis". I once again take the liberty of modifying Bion's view by suggesting that Column 1 involves only raw "wild thoughts" and/or β-elements and that it is Column 2 that renders these wild thoughts into definitory hypotheses by de-*fining* them—by subjecting them to negation, which reveals what they are *not.* Thus, from this second perspective Column 2 represents the activity of the *reality principle.*

C. I should also like to append another new hypothesis: that the operations of α-function and the Grid are either identical or at least overlapping. Both categorize, sort out, prioritize, and triage mental content—that is, β-elements as well as processed thoughts. I thus envision the following: in chapter 20 I introduced the model of the Möbius strip (discontinuous continuity), which occupies and characterizes a figure-8 configuration, the bottom portion of which dips into System *Ucs.* and the upper portion of which circumscribes System *Cs.* This Möbius strip functions as the dreaming process—that is, α-function, as well as a Grid, contact-barrier, and container for the contained.

RECONCILIATION: *the function of Column 2 represents the activity of a binary-oppositional structure that initiates the transformation-by-dreaming of wild thoughts into tame thoughts.*

Both α-function and the contact-barrier can be understood to be fractals, if not continuations, of the Grid. In other words, the Grid extends microscopically to its function as α-function and macroscopically to its function as a contact-barrier or caesura. The common function of all these levels is the screening, separating, deconstructing, and recombining of the separated elements into carefully transformed emotion–thought compounds that are selectively transferred along the mental "conveyor belt" for progressively more sophisticated abstract thinking and feeling.

In a recent unique contribution Bandera (2005) considered the probability that α-function itself should be understood as occupying a gradient or spectrum of varying container/non-container maternal styles rather than being considered to be either present or absent. While α-function is a model for transformation, it is a model that functions in human beings who have varying capacities to employ it. Thus, the concept that α-function occupies as a gradient is a valuable one. A Grid is any selective device that receives wholesale input, reorganizes it, and separates it into its components, and consequently, I believe that Bion's formulation of the Grid is incomplete.

Bion first became interested in creating a Grid during and after the Second World War, when Anna Freud and Melanie Klein and their respective followers were engaged in their Controversial Discussions in the British Psychoanalytical Society. He explained that he wanted to find a scientific language, preferably a mathematically based one, that would find common ground with analysts from any school (personal communication, 1973). At first the Grid became the analyst's handbook, whereby he thought about an analytic session *after*, not during, the analysis. I believe that Bion should have explained, as I suggest above, that the Grid can be used in the consciously purposeful way he states *after* the analytic session, but that it is unconsciously (pre-consciously) employed much of the time by the analyst *during* the session—because it is only a mathematized way of representing the *normal process of reflective (secondary-process) thinking*. Consequently, we must generalize the application of the function of the Grid to normal thinking itself for *all* thinking individuals, which obviously includes the analysand himself as he reflects on his analytic experiences.

Constant conjunction

Bion frequently refers to Hume's concept of the "constant conjunction". Its most basic meaning is the name we give to a phenomenon, person, or constant grouping of happenings in order to bind these together mentally with a designation. The constant conjunction has much in common with another idea of Bion's, the "selected fact", which he borrowed from Poincaré. The latter designates the organization or pattern that gives coherence to hitherto scattered elements or phenomena. Bion states that the constant conjunction is a function of consciousness in the observer (1965, p. 73). Once found, L, H, and K must categorize the constant conjunction, and meaning must be assigned to it. Bion states: "Once psychologically necessary meaning has been achieved reason, as the slave of the passions, transforms psycho-logically necessary meaning into logically necessary meaning" (1965, p. 73). What Bion states next is complex and all too condensed, as is typical of many of his writings, but I should like to proffer my understanding of it because of its consummate importance:

> Inadequacy of hallucinatory gratification to promote mental growth impels activity designed to provide "true" meaning: it is felt that the meaning attributed to the constant conjunction must have a counterpart in the realization of the conjunction. Therefore the activity of reason as slave of the passions is inadequate. In terms of the pleasure/pain principle there is a conflict between pleasure principle and reality principle to obtain control of reason. The objection to a meaningless universe . . . derives from fear that the lack of meaning is a sign that meaning has been destroyed and the threat this holds for essential narcissism. If any given universe cannot yield a meaning *for the individual,* his narcissism demands the existence of a god, or some ultimate object. . . . Meaning or its lack, in analysis, is a function of self-love, self-hate, and knowledge. If narcissistic love is unsatisfied the development of love is disturbed and cannot extend to love of objects. [1965, p. 73]

I take this to mean that the infantile portion of the personality ("essential narcissism") must first have hallucinatory gratification upon the assignment of the constancy of the conjunction as part of its normal narcissistic prerequisites. In other words reason, which is to be the slave of the passions, may jeopardize the narcissistic portion of the personality's rights in sharing the personal meaningfulness of the constant conjunction for its own subjectivity prior to its becoming objectified. Bion, unlike Klein and her other followers of the time, seems to be validating the concept of normal narcissism even before Kohut (1971). What is particularly at issue is the notion of a narcissistic (personal) transformation of the constant conjunction prior to an objective one. Apparently, L and H constitute the vehicle of emotionally meaningful attribution for essential narcissism, whereas K works in the service of realistic knowledge. Bion caps his previous statement with the following: "Psycho-analysis is concerned with love as an aspect of mental development and the analyst must consider the maturity of love and 'greatness' in relation to maturity" (p. 74). The point is that love and greatness spring from essential narcissism. Moreover, man's "necessary narcissism" demands meaning. He cannot tolerate meaninglessness. In default, he conjures up God.

The Grid as a form of transformation

Bion brings the preceding concepts together with the following:

> The problem is simplified by a rule that "a thing can never be unless it both is and is not". Stating the rule in other forms: "a thing cannot exist in the mind alone: nor can a thing exist unless at the same time there is a corresponding no-thing". [1965, pp. 102–103]

> The progression represented by ←↥^{4} leads to the possibility that mathematical space may represent emotion, anxiety of psychotic intensity—a repose more psychiatrically described as stupor. In every case the emotion is to be part of the progression, breast → emotion (or place where breast was) → place where emotion was. [p. 105]

The first citation confirms my earlier suggestion that the most important function of Column 2 on the Grid is *negation*—deciding what is and what is not a psychoanalytic element or thought. I have chosen to bypass the even more recondite aspects of Bion's preoccupation with geometry and its correlations with emotional life. Suffice it to say that the point, the line, circle, and the arrows are his essay into a "notation" of emotional states and their correspondence to the presence and/or absence of the object and of a mental space to contain the object, as well as the direction, in time and space, of relationships. As verbal signifiers (words) are the foundation for representations of our object world (culture), points, lines, and circles are the foundation for our conception of space—both psychic and external. Thus, these geometric signifiers constitute the formatting for the construction of the space-container as words constitute the formatting of the contained.

Bion states that the domain of thought may be conceived of as a space occupied by no-things and that the objects with which psychoanalysis deals include a relationship of the no-thing to the thing. Furthermore,

> The personality that is capable of tolerating a no-thing can make use of the no-thing, and so is able to make use of what we can now call thoughts. Since he can do so he can seek to fill the "space" occupied by the thought; this makes it possible for the "thought" of space, line, point to be matched with a realization that is felt to approximate it. [1965, p. 106]

A curious aspect of the structure of the Grid

After carefully examining the structure of the Grid, in particular its genetic (vertical) axis, the coordinate apposite for the evolution of thoughts,

I came across an apparent discontinuity.[5] The descending order of thought categories is as follows: β-elements → α-elements → Dream Thoughts, Dreams, Myths → Pre-conception → Conception, and so on. I should like to call attention to the connection between "Dream Thoughts, Dreams, Myths" and then "Pre-conception". All the thought categories antecedent to "Pre-conception" can be understood as the processing of "sensory stimuli of emotional experience"—that is, external stimuli, β-elements, and the progression of the latter into an α-element and then into an element used in dreaming. How do we account for the next jump to the Pre-conception category, however? Dr Lee Rather and I believe that *this discontinuity designates the two-fold nature of O.* The "sensory stimuli of emotional experience"—that is, external stimuli—comprise one arm of O. As soon as the external stimuli come to be registered as the intersection of "evolving O" with the individual's emotional frontier, the other arm of O activates the emergence of the inherent (or acquired) pre-conception—that is, the Ideal Forms, the things-in-themselves ("memoirs of the future"), from within the unrepressed unconscious. In other words, *O emerges in a way that gives one reason to believe that it is a conjoined twin and the human subject is caught between them!*

Other aspects of the Grid

Despite his frequent references to the Grid, Bion seems to have been dismissive of it in public. His followers, on the other hand, seemed to have taken it very seriously as a valuable aid for their theorizing and for their clinical understanding of their patients. Rose Vasta (1993) and Arnaldo Chuster (Chuster & Conte, 2003; Chuster & Frankiel, 2003) have both, independently, constructed a *negative Grid,* one that seems to be an elaboration of Column 2 that deals with evolution of lies and falsehoods. Paulo Sandler (2005), on the other hand, has devised a tri-dimensional Grid, the third axis of which reflects the emotional *intensity* associated with any particular category.

Meltzer (2000) has modified Bion's Grid by constructing two Grids: one for L, H, and K and another for –L, –H, and –K, respectively, the latter representing an extension of Column 2 (the lie column) in Bion's. In the LHK grid he replaces Bion's "Scientific Deductive System" and "Algebraic Calculus" with **G** "Aesthetic" and **H** "Spiritual". Column 2 he alters to designate "Transformations". In the –LHK grid, which itself is an extension of Bion's Column 2, he lists: **H** "Spiritual"; **G** "Aesthetic"; **F** "Concept"; **E** "Conception"; **D** "Pre-conception"; **C** "Dream

Thoughts"; **B** "α-elements", "Myths"; **A** "β-elements". In the –LHK grid Meltzer lists: **–1** "Denial of Inner Reality"; **–2** "Omniscience"; **–3** "Lies" & "Delusions"; **–4** "Misuses of Language"; **–5** "Hallucinations". It becomes clear as one surveys Meltzer's modifications of Bion's Grid that he (Meltzer) is infusing his conception of *beauty* and *aesthetics*, and his negative with regard to Column 2 seems to represent his conception of Bion's (1962b) "α-*function in reverse*" (p. 25).

NOTES

1. In analysis, Column 2 generally represents the analysand's—and/or even the analyst's—resistance to the analysis, on the one hand, and negation—that is, the attainment of logical Aristotelian thinking—on the other.

2. Bion's allusion to the Grid as a grating unknowingly prefigures my conception that α-function (as the model) and dreaming (as the actual living process) include a grating function when they sort out β-elements prior to alpha-bet(a)-ization.

3. It is my conjecture that this elusive statement may refer to Bion's recognition that, when an individual forswears the reality principle and only embraces the pleasure principle, he becomes psychotic or a liar and develops a complex world of falseness. This reminds me of Bion's (1962b) concept of "α-function in reverse" (p. 25).

4. "←↕ indicates that the object is not static" ... "and represents a force that continues after · has been annihilated and it destroys existence, time and space" (Bion, 1965, p. 101).

5. Dr Lee Rather helped me in uncovering this discontinuity.

CHAPTER 24

Fetal mental life
and its caesura with postnatal mental life

B ion, ever the imaginative explorer of both ends of the spectrum
of conceptions with the use of his technique of the reversible
perspective, began to ponder even more deeply the ultimate
headwaters of the river of life, the origin of the individual psyche
beyond and before the caesura of birth, supported by Freud's (1926d)
statement: "There is much more continuity between intra-uterine life
and earliest infancy than the impressive caesura of the act of birth
allows us to believe" (p. 138). Bion first presented his imaginative
speculations on fetal mental life in *Caesura* (1977a), where he not only
introduced the possibility of fetal mental life but also emphasized the
many facets and functions of the caesura. He asks: "Is there any part
of the human mind which still betrays signs of an 'embryological' intuition, either visual or auditory?" (p. 44).

After speculating at length about the possibility of there being such
a thing as fetal mental life and hinging his speculation largely on the
early fetal formation of the optic and auditory pits (the forerunners of
sight and sound, respectively), Bion observes:

> [T]he personality does not seem to develop as it would if it were a
> piece of elastic being stretched out. It is as if it were something which
> developed many different skins as an onion does. This point adds
> importance to the factor of the caesura, the need to penetrate what is
> recognized as a dramatic event like birth, or a possibility of success

256

DOI: 10.4324/9781003348665-25

or a breakdown. . . . We are dealing with *a series of skins* which have been epidermis or conscious, but are now "free associations". [1977a, p. 47; italics added]

Then:

The ability of the analysand to take advantage of the possibility of success which has opened out is a symptom of the penetration from the situation which Freud describes as intra-uterine, to the situation which is conscious and post-caesural. [p. 47–48]

Bion thus expands the significance of the caesura from the concreteness of its function as a boundary between prenatal and postnatal existence to its being a model, much like the contact-barrier, between the countless "onion peels", or layers, of our being, of our varied states of mind. Symptoms originate in the "prenatal" (unconscious) self and burst through the membrane to become apprehended by "the postnatal" (conscious) self. As Paulo Sandler (2005) pithily defines it: "Caesura. An event that simultaneously unites and disunites" (p. 97). To this, I would add: *defines* by separating. By constituting a boundary between two opposites, a caesura thus becomes the matrix of a *binary-opposition structure* and the defining element of the latter as *paradox*. A failure to countenance what has broken through condemns us to break up or break down.

Finally, Bion states:

Rephrasing Freud's statement for my own convenience:—There is more to continuity between autonomically appropriate quanta and the waves of conscious thought and feeling than the impressive caesura of transference and counter-transference would have us believe. So . . . ? *Investigate the caesura; not the analyst; not the analysand; not the unconscious; not the conscious; not sanity; not insanity. But the caesura, the link, the synapse, the (counter-trans)-ference, the transitive–intransitive mood.* [1977a, p. 57; italics added]

The concept of the caesura now becomes integrated with Bion's conception of the greater importance of links and connections, as compared to what and who is linked by the connections. (Bion went further in his theorizing about intra-uterine mental life in *The Dawn of Oblivion: Book 3* of *A Memoir of the Future*, 1979.)

The psychoanalytic world has yet to realize the clinical and theoretical importance of Bion's ideas about prenatal mental life and its postnatal consequences. Bion elevated the idea of the caesura to an ever-widening concept that generalized to all divisions of the personality, real and imagined. It constitutes a separating contact-barrier that, with its "selective permeability" allowing the controlled passage of elements back and forth between consciousness and the unconscious, also allows for connections. According to Lia Pistener de Cortiñas (personal communication, 2000): "Caesura is a zone that separates two regions of the personality (primitive mind/separate mind), two modes of functioning (BA and work group) and traversing this zone threatens with catastrophic change because it is where these different aspects can meet, and this meeting causes emotional turbulence. Catastrophic change is a dweller of this zone and also an indispensable factor to develop the capacity of insight, which is the only way to understand mental growth. "

In summary, Bion seems to believe that since the rudiments of sensation develop and become registered in the embryo and in its successor, the fetus, they can be considered to possess mental capacity, albeit rudimentary. If that is the case, then how do they process and dispose of these sensations, particularly troubling ones? A possible answer might lie in Bion's *Experiences in Groups* (Bion, 1961) where he wrote of "proto-mental phenomena" and "proto-mental systems" (pp. 101–104), which he later recast as "β-elements" (Bion, 1962b, p. 35). Consequently, we can imaginatively speculate that the embryo–fetus has the rudimentary capacity to register sensations and to originate responses to these sensory stimuli—as β-elements—which (1) might early on link up with their corresponding mental counterparts, the Ideal Forms (inherent pre-conceptions, "memoirs of the future", noumena, things-in-themselves) to form primitive proto-conceptions in the form of *inchoate sensory patterns* awaiting birth and postnatal development for further processing; or (2) might remain dormant as β-elements and, if there is a failure to transform them into α-elements upon birth or after birth, become projected into the body self as somato-psychic debris. Put another way, the embryo-fetus may mentally function by transformations in hallucinosis (mainly visual and auditory).

CHAPTER 25

What does it mean to dream?
Bion's theory of dreaming

"What is man?
What is man not?
Man is only the dream's shadow."

from the Eighth Pythian Ode of Pindar

Bion's extension of Freud's theory of dreaming had been quietly germinating in his earlier works (e.g. Bion, 1962b, p. 16, etc.). His interest in dreams and dreaming coincided with his formulation of the concepts of container and contained ($♀♂$) and α-function (Bion, 1962b, p. 91). The latter—a *model*, not a theory—had an interesting and complicated sojourn with his concept of dreaming under the inclusive term, "dream-work-α"—a concept that he never published, only confined to his private notebook, published posthumously as *Cogitations* (Bion, 1992, pp. 56–63). Bion finally concluded (p. 186) that the two concepts, though related, did not belong together.[1]

Freud's theory of dream-work

In *The Interpretation of Dreams*, Freud (1900a) says:

> The dream-thoughts and the dream-content are presented to us like two versions of the same subject-matter in two different languages. Or, more properly, the dream-content seems like a transcript of the

dream-thoughts into another mode of expression, whose characters and syntactic laws it is our business to discover by comparing the original and the translation. [Freud, 1900a, p. 277]

Further on, he goes on to say:

It thus seems plausible to suppose that in the dream-work a psychical force is operating which on the one hand strips the elements which have a high psychical value of their intensity, and on the other hand, *by some means of overdetermination,* creates from elements of low psychical value new values, which afterwards find their way into the dream-content. [p. 307]

Then:

[D]reams have no means at their disposal for representing these logical relations between dream-thoughts. For the most part dreams disregard all these conjunctions, and it is only the substantive content of the dream-thoughts that they take over and manipulate. The restoration of the connections which the dream-work has destroyed is a task which has to be performed by the interpretive process. [p. 312]

What Freud seems to be saying is that dream-work is necessary to *disguise* the emotional truths explicit and implicit in latent dream-thoughts. One of the way of distorting or altering them is via a *disarticulation* of the conventional links between thoughts and a *transvaluation* (p. 330) of the emotional valence attached to objects in the latent dream-thoughts. All in all, Freud emphasizes the need for dream-work to assume the role of an encoding or encrypting agency to keep latent truths *private—from their dreamer.*

To dream-work, Freud (1900a) assigns four functions: (1) condensation; (2) displacement; (3) considerations of altered representability, including the use of symbols; and (4) secondary revision. *Condensation* refers to the syncretistic process whereby a symbol may shrink or condense a limitless number of entities within its embrace. *Displacement,* the forerunner of projective identification, accounts for the transfer of attributions or qualities from one object or self to another. Considerations of *representability* require the dream-work to fictionalize the dream narrative paradoxically into a credible narrative—into a dream that works. *Secondary revision* is probably a function of the contact-barrier: it separates the Systems *Ucs.* and *Cs.* and seeks to guarantee that separation. (Secondary revision may be what Bion is referring to when he says that the analysand's free associations represent his dreaming.)

From Freud's perspective it seems that the purpose of dream-work is to *protect the conscious ego* from being overwhelmed by hidden, forbidden thoughts and impulses in the id. Bion, as we shall soon see, agrees with this rationale *and with its obverse* as well: that dream-work must also protect the unconscious from being overwhelmed by external stimuli.

Bion's theory of dreaming:
the relationship between dreaming and α-function

In notes written early on, in 1959, Bion seems to have conflated dreaming with α-function (Bion, 1992, pp. 62–101) and then differentiated between them, as I suggested above. He conceives of α-function as an *analogue model* to indicate the hypothetical process whereby the sense impressions of emotional experience become transformed from raw, inchoate, non-mental proto-emotions (impressions made by the intersection of evolving O on the subject's emotional frontier), known as "β-elements" (Bion, 1962b, p. 11), into mentalizable "α-elements". These are then relegated to notation (memory), repression, maintenance, and reinforcement of the "contact-barrier" between consciousness and the unconscious (Bion, 1962b, p. 17), and thinking itself, as well as imagistic (principally visual) supplies for dream elements: that is, supplying dreaming with irreducible dream elements for use in dream-narrative production:

> The sleeping man has an emotional experience, converts it into α-elements and so becomes capable of dream thoughts . . . and therefore of *undisturbed consciousness*. [1962b, p. 15; italics added]

Dreaming and/or α-function occur throughout the day and night. The emotional *vocabulary* furnished by α-function is used in dreaming[2] to construct imaginative, preponderantly visual narratives as *truthful* "*archival fictions*", which contain emotions that have emerged from transformed and transduced β-elements. These β-elements result from sense impressions on the subject's emotional frontier cast by intersections (interactions, confrontations) with the evolution of the "Absolute Truth" about an infinite, cosmic, *impersonal* "Ultimate Reality", "O", into a mercifully tolerable, finite, and personally acceptable truth about one's own *personal*, subjective relationship to one's objects in inner and outer reality. In other words, *impersonal O becomes transformed into personal O in a "transformational cycle"* with detours in K,[3] and, failing that, –K (falsehood). O designates an ever-expanding force field of inner *and* outer stimuli (as sense impressions) presenting as a cosmic impersonal chaos, *uncertainty*,[4] and proliferating infinity moving in the direction of increasing incoherence and absolute symmetry or indivisibility—that is, *entropy* (Bion, 1965, 1970; Matte Blanco, 1975, 1988). Britton (2006) presents the notion of the principles of "probabilism" and "indeterminacy" to encompass what Bion means by O. The ancient Greeks referred to this phenomenon as "*Ananke*" (Necessity), and I would translate it as ever-evolving, ever-approaching "raw, impersonal Circumstance". It is important to realize that O is always evolving—always in flux.

> How does a dream evade frustration? By *distortion* of facts of reality, and by *displacement* of facts of reality. In short, by dream-work on the perception of facts—not, in this context, dream-work on the dream-thoughts except in so far as the dream-thoughts are thoughts portraying the facts. Freud attributes to dream-work the function of concealing the facts of internal mental life, the dream-thoughts, only. *I attribute to it the function of evading the frustration to which the dream thoughts, and therefore the interpretation of dream-thoughts, would give rise if allowed to function properly—that is, as mechanisms associated with the legitimate tasks involved in real modification of frustration.* Consequently, since such legitimate tasks always carry an element of frustration, excessive intolerance of frustration short-sightedly leads to the attempt at evasion of the frustration intrinsic to the task of modification of the frustration.
>
> α is concerned with, and is identical with, unconscious waking thinking designed, as a part of the reality principle, to aid in the task of real, as opposed to pathological, modification of frustration. [1992, p. 54; italics added]

One can see how Bion integrates dreaming with α-function. For him α-function and/or dreaming serve "the legitimate task in . . . real modification of frustration" (not evasion). Furthermore, he thinks of α (α-function) and, thus, dreaming as serving the reality principle. He considers toleration of frustration to be pivotal in the capacity to think. Although he never formally integrated this concept with his theory of container ↔ contained, I believe that it should be.

Godbout (2004) discusses the ability to tolerate frustration:

> [T]he fact of the intolerance or "intolerability" of frustration in relation to awareness or discovery indicates how representational activity, for Bion, does not spring out of absence of gratification alone, but out of *tolerated* absence. When intolerable, this absence on the contrary *compromises* seriously representation. [Godbout, 2004, p. 1125]

Proto-emotions—that is, sense impressions of emotional experience, β-elements—are processed by α-function to yield α-elements, the irreducible elements suitable for mentalization and dreaming. The α-elements are thereupon selectively distributed to notation (memory), repression, further thought processes, and support for the contact-barrier between consciousness and the unconscious and for deployment as constructive units for dreaming. The deployed α-elements, as they proliferate and link together to form more complex structures, are like letters of the alphabet ("α–β") that combine to produce versatile images, symbols, words, sentences, and, ultimately, thoughts or dream narratives. Furthermore, for Bion the act of dreaming constitutes a paradoxical process in which two opposing masters—the pleasure principle *and* the reality principle—are mediated in a dialectical relationship. Thus P–S (pleasure) ↔ D (reality), where P–S conducts personalization and subjectivization conducts transformations—a sorting out of O—and D allows for objectification. P–S projects, and D introjects.

Bion's hypotheses about dreaming

Bion (1970), in extending Freud's ideas on the functions of dreaming, believed that, rather than thoughts emerging from the unconscious into consciousness only *sequentially*, as Freud (1900a) had suggested, (1) consciousness and the unconscious functioned *simultaneously* (Bion, 1970, p. 48) as well as sequentially, and (2) sensory stimuli had to become unconscious(dreamed) first before the subject could become conscious of them—or be able to be kept unaware of them for realistically expedient reasons. According to Bion:

> It is in the dream that the Positions [the paranoid–schizoid and depressive—JSG] are negotiated. [1992, p. 37]

> *My belief is that the dependence of waking life on dreams has been overlooked and is even more important.* Waking life = ego activity . . . the dream symbolization and dream-work is what makes memory possible. [p. 47; italics added]

> We psycho-analysts think you do not know what a dream is: the dream itself is a pictorial representation, verbally expressed, of what happened. What actually happened when you "dreamed" we do not know. All of us are intolerant of the unknown and strive instantaneously to feel it is explicable, familiar. [1977b][5]

Bion further states that the *analyst must dream the analytic session* (1992, p. 120).

Having concentrated on Bion's theories about the dependence of waking life on dreams, the progression of sensory stimuli from consciousness to the unconscious, and the simultaneity of conscious and unconscious mental processing, I now ask the question that I shall try later to answer: Why do stimuli have to be processed (dreamed) by the unconscious before consciousness can either utilize them or "choose" not to be bothered with them—that is, when they are kept unconscious? The answer that Bion offers us is that dreaming functions as a filter that sorts, categorizes, and prioritizes emotional facts that are stimulated by this incoming data, much like the motto of the *New York Times*: "All the news that's fit to print."

Suggested models

The following four models may help to explain Bion's thinking with regard to dreaming:

A. The *Möbius Strip* can, as already described, be thought of as a ribbon that is cut, given a half-twist, and then reattached. This results in a twisted continuous surface, so that in travelling along the ribbon, one finds oneself initially on the outside and then gradually on the inside surface of the ribbon—in other words, a paradoxical course of *discontinuous continuity* has been constructed. This model depicts the status of the paradoxical relationship between consciousness and the unconscious. The Möbius strip may also be represented as a *labyrinth*. The Möbius strip model depicts my conceptualization of dreaming (aka α-function) configured as a psychic–emotional immunity frontier with a figure-8 structure, like the Möbius strip—one in which one can visualize a discontinuous continuity of dreaming and its cognates, including the contact-barrier and others extended throughout consciousness and the unconscious. The figure-8 structure accounts for the intensity of "unconscious wakeful thinking" at the frontier (contact-barrier) between Systems *Ucs.* and *Cs.*

B. *Reversible perspective* (Bion, 1962b, p. 25) can be understood as an alternation for perspective dominance between foreground and background in a picture. Bion uses the picture of a vase to illustrate the "reversible perspective" (1963, p. 50). Imagine an outline of a dark vase against a light background. From one perspective, this is what one can see. From another perspective, the background becomes the foreground and one can see, instead, two light faces confronting one another. The point is that although two different pictures emerge, *one can nevertheless not observe both pictures simultaneously.* Thus when we are awake, we observe from a conscious vertex or perspective. When we are asleep, we see from the unconscious perspective of the consciousness of the dream.

C. *Binary opposition* (Lévi-Strauss, 1970) is a structuralistic concept in which two opposing forces are cooperatively opposed to one another so as to be mutually regulating of one another.

The relationship in Bion's scheme between consciousness and the unconscious is exemplified by all three of the above models. When there is consecutive movement of a stimulus from consciousness to the unconscious, the Möbius-strip model is operative. When the activities of consciousness and the unconscious function simultaneously, then the reversible-perspective or binary-oppositional model is in operation. Dreaming begins as a sequential function so as to induce a normal state of simultaneous and parallel activity in consciousness and the unconscious.

It is my belief, following my reading of Bion, that he conceives that one of the purposes of dreaming is—similarly to the function of the contact-barrier (Bion, 1962b, p. 17)—to maintain the distinction or separation and binary-oppositional functioning of consciousness and the unconscious. Rather than being obligatorily *conflictual*, which is Freud's (1915e) view, Bion conceives of them as *cooperatively oppositional*—to triangulate O, the Absolute Truth, about an infinite and indifferent or impersonal Ultimate Reality. In so doing, Bion has extended Freud's two-dimensional perspective of the relationship between the two consciousnesses to a third dimension, with O as the third vertex. O, it must be remembered, represents both the intersection of one's emotional frontier by sensory stimuli from within and without and the release by these stimuli of the inherent pre-conceptions—the Ideal Forms, the things-in-themselves. It is important to realize that dreaming converts impersonal O into personal O and then into K and that Bion (1992) ultimately substituted *"infinity"* for the unconscious. (p. 372) and *finiteness* for consciousness.

D. *Binocular perspective* (or dual-track perspective) in which any and all phenomena can be observed from two or more vertices to achieve a stereoscopic perspective.

What is *dreaming?*

I hypothesize that dreaming constitutes a "proto-language" (Fitch, 2005), one similar to the conscious and unconscious "communicative musicality" between infants and mothers postulated by Trevarthen (1999)—but with the following difference: I suggest that dreaming is the proto-linguistic communication within the System *Pcs.* between its two frontiers—the lower frontier with System *Ucs.* and the upper frontier with System *Cs.* It is communication between the "dreamer who dreams the dream" and the "dreamer who understands the dream"— that is, the "ineffable subject of the unconscious" and the "phenomenal subject of consciousness"—respectively (Grotstein, 2000a, p. 11). The relationship between the two "dreamers" is best represented by the ancient Greek "middle voice", which connotes the simultaneity of the active and passive modes of being (Greenberg, 2005; Peradotto, 1990).

Dreaming constitutes a continuous sensory (usually visual) process whereby the sensory stimuli (internal and/or external) of emotional experience undergo a transformation and an aesthetically honed reconfiguration, making them suitable for being experienced affectively, thought about cognitively, and recalled in memory. The sensory stimuli of emotional experience, O, seem initially to *surround* one until one has successfully dreamt them, after which one feels that one has some grasp of O by becoming O. In other words, dreaming acts as a narrative container (Ferro, 1999, p. 50). It is my impression from my reading of Bion that he places consummate importance on the dreaming process and strongly suggests that ultimately *psychopathology becomes an indicator of unsuccessful or incomplete dreaming.*

Dreaming constitutes an intermediary buffer zone, a veritable ozone layer, which protects us from the blinding glare of O. It constitutes an ongoing, mediating, detoxifying filter that also undertakes such transformative processes as (1) transducing the infinity of impersonal O into practical, personal, finite, third-dimensional categories (e.g. good versus bad; inside versus outside, etc.); (2) reconfiguration of its original complex meaning into personal meaning; (3) encryption into a linear narrative, and (4) the transformation of the indifference or impersonalness of O into personal O (personal meaning).

Dreaming can be thought of as a generation of ongoing "archival fictional truths" in which the Absolute Truth about an impersonal Ultimate Reality is aesthetically and kaleidoscopically reconfigured and balanced between the Scylla of the pleasure principle and the Charybdis of the reality principle—a dialectical binary-oppositional operation under the hegemony of the reality and truth principles, respectively (Grotstein, 2004b). With regard to dreaming, imagination operates in the service of the pleasure *and* reality principles as well as, ultimately, the truth principle, to extract and reconstruct the truth from its initial context and background and transform it as an invariant incognito within the dialectical functioning of the Positions (P–S ↔ D) into personal subjective truth. Dreaming, like stories, functions through its ability to achieve *vicarious* applicability, correspondence, and resonance with the subject's unconscious conflicts.

Winnicott (1971b), in one of his critiques of Klein, stated that she had been more interested in the *meaning* of children's play than in the *act of playing* itself. The same principle may apply to the practice of psychoanalysis, which has traditionally been more interested in the meaning of dreams than in the act of dreaming. According to Freud (1900a), the purpose of dreams is to preserve sleep. Bion (1962b) considers dreaming to be necessary to enhance the contact-barrier that, by effectively separating Systems *Ucs.* and *Cs.*, allows sleep to take place, so that the subject is able to distinguish wakefulness from sleep, unlike the psychotic, who cannot distinguish between them (p. 17).

To summarize Bion's theories on dreams:

A. Psychopathology is essentially the result of impaired dreaming, and this impairment is more significantly experienced by the System *Ucs.*

B. The importance of the contact-barrier is not only to protect the System *Cs.* from the System *Ucs.* but the reverse as well—and also to shield both of them from O. The contact-barrier is reinforced by α-elements donated by α-function, but the reverse is also true. Dreaming and/or α-function depend on the operation of an intact and functioning contact-barrier.

C. The significance of the analyst's interpretations of unconscious phantasies (including dreams) is not to discredit their function but to *acknowledge* their reparative mythic function and, by acknowledging them, to restore their narrative recalibrating (generalizing and abstracting) and containing functions, which run parallel with a cooperative binary opposition with the original latent content of consciousness, laying the groundwork there for *metaphor*. Put another way, the mind functions along two distinctly different but interconnected lines of operation. The unconscious functions under the hegemony of the pleasure principle (albeit with some contribution from the reality principle). There is minimal negation; thus everything is connected and symmetrical. It is the autoch- thonous (self-created) universe of objects and emotions—that is, self-created, personal, phantasmal. The second is the domain of consciousness, of a reality that has been clearly defined and refined by the application of negation. The human being needs both layers. Psychoanalysis addresses the former, both overtly and covertly. Bion (1992) states this dichotomy as one between "*narcissism*" and "*socialism*" (p. 103)—in other words, dreaming (no negation) at- tends to the personal aspects of the self and Aristotelian thinking (ruled by negation) to the more objective aspects.

D. Dreaming, unconscious wakeful thinking, *is* thinking as well as being the prerequisite to thinking, feeling, and being. Bion (1954) states: "It must mean that without phantasies and without dreams you have not the means with which to think out your problem" (pp. 25–26).

Here Bion first hints at an idea that has never been fully explored by others—that the psychotic suffers not from too much primary process but from a defectively functioning primary process—that is, *defective dreaming.* He formulated the idea that the psychotic's thought disor- der is due in part to a difficulty with phantasies (day dreaming) and dreams (by night) that would make thought possible. He will later unite and conflate the primary processes with secondary process as "α-function" (Bion, 1962b, p. 54), which, like Matte Blanco's (1975, 1988, 2005) "bi-logic", contains two complementary and opposing strands, *mythification* and *clarification.* The analyst dreams the patient's dream and thereby completes the dream.

The unconscious is, in Bion's view, the setting of an "undisciplined debate" that dreaming seeks to transform into a "disciplined debate" (Bion, 1979)—a Platonic (respectful) dialogue between the antinomies (internal objects) that comprise it. Dreams prepare the ground for the debate, thesis ↔antithesis → reconciling synthesis: ". . . Where igno- rant armies clash by night" ("Dover Beach"—Matthew Arnold, 1867).

Dreaming "licks the emotional wounds of care" to heal them. Dreaming weaves the disparate elements of experience into a tapestry of poetic, aesthetic, cognitive, and ontological coherence.

I believe that dreaming does this by virtue of its autochthonous creativity: that is, the "dreamer who dreams the dream" (Grotstein,

2000a) first narcissistically *creates* the dream narrative as it encounters the incoming O sensory stimuli. Dreaming stands between *sensation* and *perception.*[6]

"Nameless dread" (Bion, 1965, p. 79) is the experience of the destruction of the dream-work's capacity to function and to heal.

The following points integrate Bion's theory of dreaming with his ontological and epistemological metatheory for psychoanalysis, to which I add my own speculative hypotheses:

A. We dream continuously—that is, by day as well as by night (Bion, 1992, p. 63).

B. Normal dreaming is characterized by an *introjection* of the results of the dreaming process, whereas the psychotic utilizes dreaming for the *projective* expulsion of the realizations of the dreaming process (Bion, 1962b, 1965, 1992, p. 43).

C. All sensory stimuli, whether originating within the internal world or coming from the external one, must first be dreamed and relegated to the unconscious in order to be processed, encoded, encrypted, and assigned to different faculties of the mind—that is, to memory, to repression, to supply dream elements for further dreaming, for reinforcement of the contact-barrier, and to supply the ingredients of emotional and abstract thought (Bion, 1992, pp. 112, 139).

D. The contact-barrier (Bion, 1962b, p. 17), which makes dreaming possible but which also depends on dreaming for its own maintenance, is a caesura (Bion, 1977a) that effectively separates fetal mental life from postnatal mental life (Bion's imaginative conjecture) and functions as a two-way selectively permeable membrane between consciousness and the unconscious,[7] conducting transformations, transductions, and encryptions of stimuli in transit from either source and creates the effective two-way boundary that makes dreaming possible. Moreover, it constitutes a continuation of Bion's (1962b) concept of the container. The contact-barrier can be linked as an analogue with the discipline of the *analytic frame*: the need to maintain the discipline of the frame parallels the need to maintain an effective separation between analyst and analysand and between consciousness and the unconscious so that each can function separately (autonomously), complementarily, and, thus, effectively.

E. One of Bion's (1962b) tools is the stereoscopic model of "binocularity" (p. 54), which is, in turn, associated with Niels Bohr's theory of complementarity. Specifically, Bion views the relationship between the Systems *Ucs.* and *Cs.* as complementary as well as oppositional, rather than primarily conflictual. Bion also applies the binocular principle of complementarity (Bion, 1965, p. 153) to the relationship between the paranoid–schizoid and depressive positions (P–S ↔ D). Consequently, Bion is able to recruit the Systems *Ucs.* and *Cs.* and P–S ↔ D as two separate sets of autonomous and yet simultaneously oppositionally connected structures (binary-oppositional structures) to function complementarily according to the rules of their respective natures *and* at the same time to mediate binocularly or stereoscopically cooperatively and triangulate a third object, O (the "analytic object"), the Absolute Truth about an imminently intersecting and evolving infinite Ultimate Reality. In other words, as evolving O intersects the individual's emotional frontier, the latter's sentinels intercept, triage, and process its stochastic "noise" into personal, then objective, and finally transcendent meaning—"personal O"—thus completing the transformational cycle.

F. Bion (1962b, p. 56), at variance with Freud (1911b), conceived of the *inseparability*—or really the coterminousness or contiguity—of the primary and secondary processes when he postulated α-function as a transformational model. In other words, he believed that a combination of the primary and secondary processes worked intimately, cooperatively, but in different ways in the unconscious and in consciousness. Bion implied (and I hypothesize explicitly) by suggesting this juncture, but to my knowledge he never formally stated that he believed that the pleasure and reality principles were similarly conjoined normally but not pathologically. In other words, the pleasure principle and the primary processes function in complementary collaboration with the reality principle and secondary process—as subordinate functions in consciousness and as predominant functions in the unconscious, in which circumstance the reality principle and the secondary process subsume subordinate functions.

The above model finds its corollary in Matte Blanco's (1975, 1988) conceptions of "bi-logic" and "bivalent logic" (Carvalho, 2005). Matte Blanco believes that the unconscious is dominated by the principle of symmetry (the erasure of differences and the equation of opposites), whereas consciousness is dominated by the principle of asymmetry (the progressive development of differences). Yet if the unconscious were absolutely symmetrical, no signs, symbols, or dreams would be possible. Matte Blanco therefore conceived of "bi-logic" for the unconscious and "bivalent logic" (Aristotelian logic) for consciousness. Bi-logic and bivalent logic both use varying portions of symmetry and asymmetry in their respective binary-oppositional structures or systems, but bi-logic, the logic of the unconscious, is dominated by the principle of symmetry, which can be equated with the pleasure principle, and bivalent logic, the logic of consciousness, is dominated by the principle of asymmetry, which corresponds to the reality principle. Thus, these two antithetical structures of logic utilize symmetry and asymmetry dialectically but under different supraordinating organizations—along the lines of the model of conjoined twins, where the pleasure and reality principles occupy two separate structures in which they are both conjoined and separate.

Matte Blanco's scheme seems to me to be identical to Bion's concept of the dialectical binary-oppositional structures located both in the unconscious and in consciousness, respectively. In other words, *primary and secondary processes, the pleasure and reality principles, symmetry and asymmetry combinatorially comprise both unconscious α-function and conscious α-function—and find their counterpart functions in dreaming (dream-thinking) and cognitive reflective thinking.*

G. I hypothesize that α-function implies the existence of at least two mirror-image binary-oppositional structures, each consisting of dialectically opposing primary and secondary processes—and that they both subserve dreaming. (1) One binary-oppositional (binocular) structure—α-function 1—exists in the unconscious and is responsible for the transformation (mentalization—dreaming) of β-elements into α-elements, which are then relegated for use as dream thoughts, repression, memory, and reinforcement of the contact-barrier. Although this structure consists of the dialectical operations of both the primary and secondary processes, it is under the hegemony of the pleasure principle. (2) Another binary-oppositional structure—α-function 2—situated in consciousness and/or in the preconscious and under the hegemony of the reality principle, transforms (dreams) β-elements emanating from stimuli in the external world so as to render them unconscious. In other words, there is spectrum of α-functioning that extends from the most elemental to the most advanced. Ferro (2005) speaks about this gradient and uses the term "α-megafunction" for the most sophisticated aspect—the one responsible for the creation of narrative. (3) Bion implies that even the pleasure and reality principles constitute a binary-oppositional structure. I posit that this dialectical structure exists in the unconscious *and* consciousness, with the pleasure-principle "twin" predominating in the unconscious and the reality-principle "twin" in consciousness.

H. I further hypothesize that a supraordinating function oversees and mediates the multiple, complex binary-oppositional structures previously elaborated. This supraordinating function, which I call the *"truth principle"*, inaugurates the *"truth drive* or *instinct* and ultimately mediates dreaming as the messenger of truth (Grotstein, 2004b). Britton (2006) posits also the existence of an "uncertainty principle".

I. All incoming sensory stimuli, whether from the internal or external world, are considered β-elements by Bion (1962b, p. 7) and inchoate α-elements by me—that is, sensory imprints or impressions of O (O's shadow or ghost) that must be transformed and relegated to the unconscious through the apertures of the selectively permeable membrane of the contact-barrier. Yet I should like to introduce an alternative perspective, one that would modify Bion's view slightly. Ferro (2005) speaks of "balpha-element" (p. 46): combinations of α- and β-elements, such as in "undigested facts" (Bion, 1962b, p. 7). Thus, one may speculate that α-function occupies a gradient normally and pathologically. Bandera (2005) postulates a gradient of α-function in hysteria, which includes a range of categories of maternal capacities to contain their infants (Rather, 2005).

J. Bion distinguishes between mentalization and thinking. Mentalization is the process whereby β-elements—the sensory stimuli of emotional experience (Bion, 1962b, p. 7)—become transformed into mentalizable (mentally "digestible") ingredients for mental "metabolism". Thinking constitutes a more advanced process—abstraction ↔ concretization (Bion, 1962b, p. 52)—with the use of functions and categories whereby the alpha-bet(a)-ized β-elements *cum* α-elements become the irreducible components of thinking—that is, thought manipulation (analogous to glucose, fructose, fatty acids, and amino acids in gastrointestinal digestion).

K. Bion seems over time to link the following functions together in various ways in a veritable consortium: container ↔ contained (♀♂), α-function, transformation, contact-barrier, Grid, and dreaming. At one point he conflated α-function and dreaming as "dream-work-α": Bion, 1992, p. 150) but then separated them again because of his realization that he was mixing a model (α-function) with a theoretical formulation and realization (dreaming) (P. Sandler, 2005). Furthermore, α-function supplies α-elements to participate in dreaming as dream thoughts. *I*, however, postulate that dreaming, α-function, contact-barrier, caesura are all interchangeable—that is, are cognates of each other.

L. Bion also seems to associate containing, dreaming, phantasying, and mythifying along a continuum and all but equates them and their functions. When one considers the operation of α-function, for instance, one can readily see that it constitutes a contact-barrier—or creates a contact-barrier in its own image, so to speak. Furthermore, I believe that the application of α-function to β-elements constitutes a separating, triaging, classifying function.

M. Do the distortions of dreaming involve –K (negative knowledge)? According to Bion (1962a), –K is characterized by a total opposition to the analytic work or the striving for truth (pp. 96–97). A better term for the operation of disguise may be "falsification" as opposed to "Lies" (de Bianchedi, 1993). I propose the alternative term *"fictionalization"*. Whereas –K characterizes lying, falsification may constitute what the individual unconsciously believes is a necessary modification of O, Truth, in order to be able to tolerate truth, albeit altered.

N. Bion states:

> One of the points I wish to discuss is related to the fact that *the actual events of the session*, as they are apparent to the analyst, *are being "dreamed" by the patient* [italics added] *not* in the sense that he believes that the events observed by him are the same as the events observed by the analyst (except for the fact that he believes them to be a part of a dream, and the analyst believes them to be a part of reality), but in the sense that these same events that are being *perceived* by the analyst are being perceived by the patient and treated to a process of being dreamed by him. That is, *these events are having something done to them mentally, and that which is being done to them is what I call being dreamed*. . . . [italics added]. [1992, p. 39]

In other words, in so far as he freely associates, the patient is *dreaming* the latent content of his associations; correspondingly, the very way in which the analyst listens to the analysand's associations itself constitutes *dreaming*. Bion states elsewhere that the analyst *must* dream the clinical situation (1992, p. 120). Thus, *all perceptions as well as other mental transformations constitute dreaming.* By extending Bion's revolutionary idea, could we now say that all human relations, particularly loving ones like those with family and friends, function as a co-dreamer—especially when we need to share our experiences with others?

O. While I think that sensory perception of emotional experience may initially become a β-element, I also believe that the infant (of any age) has its own α-function from the very beginning, as I stated earlier. As a result I believe that the infant *communicates* with his mother via his own pre-lexical version of α-elements, which the mother's α-function processes further. It is her failure to process them adequately that renders them into what Ferro (2005) terms "balpha-elements.

P. Dreaming—both waking dreaming and night-time dreaming—are either isomorphic with or cognate with α-function, transformation, contact-barrier, caesura, the Grid (which occurs in consciousness as well as in dreams), and L, H, and K linkages. They all have the same function: triaging, sorting out, deconstructing, reconfiguring, processing, mediating, encrypting, and transducing O. I include them all under the embrasure of the *"dream ensemble"*, which finds its neurological parallel in the reticular activating system, a supraordinating system that monitors and mediates the intensity of incoming afferent stimuli for neuronal tolerability as well as for consciousness.

As an aside, scientists say they have found a code beyond genetics in DNA (Wade, 2006)—one that oversees the ultimate destiny of the gene components and vouchsafes their arrival at their appropriate destination. This genetic function sounds like an analogue for an as yet unidentified mental function of dreaming and/or α-function which oversees the syntactic future of the α-elements.

How does dreaming work?

Dreaming seems to function like a sensitive emotional computer that aligns new events, converting them into personal experiences, first through careful *de*construction and then through imaginative *re*construction, recombination, and aesthetic reconfiguration of the events, correlating them with past experiences in order to achieve personal, subjective categorization of the events and their transformation into personal—and personally *meaningful*—emotional experiences. This categorization—or, really, re-categorization—of experiences seems to be one of the chief functions of dreaming. Perhaps one can imagine that before it is dreamt, the initial event engulfs the subject's mind, whereas once dreamt, the subject's mind engulfs the event as a category. Dreaming constitutes story-telling and seems to have a remarkable and ineffable narrative-developing capacity. Dreaming is paradoxically *revelatory* and protectively *disguising*. It utilizes the function known as "triage", which constitutes an instrument for prioritization and marginalization—that is, the assignment of foreground versus background status.

One may also employ the idea of the *anagram*: A patient reported a dream in which he was asked to supply the anagram for the phrase, "problem in China". In the dream itself he came up with "incomprehensible". When one deconstructs the phrase and the anagrammatized word to which it corresponds, one can readily see that the same *letters* are reconfigured in a different sequential order, but the letters themselves faithfully maintain their invariant nature. I believe, consequently, that the anagram is a very important constituent model for dream-work.

Freud (1900a) stressed the importance of the falsification, distortion, and secondary revision of the latent content of dreams by the dreaming process (p. 488). Bion (1965), emphasizing the subject's hunger for truth (p. 38), hypothesizes that dreaming escorts the truth in disguise. Thus, the original Absolute Truth becomes altered by dream-work, but the nucleus of the Truth will endure and persist as an invariant through all its transformations in the transformational cycle, albeit encased within falsifications (fictions) until interpreted. Dreaming transforms the infantile neurosis into the transference neurosis. Dreaming disguises truth in order to protect truth and also aesthetically enhances, elaborates, and augments it.

The act of dreaming strongly suggests that the human being must be born with a propensity for story-telling, story-seeking, and story-responding, one that issues from the aesthetic vertex (Bion, 1970, p. 21). Dreaming also seems to ferret out hidden constant conjunctions (strong linkages or "marriages" of ideas) and establish new ones *in statu nascendi*. Dreaming consists in a unique and uncanny choreography of images: I (Grotstein, 2000a, 2005b) assign the role of the unconscious "choreographer", a "daimon", "intelligence", or "presence", to the "dreamer who dreams the dream". Dreaming also involves the transduction of β-elements from infinity and total symmetry, Absolute Time, and Absolute Space—acting simultaneously—to binary opposites in linear, diachronic sequence portrayed as narrative in the form of unconscious phantasy, constituting the emotional "CNN" or "BBC" of the System *Ucs.*

The human being possesses a narrative propensity, perhaps even drive, to offset evolving O's regressive destabilizing effect on the psyche. Narrative, in its linearity, binds infinite O's trajectory by offering credible rationales for the occurrence occasioned by O's intersection of one's emotional frontier. O can be thought of as a myriad unknowables lurking simultaneously and vertically (right-hemisphere mode). Dreaming realigns them longitudinally (left-hemisphere mode). The rationales may at first be fictional—in the form of dreams, unconscious phantasies, conscious daydreams, or myths. The human being seems to be a story-teller and a story-requisitioner. The purpose of the story is to bind the anxiety created by O by transforming (transferring) it into a fictive but credible narrative structure that restores the subject's sense of cosmic causality and coherence. "The Holocaust occurred because of the will of God" constitutes such a fiction, which would be credible to some and would give closure to the inexplicability of the Holocaust.

The unconscious demonstrates a narrative function—that is, a propensity or drive for narrating and narrative-seeking, which both narrates (fictionalizes) incoming events into personal experiences and seeks narratives, stories, myths, novels, and so on in order to bind the anxieties of uncertainty and chaos left in the wake of intersecting O. In the course of fictionalizing O, the narrative function is able to preserve the emotional truth as an invariant that is implicit in O's encounter with one. In the course of creating a fictional narrative, the raw data from O—that is, the infinite impersonal data within the β-elements—become initially *personified* (Klein, 1929), as in children's cartoons, into personalized unconscious dreams or phantasies, which thereupon undergo a reconfiguration of story structure, disarticulation of the object-linkages in the original cosmic event, and transvaluation of the emotional relationships to new unimportant entities for purposes of disguise.

In other words, the unconscious, along with the contact-barrier, functions in part as an emotional frontier, an immunity shield, filter, or grating, which, much like an antibody (with an inherent "memoir of the future" antigen it is destined to encounter) hastens to counterattack the antigen from O via (1) an emotional registration of O's impact, and (2) attempts to neutralize the impact by dreaming—that is, narrativization, fictionalization. The final result will be (1) a somatic *emo-*

tional categorization that anticipates being *felt* by the mind (Damasio (2003) and (2) a dream or unconscious phantasy, which has mythified, personified, and personalized the story in terms of subjective meaning for the recipient. A story has emerged from the creative process of the unconscious. Other stories will be sought from other sources (e.g. novels, plays, etc.) in order to protect the credible fiction of coherence and meaning. The subject projectively identifies with the characters in these other sources and unconsciously adjust himself and his own unique story-needing aspect to the characters and plot at hand, vicariously participating in the story.

Stories, dreams, phantasies, and myths have, as their purpose, the creation of credible fictions of coherence and plausible understanding about personal and interposing cultural events. Ultimately an unconscious phantasy must be either summoned from the analysand's unconscious reservoir of inherent and/or acquired phantasies or sought from the analyst's interpretation, to allow it to accommodate the immediate O incident that has occurred. This spontaneous or supplied phantasy (story) must, in turn, correspond to a "hidden order of art" (Ehrenzweig, 1967) that accommodates the required constraints of a universal or acquired myth, such as the Oedipus myth, the myth of Prometheus, of the Garden of Eden, of the Tower of Babel, and so on. Once confirmed by and within the authority of myth, the patient experiences a sense of an inner cosmic unity that bespeaks an acceptable personal *truth* and, with it, security.

Just as one of the functions of α-function, according to Bion (1962b), is the production of α-elements to reinforce and maintain the integrity of the contact-barrier (p. 17), so dreaming produces dreams and phantasies that proliferate to form a phantasmal network of unconscious structures, which subserve an unconscious system of predominantly symmetrical operations (Matte Blanco, 1975, 1988).

Matte Blanco (1975, 1988) conceives of the unconscious as consisting of infinite sets of all objects and as being the seat of ever-expanding symmetry as one descends into the unconscious. Bion sees the unconscious as the dialectically collaborative partner of consciousness in the apprehension and transformation of β-elements issuing from O. It may be reasonable to conceive that, contrary to Freud's (1915e) statement that the unconscious lacks structure, it does have one (albeit in terms of infinity and ever-expanding degrees of symmetry). The structure of the unconscious would consist not only of the drives, the Ideal Forms, and things-in-themselves (the latter two comprising one arm of Bion's conception of O, the other arm being the "sensory stimuli of emotional experience"), but also of mythic or dream-phantasy structures that serve as ongoing protective transformational templates to intercept, filter, triage, reconfigure, process, encode, and transduce the β-elements from impersonal O finally to one's personal fiction (dream, phantasy) about one's relationship to the O of the moment. Put another way, that aspect of the unconscious that sponsors the emergent "thoughts without a thinker" (the Ideal Forms, the noumena) constitutes *entelechy*—the activation of one's inherent (irruptive) potential—whereas dreaming constitutes one's *conatus* or *conation*.

It is my hypothesis that the unconscious becomes the continuation of the infantile state of innocence and coherence, a quality of infancy to which infant developmentalists refer as "contingency" (Beebe & Lachman, 1988; Schore, 2003a, 2003b). The concept of contingency designates a symmetrically responsive caretaker who "does not miss a beat", so to speak, in her caring and attuning of the infant. As the infant begins to separate from its mother, more and more non-contingent relations become tolerated. It is my hypothesis that as non-contingent, separating, asymmetrical interrelationships develop, the original bid for contingent symmetry goes underground and becomes an unconscious propensity guarded over by dreaming-phantasying, under the sway of the pleasure principle.

To reiterate: the unconscious and consciousness function as a binary-oppositional structure within which the functions of the pleasure and reality principles, respectively and in dialectical combination, are played out. Together, they intercept, monitor, register, encode, and transform O, raw Circumstance, "*Ananke*". Psychopathology is an indication of a rent in the otherwise seamless mythical, phantasmal dreamworld of symmetry, which exists side by side in the unconscious with scar-tissue objects—unhealed (undreamed) veterans of ancient wars with O. From this point of view all internal objects constitute unsuccessful containers of O from bygone times—awaiting the dreaming, the analysis—that can rescue and redeem them.

The visual aspects of dreaming seem to be a predominant characteristic:

> But the important and striking feature revealed by a comparison of the mental counterparts of visual with other vertices is *the superior power of the visual vertex to illuminate . . . a problem over that of all other mental counterparts of the senses.* Reversal of direction in the system of which the vertex is a part is associated with what are ordinarily known as hallucinations. *The supremacy of the visual vertex contributes*

to my belief that the solution of the problem of communicating psychoana-
lytically will have to be found through row C elements to geometrical for-
mulation and thence to row H elements [of the Grid—JSG]. [Bion, 1965,
pp. 90–91; italics added]

What is the function of dreaming?

Freud (1900a) considered the function of dreaming to be to preserve
sleep from disturbing latent content from day residues (pp. 233–234).
Bion, in extending the range of dreaming to occur throughout the day
and night, postulated that dreaming, which is at times indistinguishable in his writings from α-function, serves to process and meaningfully
transform incoming stimuli from within and without. These stimuli
are the sensory stimuli of emotional experience, as alluded to earlier.
When Bion (1962b) applies the act of dreaming to the analyst, and to
the analysand as well, he suggests yet another function for dreaming:
creative revelation or scanning of clinical as well as non-clinical phenomena (p. 105).

Bion (1970), exhorts the analyst to "abandon memory and desire"
(p. 32) so as to be conversant with the "Language of Achievement" (the
empty language dedicated for emotional revelation through intuition),
as opposed to the "language of substitution" (of representative images
or symbols), and resonate with the fundamental emotional theme, O,
within oneself as it matches that of the analysand. In other words, for
the analyst dreaming is an observational technique (perception itself)
that is uniquely qualified to apprehend emotional qualities in oneself
and the other. (I develop this theme further when I discuss the contributions of the art critic, Anton Ehrenzweig.)

The epitome of the analytic process in the analyst is "becoming"
the analysand—that is, when the analyst is able to recreate, to "give
birth" to, to "become" the analysand from within himself (Bion, 1965,
p. 146; Brown, 2006; Ogden, 2004a). *Through dreaming, the analyst "be-*
comes" his own, native version of the analysand.

The normal subject must have experienced his mother's (and father's) caring consciously as a healthy attachment and unconsciously
as the effect of their reverie, containment, and use of α-function, and
of their dreaming of his experiences in order to process them for
healthy internalization. As the infant develops, he becomes able to
exercise these functions autonomously. α-function is the servant and
supplier of dreaming, and both function continuously, day and night.

Dreaming constitutes the monitor par excellence of the subject's interface with intruding object-stimuli from the inner and outer worlds. Its function is to render all stimuli into unconscious correlated categories that allow the subject to bind the anxieties that the dreams intercept. Dreams are ingeniously conceived "archival fictions" or "novels" that maintain the integrity of Truth as an invariant in the context of a protective fictive backdrop arranged by encryption or encoding, so that the integrity of System *Ucs.* and System *Pcs.* can be maintained and continually restored.

According to Bion, first cause in both normal development and psychopathology is the success or lack of success of dreaming—that is, the containing of experiences. System *Cs.* possesses the faculty of reflective reasoning and perception, but this faculty fundamentally depends on support from the emotional foundations of Systems *Ucs.* and *Pcs.*, all of which participate in triangulating and modulating O. Dreaming repairs the protective structures and functions of all three Systems, but, above all, it *monitors and repairs the Unconscious Systems* (*Ucs.* and *Pcs.*) by reconfiguring unconscious phantasies that can collectively, as a phantasmal or mythic network, subtend and support System *Cs.* and the far reaches of our being. Bion's view of dreaming, especially dreaming-by-day, devolves into what the subject *does* to his perception of the object, which can be condensed into what perception does to the image of the object. Thus, the analyst dreams his conscious *and* unconscious experience of the analysand, and the latter does the same with the analyst. Ogden (2007a, 2007b) applies this theme of Bion's to the very act of speaking.

Finally, it is my opinion that dreaming mediates and integrates the two major streams of O and their convergence in experience. The sensory stimuli of emotional experience summon their inborn counterparts, the inherent pre-conceptions ("memoirs of the future"), and unite as the latter incarnate or become realized as conceptions and then concepts. Dreaming orchestrates this continuing union and infusion.

Ehrenzweig's The Hidden Order of Art

What Bion means by dreaming and what he seeks to achieve by abandoning memory and desire (secondary process) is shown by Ehrenzweig (1967) when he reminds us of Piaget's (1926) concept of "syncretistic vision"—a visual mode characterized by condensation and non-differentiation:

Creative work succeeds in coordinating the results of unconscious undifferentiation and conscious differentiation and so reveals the hidden order in the unconscious. [Ehrenzweig, 1967, pp. 4–5]

Unconscious scanning makes use of undifferentiated modes of vision that to normal awareness would seem chaotic. Hence comes the impression that the primary process merely produces chaotic phantasy material that has to be organized and shaped by the ego's secondary process. *On the contrary, the primary process is a precision instrument for creative scanning that is far superior to discursive reason and logic. [p. 5; italics added].*[8]

A hidden order guides soft-focusing or scanning. [p. 9] [*Bion again*— JSG]

Unconscious scanning grasps the widely scattered derivatives in a single immediate act of comprehension. [p. 10]

This recognition of objects from cues rather than from the analysis of abstract detail is the beginning of syncretic vision. Analytic vision would only obstruct the recognition of the object. [p. 15]

Undifferentiated unconscious scanning extracts from the many variable details a common denominator or fulcrum which serves as the "cue" [*selected fact*—JSG]. [p. 17]

Ehrenzweig seems to be saying that primary process is associated with syncretistic, soft-focusing scanning and is necessary for creative attention.

Autochthonous creativity, adaptive editorial transformation, and censorship as the main functions of dreaming

Bion's theory of dreaming was revolutionary. Extending and modifying Freud's dream theory, he conceived of it almost like an immune frontier that, by day and by night, intercepts β-elements, proto-emotional messages laced with primal O impressions from the Absolute Truth about Ultimate, Infinite Reality, and grades, sorts, and processes them to convert them into tolerable personal archival *fictions* about the Truth, now rendered as *personal emotional truth*. In the course of this numinous dreaming venture, the unconscious creative process of *autochthony*, which I believe to be the principal component of dreaming, is at work, artistically reordering the raw ore of β-element truths according to the "hidden order of art" that is inherent as one's aesthetic capability (Ehrenzweig, 1967). Put another way, the act of dreaming, which includes mythifying and phantasying (containing and fictionalizing), preserves the veil of innocence for the infant and child and the sense of security for the adult by effectively reordering and reconfiguring the unconscious reception and thus perception of O into tolerable yet realistic fictions—or fictional realisms that one can live with. *The fiction must, however, always contain the invariant truth.* I call this function "adaptive editorial transformation and censorship". Autochthony, the birth myth of being born from the self and the self being the creator of the universe of objects (see *Genesis*), is the unconscious phantasy of creation in all its possibilities.

The distinction that Freud (1911b) made between the primary and secondary processes is only apparent, according to Bion. Although he did not use the term, Bion leads us to believe that the primary and secondary processes normally comprise a *binary-oppositional structure* (Lévi-Strauss, 1970)—one in which each functions in cooperative or collaborative dialectical opposition to the other. I suggest, in consequence, that the pleasure–unpleasure and reality principles also function as a binary-oppositional structure. Thus dreaming is conducted by a prophylactic fictionalization of incoming β-elements utilizing the pleasure–unpleasure principle *under the hegemony of the reality principle*. If the binary-oppositional structure is impaired by challenges to the contact-barrier, the functioning of the two principles begins to go awry—they split-off from one another and go their separate ways, and delusion replaces dreams and phantasies.

This narrative fictional ploy on the part of dreaming or α-function thus fundamentally depends on the cooperative functioning of the *pleasure* and *reality principles*—and now, following Bion (1970) and Britton (2006), we add the supraordinating function of the uncertainty principle, with the former being the prime organizers in the unconscious and the latter in consciousness. In cases of severe pathology, however, this binary-oppositional cooperation does not obtain. Instead, we see that the pleasure and reality principles abrogate their alliance, as a result of which Column 2 becomes a *Lie Column*, not just a benevolently *falsifying* (fictionalizing) or *negating* Column.

I had long wondered why Bion believed it was necessary to include a category in the Grid whose function was deliberate falsification—in other words, how would falsification (–K) be *adaptive* to the individual? My first tentative answer was to suggest the obligatory operation of Freud's (1911b) pleasure–unpleasure principle, which seeks to offset and counterbalance the reality principle. Then I began to realize that α-function itself, which to me represents the model for Bion's unique conception of dreaming, must uniquely blend the operations of the reality *and* pleasure–unpleasure principle in order for a "wild thought" (a "thought without a thinker" in Column 1 "Definitory Hypothesis") to proceed through the successive categories before qualifying as a formal "thought-about" thought. This idea follows Bion's hypothesis that the primary and secondary processes are not as separated as Freud (1900a, 1911b) thought they were.

Inherent in this radical reformulation is the conception that α-function, the model, and/or dreaming, the ineffable, actual, living process, both of which imply the container ↔ contained, occur earlier in the forging of the constant conjunction that constitutes the original, emergent Definitory Hypothesis and then later in Column 2 in forging the objective, abstract thought as a more developed and sophisticated version of the original constant conjunction. To repeat, this reformulation presumes that the pleasure–unpleasure principle and the reality principle constitute a *binary-oppositional* (*dialectical*) *structure*. The intactness of the structure, which allows for an optimal dialectical tension between the activities sponsored by each principle, fundamentally depends, in turn, on the integrity of the contact-barrier, whose own intactness depends on α-function/container ↔ contained/dreaming.

It is when we follow Bion in locating the concept of the Establishment in Column 2 (Bion, 1977a, p. 38) that the adaptive function of this column is clarified:

> In recent years there has grown up the use of the term Establishment; it seems to refer to that body of persons in the State who may be expected usually to exercise power and responsibility by virtue of their social position, wealth, and intellectual and emotional endowment. . . . I propose to borrow this term to denote everything from the penumbra of associations generally evoked, to the predominating and ruling characteristics of an individual, and the characteristics of a ruling caste in a group (such as a psycho-analytical institute, or a nation or group of nations). [1970, p. 73]
>
> The mystic is both creative and destructive. I make a distinction between two extremes that coexist in the same person. The extreme formulations represent two types: the "creative" mystic, who formally claims to conform to or even fulfil the conventions of the Establishment that governs his group; and the mystic nihilist, who appears to destroy his own creations. I mean the terms to be used only when there is outstanding creativeness or destructiveness, and the terms "mystic", "genius", "messiah" could be interchangeable. [p. 74]

The function of the group is to produce a genius; the function of the Establishment is to take up and absorb the consequences so that the group is not destroyed. [p. 82]

The governing body of the society I call the Establishment; the counterpart in the domain of thought would be the pre-existing disposition or pre-conception. [p. 111]

The reaction of the Establishment is to prevent the disruption, and this it does by incorporating the mystic within itself. [p. 112]

The common features are: containment of the messianic idea in the individual; containment of the messianic individual in the group; the problem for the Establishment that is concerned with the group on the one hand and the messianic idea and individual on the other. [p. 116]

In reading Bion's comments on the concept of the Establishment, which he seems to locate both in Column 2 of the Grid and as a pre-conception, one begins to conceive of the existence of a supraordinating "homunculus" or human "gyroscope" who possesses an unerring awareness of the individual's tolerance of the "dosage of Truth" with each incoming salvo from O and its sensory descendant, the β-element. Hooke's Law, which applies to inanimate objects, states that the stress in an object is equal to the strain that exists within its structure times the modulus of its elasticity. I suggest that a human counterpart to Hooke's Law exists, and that Column 2 constitutes its operations room. Put another way, the liar seems to have a valid (for him) conception of his tolerance of truth. This agency stands behind α-function and calibrates the dosage of sorrow and truth to its hapless ward, the subject. Moreover, the Establishment must find a substitute for genius and mediate between the creative and the destructive mystic or messiah, as Bion (1970, p. 73) points out. Put another way, the Establishment serves a container function as a mediating agency, concerned with the messianic idea in the individual on the one hand and the group messiah on the other. It thus constitutes a binary-oppositional structure involving the pleasure *and* reality principles.

Final verdict: Column 2 constitutes a container–dreamer–thinker function! In chapter 22 I suggested that there are two Grids: one for the secondary process, in Freud's (1911b) terms, and another for the primary processes of the unconscious. *Negation* is the principal function in the former, and *fictionalization* in the latter.

In the final analysis we must remember that Truth (about the Reality of indifferent, impersonal O) is the cargo that is being transported by emotion, its vehicle, through the sluices of Transformation's cat-egories, as through locks in a canal. The transformational cycle is completed when it reaches its destination, not only in our filtered and adulterated version of it known as K, but in our becoming it in person-alized subjective, meaningful O.

An analysand's dream

A 76-year-old married college professor with three grown children who has been in five-times-per-week analysis for four years pre-sented the following dream in the first session of the week:

I was entering a school which seemed to be an elementary school for young children. It was being taught by a man in his forties, someone who was charismatic and spoke authoritatively—even menacingly—to the young children. The children didn't appear upset. When the teacher saw me, he grimaced and gave me a chilling look. Then he came after me. I found that I had a gun in my hand, which surprised me. I became terrified, lost control, and fired a shot, which I saw enter his abdomen. He yelled with pain and exclaimed, "Why did you do that?" He appeared to be-come unconscious and then suddenly reawakened and said that he knew how much life energy he had left and now he was going to kill me! I shot again and the same sequences repeated them-selves. He wasn't to be deterred in his plan to kill me. I noticed that all the while this was happening the children didn't seem disturbed.

I awoke in terror, then went back to sleep, and had another brief dream. *I observed young children sucking on their fingers.*

Adaptive context and associations.   These dreams occurred during the long Thanksgiving weekend break. On the day before the dream the analysand and his wife had gone to see a film—*Good Night and Good Luck*—about Edward R. Murrow and his epic television battle with Senator Joseph McCarthy. He recalled the McCarthy era and revealed how terrified he had been of McCarthy. When he saw the film clips of McCarthy in the movie, he became terrified all over again. Even though he knew that Murrow had prevailed and Mc-Carthy had been disgraced, he felt the issue to be in doubt as he watched the film. The analysand is currently writing a book that has to do with his professional field. He believes that he may be putting forth some ideas that might be considered radical and provocative to others in the field, and especially in his department. The teacher's face reminded the analysand of a younger colleague, for whom he has great respect and affection, and he was thus surprised at his demeanor in the dream.

Analysis of the dream and my reverie (my emotional and objective observations):   I had immediately experienced the analysand's own experience of terror as my own and felt a desire both to protect him (and now myself) from this deadly, maniacal teacher and to calm him so that he would not have to use the gun. It was as if the dream—actually the nightmare—was still happening, and I had personally entered into it. Later I came to realize that he had come to me for protection against the other me—the mad teacher, whom that me ultimately represented—along with his projections into me. I then spontaneously recalled how he had once informed me that the "devil" in Greek is "*diabolos*", and this means "the scatterer". I subsequently realized that the evil, charismatic teacher represented O, an evolving, scattering force-field (paranoid–schizoid anxiety), which got steadily worse over the prolonged break. Senator McCarthy was a signifier who represented incompletely dreamed aspects of the analysand's personality relevant to that period of time. I remembered that I, too, had feared Joseph McCarthy: I had been compelled to sign a statement of my loyalty to the State of California when I became a psychiatric resident at the UCLA School of Medicine. I "became" (my internal version of) his anxiety—his anxiety and his demon became mine.

That evening I had a nightmarish dream in which a McCarthy-like figure was chasing me. Between hearing the patient's dream and dreaming my own dream, I had encountered another colleague at a restaurant whom I had not seen in almost 40 years. He had been on the opposite side in a bitter dispute at my analytic society when the Kleinians—of whom I was one—had been in great peril of expulsion. In my nightmare I conflated my patient's image of Joseph McCarthy with a signifier of my own personal demons from long ago. In so doing, I "became" the patient and dreamed him into life within my unconscious (Bion, 1965, p. 146; Brown, 2006; Ogden, 2004a).

Put another way, as the analysand shared his dream with me, it had been incompletely dreamed. As I listened to him, I unconsciously entered his continuing dream and "became" his "dreaming co-pilot" in order to complete the dream.

The demonic teacher also represented me, his "analytic teacher", who had become unconsciously filled with the analysand's hate—because of his having been "abandoned" over the long weekend—and had also become a harsh "superego editor" who enviously attacked and disapproved of his forthcoming book.

The analysand then recalled in the dream that he had shot the teacher four times (the number of days of the analytic interruption), and the last three times he had had a difficult time aiming at the teacher because of his fear of hitting one or more of the children. He wondered why the children seemed not to have been upset. I interpreted that perhaps the children were mine—who did get to spend the holiday weekend with me—and that they may have been under his or my special protection. (Here I was thinking of Klein's [1928] concept of the special, "unborn children" who are privileged to remain inside the mother's body.)

The analysand, who is Jewish, then recalled that the teacher had reminded him generically of the young gentile men he had known in his earlier life. He recalled a charismatic anti-Semitic Baptist minister. His parents are Holocaust survivors. Thus, another of the determinants of the dream was his dread of another Holocaust, with someone like Joseph McCarthy creating it. In addition, it appeared that the mad teacher also represented the omnipotent and cruel authority of his own envious and moralistic superego.

The second dream, which was apparently dreamed to patch the first unsuccessful dream, represented an awareness of childhood times when he had had to soothe himself by licking his thumb and fingers.

Note: Space limitations prevent me from presenting all the patient's associations to his dreams. He did mention that the dreams were far more elaborate and detailed than he could reveal, suggesting secondary revision. It is perhaps secondary revision that Bion is referring to when he says that when the analysand freely associates, he is dreaming. Furthermore, all the hypotheses I enumerated above came to me while I was "dreaming" the session and seeking to complete the analysand's dream by entering it as a "co-pilot dreamer".

One can see the effects of condensation and displacement in who it was that the mad teacher came to represent. Conditions of representability can be noted in the way the plot—especially of the first dream—was laid out. His fear that he could not kill the mad teacher before the latter killed him represents his unconscious awareness that I was the teacher and that he did not really want me to die. The ultimate mythic templates that subtended the analysand's unconscious phantasies were archaic oedipal ones with the addition of Bion's conception of the hyper-moralistic "super"ego (1962b, p. 97).

About this murderous, moralistic "super"ego, Bion says:

> I shall assume that the patient's fear of the murderous super-ego prevents his approaching the Positions. This in turn means that he is unable to dream, for it is in dreams that the Positions are negotiated. [1992, p. 27]

> His statements that he feels anxious—"I don't know why"—may, in addition to being denials, support very strongly, in view of their constant reiteration, my idea that there is a breakdown of dream-work-α, which makes it impossible for the feelings to be ideogrammaticized and so verbalized. This breakdown is due to the need to prevent the synthesis, in the depressive position, of a frightening super-ego. [p. 59]

Dreaming prepares the individual to accept modulating the paranoid–schizoid position so as to attain the depressive position. It is then that the analysand must face being confronted of the horror of his creations in P–S—that is, the murderous, hyper-moral "super"ego.

NOTES

1. The reader is referred to P. Sandler's (2005) in-depth review of the many changes in Bion's thinking about the relationship between α-function and dreaming. The relationship between "α-function" and "container $\leftrightarrow$ contained" has come to be better known. That between *dreaming* and container $\leftrightarrow$ contained has only been touched on recently by Grotstein (1981c, 2000a, 2002), Ogden (2004a), Paulo Sandler (2005), Schneider (2005), and others.

2 Further on in this chapter I conjecture that dreaming subsumes α-function, that it may *be* α-function and/or its cognate, a characteristic it shares with contact-barrier, transformations, containment, the Grid, and L, H, and K linkages.

3. The mystic does not need to take this detour.

4. O is not uncertain: our emotional experience of it is.

5. I am grateful to P. Sandler (2005) for these citations.

6. Weisberg (2006), speaking of Nicholas Humphrey's (2006) work on perception, states: "Humphrey holds that blind sight demonstrates the dissociability of sensation (the feel of experience) and perception (our awareness of the world). He adopts the bold suggestion that sensation is not part of the casual chain leading to perception. Instead, he argues, sensation makes up a separate, more primitive system that plays no direct role in our perception of the world. Sensation is self-contained evaluative activity . . ." (Weisberg, 2006, p. 577).

7. Freud (1915d) conceived of a repressive barrier that defends consciousness from the unconscious but not the reverse. Bion's concept of the contact-barrier, which he derived from Freud's (1950 [1895]) "Project for a Scientific Psychology", functions as a mediating protective barrier in both directions.

8. This idea is totally congruent with Bion's view of dreaming.

CHAPTER 26

Dreaming, phantasying, and the "truth instinct"

I n this chapter I seek to throw new light on the nature and function of unconscious phantasies. Freud (1914d) wrote that

> Phantasies were intended to cover up the autoerotic activity of the first years of childhood, to embellish it and raise it to a higher plane. And now, from behind the phantasies, the whole range of a child's sexual life came to light. [Freud, 1914d, p. 18]

I pose the question: Does a validated interpretation mitigate the effect of the operant unconscious phantasy in favour of reality, and/or does it release a troubled or obstructed—and therefore clinically failing—phantasy from its obstruction so that it can then proceed on its way and re-enter the mythic stream or phantasy cycle of the unconscious? Behind this question lies yet another: May not psychopathology be due, from one perspective, to defective or inadequate phantasying and/or dreaming, as Bion suggests in his radical theory of dreaming? If that is indeed the case, then the effect of validated interpretations may be, in part, to assist, correct, reinforce, supply, or free-up extant troubled phantasies or dreams (phantasies/dreams that themselves are in trouble: that is, not properly functioning). Behind this line of thought is Bion's hypothesis that all experiences (external and internal) need to be dreamed (phantasied) in order to be processed, and

DOI: 10.4324/9781003348665-27

that psychopathology may be due—if not totally, then in part—to a defect, the source of which lies in defective "α-function" or "dream-work-α" (Bion, 1962a, 1962b)—that is, defective or inadequate phantasying or dreaming.

Alpha-function combines the primary and secondary processes. These premises derive from the cooperative bimodal "binocularity" (stereoscopy) that he posits to exist between the Systems *Ucs.* and *Cs.*, which he considers to be in collaborative dialogue—in opposition but not in conflict with each other, provided that the contact-barrier that separates and mediates them is intact, which fundamentally depends on the operation of α-function to supply α-elements to maintain and restore it.

Bion's psychoanalytic epistemology

The analyst must abandon memory and desire, the derivatives of sensation, so as not to be misled by images or symbols of the object, which, though they *represent* the object, are *not* the object (Bion, 1962b). Only then can the analyst, with much patience—the patience of tolerating uncertainty and doubts—be qualified to *"become"* the analysand or, more precisely, "become", through immersion and absorption, the analysand's distress, O (β-elements) (Bion, 1965, 1970). In this state of reverie, the analyst has become the container for the analysand's projected mental content (contained) (Bion, 1962b). Bion calls this *thinking* and also *dreaming*. As the mother does for her infant, so the analyst absorbs the analysand's pain by partial or trial identification ("becoming") and allows it to become part of himself. In his reverie he then allows his own repertoire of conscious and unconscious personal experiences to be summoned, so that some of them may be symmetrical to or match up with the analysand's still unfathomable projections (β-elements, O). Eventually, the analyst sees a pattern in the material—that is, the pattern becomes the selected fact that allows the analyst to interpret it (create a permanent constant conjunction of the elements).

The analyst's function as *container* seamlessly blends with Bion's (1965, 1970) notions of *dreaming, thinking, α-function*, the Grid, and the *contact-barrier* between the Systems *Ucs.* and *Cs.* Alpha-function (dreaming) intercepts the β-elements (O) of raw, unmentalized experience and transforms them into α-elements that are suitable for memory and thought—but also for reinforcing the contact-barrier. The sturdier the contact-barrier, the more the analysand can learn from his experience because he is better able to think—because he is more able to distinguish (separate). One must first be separate in order to separate mentally. For Bion, *thinking* (*dreaming*) occurs after thoughts first arrive as "thoughts without a thinker" ("β-elements", O"), awaiting a thinker (thinking mind) to think them. The mother's α-function is the infant's first thinker/dreamer. When the infant introjects mother's α-function, he is then able to think/dream his own thoughts. The projective identification of β-elements into the container (first the mother, then within the self) is the origin of thinking and dreaming.

Thus, the better the container with its (his) α-function, the better the analysand can think. What does thinking mean here? For Bion, thinking has two forms. The first, "becoming", the non-Cartesian form, the one just discussed, consists of dreaming (phantasying, α-function), much of which is involved in reinforcing the selectively permeable contact-barrier. The better the containment by the object or the self, the more effective is the selectivity of the contact-barrier in its capacity to define, refine, and guard the frontiers between *Ucs.* and *Cs.* and allow through "wild thoughts" (inspired) from *Ucs.* to *Cs.* and irrelevant thoughts from *Cs.* to *Ucs.* In other words, in this form of thinking, the subject *becomes* what he is processing as an experience.

The second form of thinking is Cartesian (subject–object differentiation) and is characterized by abstraction, reflection, correlation, publication, and shifting of perspectives. The second form of thinking can be seen in Bion's Grid (1977a), which is a polar-coordinated table in which the left-hand column, the genetic axis, designates, from top to bottom, the progressive sophistication and abstraction of thoughts. The horizontal axis designates thinking itself—how the thoughts are being thought about.

Interpenetrating Bion's ideas about the first and second forms of thinking is his notion of the contact-barrier or caesura (1965, 1977a) and its flexible function of dividing and reuniting different elements. He refers to this in his formula P–S ↔D, where the former divides (splits) and the latter unites in improvisational combinatorial virtuosity (creative or inventive thinking). The Oedipus complex represents one aspect of the barrier. Abstraction refines the essence of the common denominator in any element. Correlation represents the comparison function. Publication is the ability of the mind to be receptive to its own "wild thoughts". Shifting of perspectives from multiple vertices represents the ultimate ratiocinative reflection on data obtained from within or externally. In *A Memoir of the Future* (1975, 1977b, 1979, 1981) he referred to it as "disciplined debate".

Phantasy as the obligatory counterpart or accompaniment to reality (binocular vision)

In *Learning from Experience* Bion presents his next major difference with Freud, that of the latter's distinction between the primary and secondary processes (Freud, 1911b):

> The weakness of this [Freud's—JSG] theory of consciousness is manifest in the situation for which I have proposed the theory that α-function, by proliferating α-elements, is producing the contact-barrier. . . . The theory of consciousness is weak, not false, because by amending it to state that the conscious and unconscious thus constantly produced together do function as if they were binocular therefore capable of correlation and self-regard. . . . For these reasons . . . I find the theory of primary and secondary processes unsatisfactory. [Bion, 1962b, p. 54]

Here Bion, who had already challenged Freud on the primacy of the wish-fulfilment hypothesis that Freud (1900a) had assigned to the motive of dreams, was now challenging him again in terms of the autonomy of the wish-fulfilling notion of the unconscious as well as of the primary processes. Eventually, Freud's wish-fulfilment hypothesis seems, in my opinion, to have ended up in Column 2, the "psi column", of Bion's (1977a) famous Grid, as the saturated element that attacks and challenges the truth that inheres in the emerging definitory hypothesis of Column 1.[1] The implications of this for psychoanalysis were to become so far-reaching that to this very day they have not been fully realized. Bion believed that the unconscious emits the Absolute Truth about Ultimate Reality (which he would later call O—1965, 1970) *vis-à-vis* what *I* call the "truth instinct", not wish-fulfilling drives primarily.

Dreams mediate and facilitate the acceptance of Truth in transformations initiated by what Bion (1962a) was to call "α-function" ("dream-work α"—Bion, 1992). Thus, he stood the psychic apparatus and the theory of the unconscious on its head. His conception of the binocular complementarity and reciprocity between the Systems *Ucs.* and *Cs.* became a radical revision of Freud's view of their being in adversarial conflict. Bion views them as oppositional partners situated in different vertices, each responsive to and participating in mediating O (β elements, the Absolute Truth about Ultimate Reality, noumena, things-in-themselves, godhead). Bion was to do the same with Klein's (1940, 1946) concepts of the paranoid–schizoid and depressive positions—that is, reinterpret them as being cooperatively and complementarily dialectical in confronting and processing (transforming) O (P–S ↔D).]

The Raw, Absolute Truth had to be mitigated by being subjected to dreaming (phantasying) according to aesthetically creative considerations, so that two masters had to be accommodated: (1) the reality principle primarily, and (2) the pleasure principle secondarily. Implicit in this conception is the notion of a binocular function of the two principles in which the reality principle is predominant and mediates the operation of the pleasure principle. We witness this idea in dreams. Like miners sifting for gold, we analysts respect the truth that is implicit in dreams, thanks to the reality-principle aspect of α-function, and carefully sift through their manifest content, replete as the latter is with protective censorship and distortion, thanks to the operation of the pleasure-principle aspect of α-function (see Ehrenzweig, 1967; see also chapter 25). Thus, by using binocular vision, Bion places dreaming (phantasying) and cognition on parallel, dialectically interacting courses. According to Albert Mason (2000), who had been in training supervision with Bion in London:

> I have often likened analysis to riding a bicycle. Recalling the process, I first had to learn to hold the handlebars and use the brakes, then to balance, and to learn all the rules of the road. When these were mastered, Paula Heimann told me to take my hands off the handlebars and let my countertransference take over. Finally, Bion removed the front wheel and told me to steer with that intuitive binocular mind, which I hoped was a distillate of all that I had learned and had now forgotten. While it appears to have no memory or desire, the binocular mind has digested its experiences and now faces the unknown enemy outside in the patient, as well as the saboteur within itself. [Mason, 2000, p. 988]

The breakdown of "binocular vision"

The protocol described above applies to the normal situation of the unitary self—or to the normal or neurotic aspect of a troubled personality. As for the troubled, split-off, dissociated aspect of the personality, Bion variously dealt with this aspect as "The Imaginary Twin" (1950) and "Differentiation of the Psychotic from the Non-Psychotic Personalities" (1957b). Both here and in his other early case descriptions in *Second Thoughts* (1967c), he attributes this to an "infantile catastrophe" that had occurred in many of the cases, resulting in a major cleft in the personality.

As the personality divides, the binocular vision disappears, and each split-off self becomes concretistically monocular. As a result, the pleasure principle functions no longer under the hegemony of the reality principle but almost entirely along the principle of avoiding unpleasure at all costs. This is what Bion (1956, 1957b, 1958, 1959, 1962a) calls "psychotic thinking". It is characterized, *inter alia*, by an avoidance of reality, an intolerance of frustration, excessive protective identification (as opposed to introjection) in order to rid the psyche of painful thoughts and feelings, hallucinosis as a substitute for dreaming, and a reversal of α-function. Today I believe that we can apply what Bion ascribed to the psychotic to the split-off aspects of primitive mental disorders and to pathological organizations or psychic retreats (Steiner, 1993).[2] If Bion is right, then Freud's (1911b) distinction between the primary and secondary processes applies only to psychopathology where a split or dissociation has occurred, the secondary process loses its dominion over the primary process, and the latter becomes pathologically autonomous as a psychic retreat (Steiner, 1993) or is transformed into "α-function in reverse" (–K) (Bion, 1962b, p. 25).

In these cases a seemingly separate pathological personality evolves that functions—solely along the pleasure–pain principle—to abrogate the reality principle and to sabotage progress. Bion (1962b) wrote about "α-function in reverse" (p. 25), where the psychotic personality had purloined the healthy personality's α-function for itself and had thereby developed "method in its madness". Bion's other way of formulating this rupture of the personality is to consider the dreaming or phantasying process itself as being impaired.

We now turn to Bion's hypothesis about defective dreaming—the origins of dreaming itself in the container (1962a, 1962b).

The "truth instinctual drive"

Behind these assumptions is Bion's (1965, p. 38) belief that the psyche requires truth in the way the soma requires food. *This and his conception of O* (which he associates with the Absolute Truth about the Ultimate Reality of raw Circumstance[3] and which he also associates with β-elements—that is, unprocessed mental elements), *transcends Freud's* (1911b) *concept of the hegemony of the libido principle and Klein's* (1933) *concept of the primacy of the death instinct in unconscious mental life by postulating the activity of a "truth instinct"* (Bion, 1992, pp. 99–101, 299–300; personal communication, 1979).

Having transformed Freud's (1905d, 1920g) drive theory and added Klein's (1930) emphasis on the epistemological part-instinct, Bion conceived of the L, H, and K basic and inherent links between self and object (1962b). Though he speaks of them individually, he implies that they are inseparable when experienced—that is, one "knows" the object by how one feels (L and/or K) about it. In other words, these links conflate affects and drives and reorganize them as personal and emotional ways of knowing how one feels about an object. They represent emotional (loving and/or hateful) knowing. Bion (1965, p. 38; personal communication, 1979) then extended K to include the "truth instinct" and linked its operation with the evolutions of O and its intersections with the individual's emotional frontier.

One learns (gains) from experience by being able to tolerate its uncertainty and/or severity and by being able to process it into its personal (subjective) and object meaning, according to Bion (1962b). This processing is originally performed jointly by mother and infant, using the mother's reverie and α-function, and later by the infant alone as he incorporates the experience of mother's α-function for himself. The "Absolute (impersonal and infinite) Truth about Ultimate Reality", if initially tolerated and accepted, becomes transduced, first, into "personal truth" (K) about oneself *vis-à-vis* how one responds to O's impact (paranoid–schizoid position) and, second, into "objective (realistic) truth" (depressive position).

"The truth of the matter is that I cannot face the truth!"

Bion (1970, p. 98) distinguishes between falsehood and lies. The former relates to well-known defence mechanisms that operate so as to censor, alter, or disguise the truth for palatability. Lies, on the other hand, utterly disavow truth in favour exclusively of the pleasure–pain principle. Paradoxically the liar, like the psychotic, is closer to the truth than is the neurotic, whose defence mechanisms are such that they partially falsify the truth. The liar and the psychotic seem to have a more genuine estimation of their vulnerabilities regarding their inability to face truth as well as of the broader implications of the truth that they feel fated to confront.[4] Psychotic patients, those with character disorders, and those suffering from other primitive mental disorders all claim, if I may summarize their beliefs in a collective statement: "The truth of the matter is that I cannot face the truth because I know the truth all too well, having not been sufficiently shielded from it, and I know the limitations of my inner resources (my α-function) to deal with it—and that's the truth." This "truth" may explain why so many of the psychotic patients discussed by Rosenfeld (1965) and Bion (1967c) experienced negative therapeutic reactions when they encountered the threshold of the depressive position—that is, the "moment of truth". Yet another perspective of their plight *vis-à-vis* truth is their apparent forfeiture of their "entelechy"—their hopes for future development. It is as if they had early on made a veritable pact with the devil (their death instinct[5]) to eschew promise and progress in order to maintain the illusion of safety, a safety "vouchsafed" by their "protective" psychic retreat (Steiner, 1993).

Parenthetically—following Fairbairn's (1943) conception, with which I agree, that only bad objects are internalized, not good objects (p. 63)—one might hypothesize that all internal objects constitute defective containers of O.

"Binocular vision": α-function conflates *primary* and *secondary processes*

Central to Bion's (1965) thinking is the concept of "binocular vision" or "mental stereoscopy"—a dual-track model in which polar opposites conjoin collaboratively for a common goal, much like the operation of the two cerebral hemispheres. Bion's view is that the primary and secondary processes combine as a binary-oppositional structure (α-function) to constitute a binocular vision of internal and external mental life. Similarly, the Systems *Ucs.* and *Cs.*, rather than being in conflict with one another, constitute a binocular vision of O. To apply this to the clinical situation: when an interpretation is validated (by the analysand's unconscious), this means that: (1) a truth has been acknowledged and accepted by the analysand, with corresponding emotional growth; and (2) the truth was acceptable because it was not the *whole truth*—that is, the Absolute Truth about the Ultimate Reality of raw Circumstance. Dreaming (phantasying) attenuated its impact. Some fictionalization must always accompany the truth—except in the case of the mystic—according to Bion (1970).

The container and the contained (♀♂) and their coalescence with dreaming and phantasying

Bion (1956, 1959, 1962a) began to realize that the psychotic patients whom he was analysing had lacked the childhood experience of having competently caring mothers who could "contain" their infants' cries of distress, which Bion interpreted as projective identifications into them of their fear of dying (Bion's way of referring to the death instinct). He then formulated—independently of Winnicott's (1960b) "holding environment"—the concept that in normal development the infant experiences intolerable (for the moment) emotions and experiences that require the mother, in a state of *reverie* (thoroughly immersed in her infant's experience to the exclusion of self) to allow her α-function to enhance her "dreaming her infant". This "dreaming" can be compared with Stanislavski's (1936) "method acting", in which the actor, rather than attempting to understand the role he is to play, allows instead his own inner repertoire of life experiences to match up symmetrically with the part.[6] The principle is virtually the same with the mother as container with the infant and the analyst with the analysand. Bion then enjoins the mother, as well as the analyst, to "abandon memory and desire" (as well as preconceptions and understanding) so that the container–mother-analyst can "cast a beam of intense darkness into the interior so that something hitherto unseen in the glare of the illumination can glitter all the more in that darkness".[7] As Bion (1970) states: "Freud said that he had to 'blind myself artificially to focus all the light on one dark spot'" (p. 57; see also p. 43).

Bion (1962a, 1962b) goes on to suggest that the normal infant projects into its mother as container, who, in her reverie, willingly receives, absorbs, and processes her infant's projections. "Processes" means allowing them to settle within her and allowing her internal world to match up symmetrically with the content (unconsciously). At first she may experience uncertainty or anxiety, or even chaos or randomness. After a while her patience is rewarded with an intuition of sudden awareness about a coherence in all the chaotic data she has experienced. Freud called this the moment of "*aha Erlebnis*" and Bion the "selected fact". One may also think of it as the "strange attractor" of chaos theory.

It must be remembered, however, that the containing process is equated by Bion with dreaming. The mother as container must *dream* her infant (as well as her infant's content—that is, "contained"). This maternal dreaming function includes: (1) a renal-dialysis-like function in which a "detoxification" of the emotional projections occurs; (2) a sorting-out and matching-up with unconscious, and then conscious, aspects of the mother's own repertoire of experiences; (3) a repression of those elements that the infant is not prepared to "digest" at this time (issues of timing and dosage); and (4) corrective action of one kind or another that would amount to doing something appropriate—or giving an interpretation, if one is an analyst.

Bion theorizes that as time goes on, the normal infant introjects the mother's use of her α-function for himself and thereafter begins to project internally. *Bion considers this operation to be the foundation of thinking, which he distinguishes from thoughts proper.* The latter were the β-elements, the content of the infant's projective identifications, which Bion (1992, p. 325) also terms "thoughts without a thinker" awaiting a thinker (a container) to think them.[8] Thus, the capacity for "successful dreaming and/or phantasying is directly dependent on the individual's own self-"containing" capacity, which is, in turn, dependent in great measure on the legacy of having been successfully contained—that is, dreamed—by caretaking objects. Lest these ideas appear to be too recondite, let me approach them in another way. *The infant looks at reality through the veritable periscope of his mother's eyes. If mother (and father) can countenance their own experience of O, then the infant can. Tolerating O is made possible only by virtue of dreaming-containing.*

The contact-barrier and dreaming

One of the functions of dreaming is to render a continuing supply of α-elements to the contact-barrier, according to Bion (1962b, p. 17). This seems almost identical to Freud's (1915d) repressive barrier, but it differs in one significant way, as we shall soon see. The purpose that lay behind the need to maintain the integrity and functioning of the contact-barrier is to guarantee its operation as a gatekeeper in separating the System *Ucs.* from the System *Cs.*—*and the reverse.* It seems to have been Freud's idea that the System *Cs.* needed protection from irruptions from the System *Ucs.* but not the other way around. Bion, however, sees both systems as constituting a cooperative, binary-oppositional (not necessarily conflictual) complementarity in which both scan O and inform one another of their respective findings—a triangulation of observation.

> The contact-barrier may be expected to manifest itself clinically—if indeed it is manifest at all—as something that resembles dreams. [1962b, p. 26]

We have just seen that Bion equates dreaming with containing. Now we shall see what I believe to be a seamless chain of continuity between dreaming, containing, and other entities, such as: (1) dreaming or phantasying itself; (2) the "caesura" between fetaldom and birth; (3) "negation" (as a necessary aspect of Aristotelian logic), (4) the "Oedipus complex" (both Kleinian *and* Freudian versions[9]); (5) the "analytic frame"—itself an ongoing temptation to the analysand to challenge and an obligation by the analyst to vouchsafe; and (6) the "container" (Bion, 1959, 1962b) whose task it is to absorb, process, transform (transduce and translate) some aspects of the subject's distress—as the "contained"—into tolerable meaning as interpretation and hold on to other aspects that the subject is not yet ready to bear (repression, dosage, timing, the destiny of the "return of the repressed").[10]

The contact-barrier can be likened, to some extent, to a *cell membrane*, which must contain and define the cell within the tissue of its location *and* at the same time be able to allow nutrients into and waste-products out of the cell. In other words, it must function as a *selectively permeable* membrane.[11] Dreaming is equivalent to α-function, which, in turn, is equivalent to an ongoing contact-barrier, and it functions to maintain the intactness of the boundary between the Systems *Ucs* and *Cs.* while at the same selectively allowing certain "qualified" elements across its frontier—each way. Moreover, not only does dreaming supply α-elements to reinforce the contact-barrier, but the contact-barrier itself, by virtue of its ability to separate the Systems *Ucs.* and *Cs.*, makes it safe for dreaming to take place. In other words, a closed loop seems to exist between them.

Bion (1965, p. 38) also considers the function of the Systems *Ucs.* and *Cs.* to be to reveal truth (as a mercifully diluted and processed version of the Absolute Truth about the Ultimate Reality of raw Circumstance, O, β-elements). Freud (1915e), on the other hand, views the System *Ucs.* as a "seething cauldron" and unadulteratedly hedonic (only desiring fulfilment of its wishes). Bion states that psychotics (or the psychotic portion of the personality) seek to evade truth and therefore use splitting and projective identification not only to rid their minds of intolerable emotions but also to rid themselves of the mind that could potentially harbour these feelings. They follow the pleasure–pain principle to the exclusion of the reality principle, according to Bion.

Notes on unconscious phantasies

Isaacs (1952) wrote that Klein's theory of phantasies constituted the mental representations of instincts. In a more recent contribution, Spillius clarified the differences between Freud's and Klein's understanding of phantasies:

> In Freud's view, although there *are* phantasies in the *system unconscious*, the basic unit of the *system unconscious* is not phantasy but the unconscious instinctual wish. Dream-formation and phantasy-formation are parallel processes; one might speak of "phantasy work" as comparable to the "dream work"; both involve transformation of primary unconscious content, and dreams are a transformation of it. For Freud, the prime mover, so to speak, is the unconscious wish; dreams and phantasies are both disguised derivatives of it. For Klein the prime mover is unconscious phantasy [Spillius, 2001, p. 362]

> Klein developed her idea of phantasy gradually from 1919 onwards, stressing particularly: the damaging effect of the inhibition of phantasy in the development of the child; the ubiquity of phantasies about the mother's body and its contents; the variety of phantasies about the primal scene and the Oedipus complex; the intensity of both aggressive and loving phantasies; the combination of several phantasies to form what she called the depressive position ... the paranoid–schizoid position was to come later. ... Essentially, I think that Klein viewed unconscious phantasy as synonymous with unconscious thought and feeling, and that she may have used the term *phantasy* rather than *thought* because the thoughts of her child patients were more imaginative and less rational than ordinary adult thought is supposed to be. [p. 364]

From Spillius' account it would seem that Klein gave a more central role to unconscious phantasies. She believed (1) that they constituted *unconscious thinking*, (2) that all fundamental communications and relationships between self and self (internally) and self and others (internally *and* externally) are conducted through unconscious phantasies, and (3) that even all defence mechanisms—schizoid mechanisms (splitting, projective identification, idealization, and magic omnipotent denial), manic defences (triumph, contempt, and control), or obsessional defences, and even repression—are themselves more nearly permanent (concretized) phantasies.

"Daddy, tell me a story": psychoanalysis as a "dream mender"

We are now in the age of *Harry Potter* and need not wonder why this wonderfully crafted phantasmagoria is enjoying unparalleled popularity and acclaim. Those of us who are parents know well the timeless plea of children: "Daddy (or Mummy), tell me a story!" Stories, legends, fairy tales, fables, parables, and myths are all different versions of dreams or phantasies. They are all narratives that give meaning to the chaotic outpourings of the unconscious.

More specifically, if we employ Bion's binocular model, as alluded to earlier, we can come up with the following image: If we conjecture that the paranoid–schizoid position constitutes one pincer that intercepts O and the depressive position another, and also that the former functions to lay down a barricade of unconscious phantasy or myth to hold back the β-elements of O and the latter seeks to give a more realistic version of Truth in tandem with (following) the initializing phantasmatization (mythification) of Truth, we acquire a model of the importance of stories for unconscious well-being and for the well-being of the individual. Stories, phantasies, or dreams are the first line of defence against being overwhelmed. We must first be able to falsify (alter) or attenuate Truth in order to tolerate it, after which we must personalize it as our own subjective experience that we (re-)create from within ourselves in order to vouchsafe our sense of agency. Thanks to the objectivity offered by the depressive position, we can then objectify its Otherness.

To restate this from another angle, traditionally, when psychoanalysts interpret unconscious phantasies to analysands, the predominating point of view has been that from an external factual reality—"When you were in the waiting room and heard me on the phone, you thought that I was talking with my mistress" (in fantasy[12])—I imply that, in reality, I was not. In other words, phantasies were understood as the prime cause of pathology, and a debunking of the phantasy by a safe restoration of reality was the cure. I believe that while that premise *may* be valid, there is another, obverse way of understanding the role of phantasies. I conceive of them as the first line of defence against the evolution of the β-elements (unprocessed non-mental proto-experiences, O). Phantasies arrest their impact by mythifying them and converting them into personal narratives that flow and cascade in the ongoing mythic stream of the unconscious.

By interpreting phantasies, we are validating their importance and their inner truth in preparation for the succeeding process—that of allowing the mechanisms of the depressive position to conduct transformations of the phantasies into statements of objective (separate) reality. Thus, an interpretation about an unconscious phantasy verbally *completes* and therefore *validates* the phantasy by allowing for a transformation from the sensual image to the verbal abstraction, in addition to a verification of its function by the analyst. In other words, there must be an *alignment* between the unconscious *phantasy* and its conscious descendant, the *thought*. Furthermore, when Shakespeare said, "Sleep knits up the ravelled sleeve of care", he could just as well have said "dreams and/or phantasies knit up the ravelled sleeve of care"—in preparation for an emotional processing and mental digestion that will happily culminate in abstract thought about one's emotions.

All the above is probably well known to infants and children in terms of their preoccupation with fairy tales and fables, which they need to have repeated over and over again. Dreams, fables, legends, myths, and/or phantasies are the lost primal tongue of imagery that has dominated the preverbal life of infants. They washed away the tears of grief and care and preserved the innocence of the infant. They subsequently submerged and surrendered to the overlord of word symbols, but they can still be located in the nether world of our being as our "silent service", imagistically licking our wounds and being at our beck and call for all our rites of passage and wrongs at the hands of circumstance.

NOTES

This chapter is an abbreviated version of a longer annotated contribution that explored virtually all of Bion's contributions on the subject of dreaming. Editing was undertaken here in order to reduce redundancies.

1. I should state that this is my own opinion as I reflect on the implications of the extensions of Bion's conception.

2. With regard to "psychotic dreaming", I believe that Bion's case material on the subject would perhaps be better explained by hypothesizing that the psychotic, rather than being able to dream, becomes "dreamed" by a persecutory object, as suggested in Tausk's (1919) "influencing machine".

3. This arrangement is strictly my own way of editing Bion to make sense of these items. He himself lists them separately as "Absolute Truth", "Ultimate Reality", "β-elements", inherent pre-conceptions", "noumena", "things-in-themselves", and "godhead". I believe that my edited version does greater justice to his views. The simplest way of understanding O would be pure, raw experience before we process it.

4. This self-recognition of unconscious inner incompetence is noteworthy among schizophrenics, who seem to carry with them constitutional flaws in mental processing of emotional information. They are afflicted, *inter alia*, with a tendency towards overinclusion of sensory stimuli, a sensory-gating problem that closely correlates with Bion's concepts of the contact-barrier and the Grid.

5. It is noteworthy that Kleinians, including Bion, never contemplated the adaptive (Hartmann, 1939) aspects of the death instinct. Bion himself, whose O

transcends it, seems never to have come to realize that the death instinct may be an adaptive defence for those whose defective α-functions had failed them, and who thus default into the use of the death instinct as their only hope.

6. Francesca Bion informed me that Bion had been familiar with Stanislavski's ideas.

7. This is an exact quote from Bion during my analysis with him in 1976. He mentioned that he had obtained it from one of Freud's letters to Lou Andreas-Salomé (Freud & Andreas-Salomé, 1966).

8. I differ somewhat from Bion on this issue. I believe that the infant is "hard-wired" from the beginning with its own rudimentary α-functions as a Kantian primary category; this would explain why infants can communicate with their objects nonverbally from the beginning and are apparently able to dream from the beginning. I believe, however, that the mother's α-functions are, nevertheless, necessary.

9. The barrier or taboo in the Kleinian version refers to the sanctity of the in-sides of mother's body (part-object). In the Freudian version the barrier or taboo refers to the incest object *qua* whole object.

10. The contact-barrier designation may also apply to the concept of the "pas-sive stimulus barrier" (Freud, 1920g) which itself is related to Hartmann's (1939) concept of inborn "stimulus threshold" as an apparatus of primary autonomy.

11. I suggest that the contact-barrier's capacity for selectivity predicates the operation of a cryptic, numinous, and vitalistic presence or intelligence within the structure.

12. Here I spell *"fantasy"* with an "f" rather than a "ph" because in this usage it is conscious or preconscious, not unconscious.

CHAPTER 27

"Become"

The reader will have noted that I repeat myself often in this work. My rationale for doing so is that Bion did so himself in his writings—but he repeated himself in different contexts each time, and so do I. Lacan (1966), in addressing the problem of the repetition compulsion, stated that in every session the patient repeats himself—differently! "Become" is such a profound and important component of Bion's episteme that I could do no less than give it a separate treatment.

Bion uses the verb to "become" in two ways. Both uses derive from Plato (the *Theaetetus*, for one). The first use is synonymous with "evolve". Plato stated: "That which is is always becoming." The second use is clinical: the analyst must become the analysand. Lest this statement sound too mystical, let me put it this way: Just as we are destined physiologically to become the food we digest and assimilate, so we must allow ourselves as analysts to digest—assimilate, *become*—the emotional experience the analysand is unconsciously as well as consciously conveying to us. "Become" constitutes an ontological, epistemological technique of emotional knowing. The better-known epistemological (but not ontological) technique is Cartesian, in which a separation is required between the mind and the mind's object.

Bion undoubtedly found the first meaning of "become" in the *Theaetetus* (*Dialogues of Plato: 2*—Jowett, 1892).

DOI: 10.4324/9781003348665-28

Socrates: I am about to speak of a high argument, in which all things are said to be relative; . . . there is no single thing or quality, but out of motion and change and admixture all things are *becoming* relatively to one another, which *"becoming"* is by is incorrectly called being, but is really becoming, for nothing ever is, but all things are *becoming.* . . . Summon the great masters of either kind of poetry—Epicharmus, the prince of Comedy, and Homer of Tragedy; when the latter sings of . . . does he not mean that *all things are the offspring of flux and motion?* [Jowett, 1892, Vol. 2, p. 154]

Socrates: Or that anything appears the same to you as to another man? . . . Rather would it not be true that it never appears exactly the same to you, because you are never exactly the same?. [p. 155]

Everything *becomes* and *becomes* relatively to something else. [pp. 158–159]

As for the second meaning of "become" consider the following:

Soc. When I perceive I must *become* percipient of something—there can be no such thing as perceiving and perceiving nothing; the object . . . nothing can become sweet which is sweet to no one. . . . The inference is, that we [the agent and patient] are or *become* in relation to one another. [p. 162; italics added]

[T]he soul views something by herself and others through the bodily organs. [p. 188]

Soc. Then perception, Theaetetus, can never be the same as knowledge or science? [p. 190]

And now, my friend, . . . having *wiped out of your memory* all that has preceded, see if you have arrived at any clearer view, and once more say what is knowledge. [p. 190; italics added]

It is clear from Bion's writings that he believed in the flux and motion of all things, including all aspects of life itself. He was fond of citing Heraclitus' dictum that one can never enter the same stream twice. A corollary of this idea is that of *transience.* Memory is the place where truth has once transiently been but is no longer. In order to perceive an object, I have to enter into a rhythm-in-flux with the object, and in that rhythm (my word), I *become* the object.

There is a deeper meaning to the concept of becoming the object, however. It is easy to mistake becoming with fusion with the object. This is clearly what Bion does *not* mean. If one fuses (in unconscious phantasy) with the object, one has surrendered one's ego boundaries and can no longer function as an integrative or percipient self. I believe that what Bion means by "becoming" in the clinical situation is that the analyst, while in a state of reverie, is receptive to his patient's emotional communications by being in exquisitely sensitive contact with *his own inner self*—that is, *his own* unconscious reservoir of *counterpart* emotions, experiences, phantasies, and so on, which match up with those of the patient. Thus, the analyst's unconscious *resonates* with that of the patient. This act constitutes "becoming" or what I would call, following Plato, the "flux" or the "rhythm of becoming". This act is aided by our inherent possession of "mirror neurons" (Gallese, 2001; Gallese & Goldman, 1998), the neuronal basis for the quality of empathic observation (Grotstein, 2005). (Parenthetically, as I have stated earlier, "become" exemplifies the ancient Greek "middle voice"—a grammatical construction that unites the active and passive voices.)

The advice offered to his acting students by Stanislavski (1936), one of the founders of "method acting", poses an interesting parallel with Socrates' and Bion's "becoming". Stanislavski renounced the traditional classical acting technique whereby the actor identifies (projectively and then introjectively) with the appointed role. Instead, he advises the student to look within himself to locate those internal experiences and memories that match up with or correspond to the role to be played.

From a more practical perspective, the concept of "become" can be applied to infant development and the clinical situation as follows: as the infant evolves from the paranoid–schizoid to the depressive position, one of his tasks is to accept—that is, to "become", to own—his experience of neediness, including the drives. The same is true for the clinical situation in which the analyst seeks to help the analysand "own: that is, "become" their emotions by feeling them.

CHAPTER 28

P–S ↔ D

The P–S ↔ D formula represented another change in Klein-ian thinking. Until Bion's reformulation, Kleinians tended to pathologize the paranoid–schizoid position and privileged the attainment of the depressive position. Bion saw them both from the vertex of binocular vision—that is, dialectically. P–S exerted a mediat-ing function on D, as D exerted a mediating function on P–S. D is in danger of becoming an ossified Establishment signifier, whereas P–S is in danger of too much scattering or fragmentation. Bion finally, and ingeniously, placed P–S ↔ D into a configuration of triangulation with O through a process of binocularization whereby P–S and D both me-diate O, but from differing vertices. He was to do the same with the relationship between consciousness and the unconscious *vis-à-vis* O.

One of the implications of Bion's depicting the double and reversed arrows between P–S and D is that they occur and function simultane-ously and presumably have done so from the beginning. This is not to gainsay that there could also exist a seemingly epigenetic develop-ment from P–S to D—a phenomenon we do see clinically. P–S and D being parallel and simultaneous is reminiscent of Klein's (1935) original description of the depressive position, which included what she would later term the paranoid–schizoid position (Klein, 1946). Bion's mathematical categorization of P–S ↔ D also implies an active,

DOI: 10.4324/9781003348665-29

reciprocating, dialectical relationship between the two positions, as he suggests in *Transformations*:

> Melanie Klein's theory of the part played by intolerance of depression illuminates the problem presented by the chain of causation I have reported. The patient is persecuted by the meaning of certain facts that he feels to be significant. Further, he is persecuted by the feelings of persecution. This is explicable if we accept that the patient is intolerant of depression and that this hinders the Ps ↔ D interchange. The proposed chain of causation can be seen as a *rationalization of the sense of persecution*. [1965, p. 57]

Essentially, P–S ↔ D is the notation that signifies "learning from experience"—the emotion, O, in its unmentalized sense-impression as a β-element, has become transformed into a mentalizable α-element, which is suitable for mental digestion and distribution to the rest of the mind:

> The process of change from one category represented in the grid to another may be described as disintegration and reintegration, Ps ↔ D". [1963, p. 35]   [*That is, from scattering or splitting to coherence.*]

> It would seem that there is a connection between P–S ↔ D and ♀♂ yet the dissimilarity makes it hard to see what form the connection ... would take, The bringing together of elements that apparently have no connection in fact or in logic in such a way that their connection is displayed and an unsuspected coherence revealed ... is characteristic of P–S ↔ D. [1963, p. 37]   [*P–S ↔ D and ♀♂ function complementarily and in parallel to engender coherence.*]

> [B]efore ♀♂ can operate, ♀ has to be found and the discovery of ♂ depends on the operation of P–S ↔ D. It is obvious that to consider which of the two ♀♂ or P–S ↔ D is prior distracts from the maim problem. I shall suppose the existence of a mixed state in which the patient is persecuted by feelings of depression and depressed by feelings of persecution. [1963, p. 39]   [*Here Bion is proposing the concept of the "Positions", a combination or mixture of both P–S and D.*]

> The first problem is to see what can be done to increase scientific rigour by establishing the nature of minus K (–K), minus L (–L), and minus H (–H). . . . [I]nstead of an interaction involving dispersal of particles with feelings of persecution . . . and integration with feelings of depression we have in –PS ↔ D disintegration, total loss depressive stupor, or, intense impaction and degenerate stuporous violence. [1963, p. 51–52]   [*P–S ↔ D is now considered in its negative functioning in parallel with –L, –H, and –K.*]

Bion's concept of P–S ↔ D elevates Klein's positivistic, cyclopean (one point of view), one-dimensional (either/or) linear (sequential) pathway into a series of dialectics. A dialectic is implied in Klein's P–S in terms of "good-breast" versus "bad-breast". Then, when the depressive position comes into view, another dialectical encounter develops between P–S and D, presumably with progressions and regressions. Just as Bion's container ↔ contained intersubjectivized the infant in P–S with a mother who must simultaneously be in the depressive position in order to be an appropriate container, so his P–S ↔ D implies that the depressive position has been there in a dialectical relationship with P–S all along (since birth), but it only reaches prominence with its later ascendancy.

Put another way, the infant can be understood to be born in the most inchoate form of the depressive position—*insofar as this position predicates the experience of object loss,* the first instance of which is the birth situation. However, since the depressive position also predicates maturity, self-identity, acceptance of one's dependency on the object, and whole-object (intersubjective) relations altogether, requirements for which the neonate is totally unprepared, it must first traverse developmentally through P–S in order to screen, process, and "alpha-bet(a)-ize" the random data of its emotional experience, first by categorizing them into "good" and "bad" through splitting differentiations that pend future integrations in the *successive ascendancy* of the depressive position. (NB: according to Bion's revision of the concept, the depressive position also exists and functions simultaneously with P–S.)

CHAPTER 29

L, H, and K and passion

Bion (1962a, 1963, 1965, 1970) used L, H, and K as abstract nota-
tions and elements to designate emotional links between self
and objects and between objects themselves. They also constitute psychoanalytic elements. The terms from which they are abstract-
ed were formerly considered to be drives. While still maintaining the
integrity of the drives, Bion has taken liberty with them to select out
their strictly emotional component and linking or joining capacities.
Most elementally, one could consider that they are inseparable and
mutually interchangeable. For instance, x K y because he is aware that
he L y but also H y. In other words, we emotionally *know* someone by
our awareness of our *love* and/or *hatred* of him or her:

> [T]he signs can be related to fact in a way that saves them from
> becoming meaningless symbols and can at the same time be suf-
> ficiently abstract to ensure that they are generally and not merely
> accidentally applicable to real emotional situations. . . . The analyst
> must allow himself to appreciate the complexity of the emotional
> experience he is required to illuminate and yet restrict his choice to
> these three links. He decides what the linked objects are and which
> of these three represents with most accuracy the actual links between
> them. [1962b, p. 44]

To sum up an emotional episode as K is to produce an imper-
fect record but a good starting point for the analyst's speculative

DOI: 10.4324/9781003348665-30

meditation. . . . [It] possesses the rudiments of the essentials of a system of notation—record of fact and working tool. [p. 44]

Here Bion is justifying and rationalizing the use of a limited number of abstract, unsaturated icons as models. Each of them and all of them together collectively can syncretistically expand to include a vast array of qualities and quantities of emotion. This is an aspect of Bion's ambition to impart mathematical precision to psychoanalytic theory and practice. The ultimate aim is to find an emotional *notation* system. Later in the same section Bion points out that the L, H, and K notation systems are to be used exclusively for living beings. They do not apply to non-living being beings—only "science" does.

Bion (1963) links L, H. and K with "passion".

By "passion" or the lack of it I mean the component derived from L, H., and K. I mean the term to represent an emotion experienced with intensity and warmth though without any suggestion of violence. . . . Awareness of passion is not dependent on sense. For senses to be active only one mind is necessary: *passion is evidence that two minds are linked* and that there cannot possibly be fewer than two minds if passion is present. *Passion must clearly be distinguished from counter-transference*, the latter being evidence of repression. [1963, pp. 12–13; italics added]

L, H, and K are the components of passion. Passion must be shared in order to qualify as passion. Passion conveys the emotion of suffering as well as that of warmth. It is the *sine qua non* of the analyst's capacity to contain. Bion's description of it approximates the Passion of Christ. To me it also closely approximates the mystical act of *exorcism*, the transfer(-ence) of emotional pain from one person to another (Grotstein, 2000a, 2005, in press-a; Meltzer, 1978). I believe that L, H, and K function inseparably, but at any given moment one of them can become prominent as the others seem to recede. Fundamentally, we can only K an object by knowing how we feel (L ↔ H) about it. Bion often stated that we cannot love without hating and cannot hate without loving. K is more often mentioned by Bion scholars and others, but it is my opinion that there can be no K without L and H, only attempts at pretence of their absence. True K is always transient (in flux) and incomplete—even heralding its unknown counterparts in the future. As the analysand accomodates to K, catastrophic anxiety is produced as K's future counterpart, O, beckons it. If the K interpretation is taken as fact, on the other hand, K becomes transformed into –K (falsehood).

Minus L, H, and K (–L, –H, and –K)

In *Elements of Psycho-Analysis*, Bion discusses K and –K:

> The conflict between the view of the [psychotic—JSG] patient and the view of the analyst, and in the patient with himself, is not therefore a conflict, as we see it in the neuroses, between one set of ideas and another, or one set of impulses or another, but between K and minus K (–K). . . . [1963, p. 51]

Bion goes on to suggest that –K activity on the part of the patient may account for predictable analytic discourses so as to prevent deeper spontaneous exploration. The role of –K is due perhaps to the need for a negative faith to replace the one that either never appeared in sufficient force or defaulted because of the loss of innocence (due to the putative results of negative containment) and the original faith that was necessary to join it in a covenant. Put another way, –K can be thought of as the maladaptive operation of the death instinct, which seeks to annihilate growth that is felt to be progressively unsupportable and also the Lie aspect of Column 2 of the Grid. Here I am alluding to the demoralization that accrues from a failure to develop a background presence of primary identification (Grotstein, 1981a, 2000a) as the initializing experience of containment, otherwise known as being *blessed*. A foreclosure on this entity presupposes that the infant had prematurely plummeted into the Real (O) before being baptized by the blessed protection of the covenant of parental imagination and conception. He is therefore now the hapless one, predisposed, I believe, to a cataclysmic "orphandom" of the Real (O) where he feels impelled to swear a new allegiance to the dark (and only) saviour, –K. Bion describes this phenomenon as the postnatal persistence of fetal existence in which the fetus becomes prematurely aware of pain and then closes off, and thereby forfeits, some aspects of its developmental and maturational future. –K designates "lying "in the first degree" (deliberate and disingenuous). It should be distinguished from "falsification", which, according to Bion, characterizes all forms of thinking and dreaming, (see de Bianchedi et al., 2000).

In *Transformations* Bion defines the limitations of L, H, and K:

> [M]y reason for saying O is unknowable is not that I consider human capacity unequal to the task but because K, L, or H are inappropriate to O. They are approximate to transformations of O but not to O. [1965, p. 140]

About the patient's dread of undergoing a transformation from K to O Bion states:

> Interpretations are part of K. The anxiety lest transformation in K leads to transformation in O is responsible for the form of resistance in which interpretations appear to be accepted but in fact the acceptance is with the intention of "knowing about" rather than "becoming". [1965, p. 160]

I think Bion is discussing the difference between intellectualizing and experiencing interpretations.

Whereas –K denotes falsification of linkages with objects, –L may imply, among other feelings, false, pretentious, narcissistic love, and –H indifference rather than hate.

CHAPTER 30

Faith

F aith first appears in Bion's *Attention and Interpretation*:

If he [the patient—JSG] is able to be receptive to O, then he may feel impelled to deal with the intersection of the evolution of O with the domain of objects of sense or of formulations based on the senses. Whether he does so or not cannot depend on *rules* for O, or O →, but only on his ability to be at one with O. . . . My last sentence represents an "act" of what I have called *"faith"*. It is in my view a scientific statement because for me "faith" is a scientific state of mind and should be recognized as such. But it must be "faith" unstained by any element of memory or desire. [1970, p. 32; italics added]

As I read this passage, I became aware of Bion's occasionally stentorian rhetoric and could not help thinking of Moses descending from Mount Sinai with the ten tablets (O) and encountering the Israelites worshipping the golden calf (K). For Moses, as for Bion, faith lay in a belief in the existence or presence ("holy ghost") of an ultra-sensual object. In the daily practice of psychoanalysis we take this kind of faith for granted, but we rarely ponder its mystery as Bion did. Specifically, when a weekend or holiday break is looming or has taken place, our analysis of it often centres on the patient's transformation of the analyst's image over the break—that is, whether during that time the analyst's image "morphed" into the internal image of a bad object (no faith or negative

DOI: 10.4324/9781003348665-31

faith), or whether there remained a continuing presence of the legacy of the patient's experience with the analyst. The first (no faith) is due to the tendency of the desperate infantile portion of the patient's personality to blame the analyst for departing and thereby creating, in his unconscious phantasy, the image of a bad, hateful, persecutory object. The infant who cannot tolerate frustration—and/or his adult counterpart, the analytic patient—may become so terrified because of what feels like a breach of faith by mother (analyst) that he abrogates his faith and transfers it to the dark but "trustworthy" force of permanent disappointment (–F), which can always be relied upon.

In the case of the patient who has entered the depressive position, he now has the capacity to mourn the object in its absence and has developed the grace to be able to feel the good effects of the object in the latter's absence. This is faith. Frances Tustin (personal communication, 1985), citing Ernest Hemingway's novel, *The Sun Also Rises* ("after it sets"), called attention to a valuable milestone in development when the infant is able to move from the image of the line (always of departure of the object down the line) to the circle (of the object's return up the line). This is how I envisage Bion's conception of faith *vis-à-vis* the infant (and patient). The infant is born with an inherent pre-conception of a breast. In the absence of the breast, the infant is constrained to have faith that in the external world a real breast exists that corresponds to his pre-conception. He must consequently have *faith* in its arrival as an *incarnation* or *realization* of the breast, at which point the realized breast becomes a *"conception of a breast"*. Perhaps this is what Bion, after Bishop George Berkeley (*The Analyst*, 1734), means by "the ghosts of departed quantities" (Bion, 1965, p. 157). An important factor behind the infant's capacity to have Faith is his ability to mourn the breast-mother in her absence. This idea derives from Bion's belief that the infant is born into "the Positions"—that is, simultaneously into D as well as P–S (P–S$\leftrightarrow$D).

> The discipline that I propose for the analyst, namely avoidance of memory or desire, in the sense in which I have used those terms, increases his ability to exercise "acts of faith". An "act of faith" is peculiar to scientific procedure and must be distinguished from the religious meaning with which it is invested in conversational usage. ... The "act of faith" has no association with memory or desire or sensation. It has a relationship to thought analogous to the relationship of *a priori* knowledge to knowledge. It does not belong to the +– K system but to the O system. ... An "act of faith" has as its

background something that is unconscious and unknown because it has not happened. [1970, pp. 34–35]

A bad memory is not enough. . . . [p. 41]

I have emphasized the technical importance on the part of the analyst to analyse his *patient's* incipient lack of faith during absences. Bion here considers an "act of faith" an absolute requisite for the analyst's technique. The "discipline" required by the analyst is *"negative capability"* (Bion, 1970, p. 13). Abandoning memory and desire clears the way for the operation of faith in allowing the analyst to "become" his analysand's passion *from within himself*. The analyst must have the faith that his inner repertoire of unconscious emotions, memoirs, and inherent pre-conceptions (Ideal Forms, noumena) exists and can be spontaneously and appropriately summoned and retrieved so as to match up with those in the analysand.

The "selected fact" and the "act of faith"

Bion exhorts the analyst to abandon memory and desire (and all the fruits of the sensory apparatus) so as to be able to enter into reverie—a meditative state of absence of thought" ("cerebral noise"). As the analyst *listens* to the patient—and simultaneously *listens to himself listening* to the patient—he is at first a passive dual observer ("sense") and receptor-container ("passion") of the patient's free associations. Because of the latter's alleged freedom, they may at first seem random and incoherent. The analyst must wait for a *pattern* to appear that would give them a meaning, one that the analyst could then transmit to the patient as an interpretation. The incipient appearance of incoherence or non-coherence of the patient's free associations, which then develops, in the analyst mind, into a pattern, is itself an analytic pattern. What the analyst is awaiting is the "selected fact"[1] (Bion, 1962b, p. 67; Poincaré, 1963, p. 3), and he must have faith that the "selected fact" will arrive. This faith of the analyst is due to his own at first *inherent* and then later *acquired pre-conception* (from analytic training) that such a thing as a "selected fact" exists. Bion alludes to this belief in his concept of the gnomon (Bion, 1965, p. 94) and the godhead (Bion, 1965, p. 139), which to me represent the unconscious phantasy of an "ineffable presence", the "numinous librarian" of the Ideal Forms (inherent pre-conceptions) and noumena, the one who "knows" the infinity of the unconscious, the one who constitutes the supraordinate inherent pre-conception or anticipating counterpart to the "selected fact". When the two meet, infinity and symmetry become asymmetrically comprehensible as conceptual realizations. In other words, *for Bion the inevitable arrival of the selected fact is Faith* (F)!

A problem emerges in terms of the locale of the selected fact, as I have mentioned earlier. Do I, as the analyst, faithfully await the arrival of the selected fact from within my own mind as the reward for my patience, or does the selected fact emerge from outside (within the context of the analysand's seemingly disconnected associations), or both? The chaos of infinite O is organized, not random. The godhead of O would seem to be its hidden order. Consequently, I have come to believe that the selected fact, like O, has two locales. They are like two separated twins who repeatedly part and then, after searching for one another, with Faith, reunite.

CHAPTER 31

Bion's discovery of zero ("no-thing")

From the very beginning of his career, when as a psychoanalyst Bion first treated psychotic patients, he realized —that their thinking constituted a pattern unto itself that was qualitatively, not just quantitatively, different from that of neurotics. As he made efforts to ferret out these distinctions, however, he broadened his research to normal thinking as well.

First, Bion drew an important distinction between thoughts and the thinker who thinks the thoughts—thinking being a function of a mind that had to be created to absorb and to transform the traffic of "thoughts" emerging from the process of experience. Bion cited the model of the alimentary track to suggest that, like the gut, the mind must accept food (for thought), must be able to sort it out by separating it into its indivisible elements, must consequently have the capacity for certain functions that permit this refinement into elemental ingredients, and must then pass on these irreducible elements into the interior of the body (mind) for absorption and then storage (metabolism) and/or evacuation of those elements that are not useful or did not achieve proper prioritization in the transformation. Growing from experience depends upon learning from experience, and the latter depends upon the existence of functions that can accept experience and deconstruct it into its elements in preparation for absorption and metabolism. The thinking mind is characterized by the development of functions that harvest and digest experience, deconstructing it into elements capable of being "chewed on" and then encoded for storage and further processing.

The mind of the analyst must be capable of suspending memory and desire (L, H) in order to experience a transformation (T) in O, in order, in turn, to be able to establish the selected fact—an emotional capacity that binds what seem to be unrelated elements in a series of free associations. Thus, the mind of the analyst must approach the zero (null) state in order to be able to free itself from pre-conceptions (residues of memories and other attitudes) that would otherwise obscure the capacity to "hear" the analysand's associations "freely". The analyst must, in other words, aim for unsaturation in order to have an experience in O—not to achieve O, but merely at a maximum to approach *being* O. In this way the analyst is able to employ α-function to be able to absorb the analysand's associations—that is, bear them emotionally prior to attempts to give them meaning—and then to translate them, using the processes of abstraction and generalization, the former to elementalize them into their lowest common denominators or elements and the latter to sort out new connections: conceptions, concepts, hypotheses, theories, and so on.

The analyst's emotional capacity to tolerate the zero state (the absence of memory and desire) allows him to process these data insofar as he is able to employ the selected fact—that is, the ability to intuit connections between these elements that would allow them to coalesce in ways that could not have been anticipated in their predigested form. Thus the zero state of mental expectation—the absence of memory and desire—is necessary as the foster ground for the emergence of the functioning of the selected fact following the analyst's absorption of the analysand's associations.

However, the analyst as thinker, who approximates zero in order to attempt the achievement of the experience of O, must ponder the free associations of the patient as if they were something quite different from zero or nothingness. At the same time, the patient would have been unable to express, let alone experience, the elemental ingredients of his feelings—and to formulate conscious and unconscious thoughts about them—without himself being in the zero state from one point of view. Bion believes, in other words, that not only does the analyst require the employment of α as a function to translate the patient's associations, but the patient himself must employ α in order to generate free associations. The capacity to generate free associations—that is, α-elements—presupposes the existence of a contact-barrier that separates conscious from unconscious. The capacity to dream while asleep presupposes that the day residues of consciousness must be nullified—effectively turned into the domain of zero—by the contact-barrier, which allows sleep to take place and allows dreaming as its consequence. Dreaming, in turn, has as its function the further development of the contact-barrier, which divides consciousness and unconsciousness. The ultimate value of this contact-barrier—and of the dreaming that supplies it and reinforces its functioning—is to prevent one domain from interfering with the functioning of the other. In other words, consciousness should not interfere with unconsciousness—ultimately so that the person can effectively be awake when not asleep and effectively asleep when not awake. Therefore each domain must be zero to the other, and it is the function of the contact-barrier to maintain this distinction of mutual nullification.

However, the capacity to dream and therefore to have this contact-barrier upon which α-function depends—not only the α-function of the analyst, but also the α-function of the patient, which generates significant, meaningful free associations for translation by the analyst—depends upon the patient's capacity to tolerate the experience of zero, the experience of no-breast. In other words, the patient has to allow for a space in which he can contemplate the presence of an absent breast alongside the desire to get rid of the presence of the painful experience of a bad breast. The patient must, in other words, tolerate zero, and from that zero, in consort with the mother's capacity to help him tolerate that zero by virtue of her own capacity to tolerate zero—to forge what Winnicott was otherwise to call a potential space where concrete somatic phantasies (which Piaget advises us are stimulus-bound—that is, sensorimotor prisoners of the percept) can now evolve in this potential space into spontaneous illusions of a newly enfranchised imagination. In other words, in infancy the neurotic acquires the capacity for α-function from the mother when the mother's capacity for negative capability—otherwise known as reverie and/or primary maternal concern—affords a model to the infant of the capacity to tolerate zero.

Alpha-function emerges from a sense organ that is sensitive to consciousness and to unconsciousness. Bion believed that his concept of α-function had an advantage over Freud's concept of primary process and secondary process, insofar as the latter seem to be agencies of independent origin, whereas in the case of Bion's α-function, the two emerge from a common source and are in a dialectical relationship—that is, an opposing partnership, each defining the other.

Although Bion rarely refers to nullity or zeroness as such in his work, it can obviously be inferred that the concept of zero came to have greater and greater importance for him. His second major use of nullity refers to the experience of the psychotic who, unable to tolerate the experience of emotional events because he lacks an α-function and/or he uses his α-function in reverse to evacuate awareness of them, therefore endures them rather than suffers them. This may be due to the psychotic's own mother having lacked an α-function to give him in infancy as an internalized legacy, compounded by her transformed presence as an obstructive object that internally attacks whatever links he tries to make between self and object and between object and object. Therefore we can see that nullity applies to the denudation that characterizes the psychotic's mind after he has evacuated his unprocessed (undigested) potential elements of experience—β elements. The psychotic evacuates not only his experiences, reinforcing their evacuation via the use of his already diminished α-function in reverse, but also the very mind (including this diminished α-function) that can experience mental pain, into whatever objects are available that correspond to his projections. Following that massive evacuation of experience and mind, the psychotic's mind is denuded, transformed into hallucinosis, and disconnected from his ownership.

Another interesting component of this massive exodus of thinking capacity is the exodus of the inherent and acquired pre-conceptions that, according to Bion, exist within the normal mind—the inherent and acquired capacity to anticipate experience—"memoirs of the future", as he more poetically terms them. When these pre-conceptions are projected into objects, the objects become numinous, which is the quality of pre-conceptions before they have mated with experience. It is perhaps this numinous quality imparted by the detached and projected pre-conceptions that gives psychosis its peculiar, bizarre, awesome appearance. Parenthetically, I believe that it is important to distinguish between omnipotence and numinousness. Omnipotence is the nature of cosmic interaction within the domain of the unconscious internal world. It is dangerous when it has seemingly invaded the domain of thinking—of consciousness. Numinous is awesome, eerie, with a quality of *déjà vu*, the uncanny preter-matured.

In modern semiology we could say that Bion understood the psychotic's dread of the pain of experience by understanding that the psychotic must de-signify what he already anticipates (via pre-conceptions) to be the meaning of the experience, were he to allow himself to experience it. The psychotic de-signifies not only the potential meaning of the experience—in order to eliminate the signified—but also his own mind, which can give signification and derive meanings from these significations. The desired result is a state of meaninglessness, nullity, concrete mindlessness.

Following the evacuation of mental content, mind, pre-conceptions, α-function, and so on, the psychotic's mind is denuded—nullified into zero capacity—and is consequently unable thereafter to continue the projective identificatory progression, because the space of the psyche of the psychotic and the nature of the bizarreness of the objects available to him offer progressively less opportunity to project and/or to translocate identities and identifications. Consequently, the psychotic resorts to fragmentation, which to the outsider appears to be projection or projective identification but is really the catastrophic residues of a mind withdrawn from itself, numinously haunted by its former self, but which has really not moved—only the mind that disavowed it has moved further and further away, as it moves further and further within what used to be itself.

The psychotic attempts both to retreat into zero subjectivity—that is, zero awareness of experience—and to nullify the objects of experience by throwing them away, along with the mind that can know them. These latter transform into numinous bizarre objects. In other words, the psychotic cannot ultimately project because he has no object to contain—that is, to correspond—to the feeling; instead, there is fragmentation—which looks like projection. The psychotic tries to create zero—to be in zero—and, having fled from meaning, finds only painful bizarre *Meaning*. The psychotic may experience emptiness or deadness or nothingness, all of them a final common pathway of retreats from meaning and significance.

Nothingness, meaninglessness, is at first the goal of the psychotic to escape from painful experience, but it becomes, instead, a "living", external hell of insufferable (because they would not be suffered) but painfully endurable elements of nothingness. The nothingness of psychosis is the experience of randomness, entropy, meaninglessness, unpredictability, the first recourse against which is paranoia. It was perhaps one of Klein's most important achievements to chart the topography of the paranoid–schizoid and depressive positions as the irreducible states of primitive mental life. From Klein's point of view, in the normal and the neurotic mind there is never nullity at the beginning. When the good mother leaves, the bad mother instantly appears as her ineluctable counterpart. They are exact reciprocals of each other. The internal world of Klein—like the internal world of Freud, which was characterized by a seething cauldron of instinctual drives—comprises a state of volatile, irruptive positivity elements. Klein's paranoid–schizoid position gives organization to Freud's concept of instinctual drives, so that the latter are reborn as phantasies that link biological–psychological experiences within the infant to the mother's coming and going.

There is no nullity in Freud or in Klein. It is here that Bion made a leap. In his own explorations of the psychotic mind, Bion has taken the paranoid–schizoid position to a deeper level, where no meaning takes place. Although this state is only contemplatable in the psychotic who has undergone an infantile catastrophe of severe emotional turbulence, it is a hypothetical construct for the normal infant as well. Elsewhere I offered the notion that what Bion had discovered was not only a dual track in terms of α-function (combining Freud's primary process and secondary process) but also an earlier origin for a primitive depressive position, so that the infant, when mentally born (this may be intrauterine), first experiences randomness or entropy—that is, absolute meaninglessness—much as does the psychotic, but is saved from this experience by mother's reverie (α-function), which then allows the infant to exploit the paranoid–schizoid position as an adaptive detour from his inchoate depression (primary object loss, first disruption of primary narcissism) in order to give narrative meaning to this random experience of painful aloneness. The consequence is an evolution from the zero dimension of meaninglessness and randomness or of entropy or of nothingness to the first dimension of either/or—that is, of good versus bad. This capacity for separation between two entities is a primitive Grid, which allows for separation of one element from others in the morass of the multiple elements of randomness and allows the infant to return the mother's signification of him by designating a signification of her in the positive and in the negative, originally in terms of good and bad and later in terms of present and not present. When Bion formulated his concept of the container and contained, he stated that the mother's reverie is necessary to absorb and detoxify her infant's fear of dying, which the latter projects into mother's container capacity. Note that Bion uses the term "fear of dying", not fear of persecution of bad objects. Here, I believe, he is in touch with the first infant experience of separateness—not yet one of persecution, but one of randomness, of entropy, of irrupting nothingness, of "fearful symmetry", as Blake terms it.

In his later work Bion reverted to an early interest in Milton's *Paradise Lost,* from which he frequently quoted the phrase "the deep and formless infinite", designating "the face of the deep" of *Genesis.* Bion was now consolidating his conception, already arrived at by Existentialists such as Boss, Binswanger, and others, that the most frightening state in the individual is that of zeroness. But there are two zeros, as I have tried to demonstrate above: the nullity of optimum expectation on the one hand, and the nullity of the assassination of meaning on the other.

Bion was deeply interested in mathematics and sought to employ mathematical concepts and paradigms to psychoanalysis, not only to avail himself of the precision that mathematics offers, but also because mathematical integers lack memory and desire—that is, they are unsaturated and are therefore more versatile as symbols that can represent elements of meaning. Bion was especially alert to the fact that mental or psychoanalytic objects were more difficult to conceptualize than were material objects of the scientific world. He stated that we know things through K because of the capacity of our sense organs to achieve a common sense about the objects they perceive—but this is only within the sensual waveband. There are experiences with psychoanalytic objects that are in the ultrasensual band of experience, and language as we know it seems unsuitable as a representational medium for those ultrasensual experiences. Even mathematics, in its own development, suffered from "sensual" limitations until it developed the concept of zero—and the reciprocal of zero known as infinity—the latter two conceptions enabling mathematicians to transcend the world dominated by the senses and to travel into domains and perspectives that were contemplatable by intuition alone. Bion entered the galactic vastness of the deep and formless infinite, the domain of the cosmic nothingness of outer space, of no-thingness, to obtain two of his most important figurative concepts, already well-known entities in astronomy. Bion, in using theoretical and applied mathematics, was exploring the dialectic between loneliness and aloneness, between nothingness as unsaturation and nothingness as the saturation of meaninglessness. He was the intrepid explorer of the meaningfulness and meaninglessness of the zero experience.

Postscript

Samuel Beckett may once have been a patient of Bion's. As a matter of fact, there has been some speculation that Bion and Beckett were existential alter egos (Bennett Simon, personal communication). Could it be that Beckett's *Godot* is the counterpart to Bion's "God–O"?

Epilogue

W hat is the essence of Bion's works? What are the points or vertices of his compass? Bion has created a psychoanalytic metatheory that fundamentally involves how we come to know (real-ize) what we know, how we *"learn* (and evolve—that is, transcend) *from experience"* by *"becoming (feeling) our emotions"*—and, as a result, how we are enabled to think cognitively and reflectively. Emotions form the template for thinking. *Dreaming*—and the vast retinue of its subordinate functions: *containment, α-function, transformation,* Grid, and *contact-barrier,* which are all, I have come to believe, either synonyms for each other but with different names to designate their respective *vertices* of operation or are intimately connected and/ or overlapping functions—is the obligatory twin and helpmate that makes *thinking* possible. This is the symbolic model for the relationship between our being able to feel our emotions and then categorize (think about) them. Put another way, Bion's metatheory propounds the consummate significance of O as the constellating force that confronts the individual internally *and* externally—that is, the human subject is existentially imprisoned between the two arms of O. *Dreaming, thinking,* and *becoming* allow for an exit.

In the course of creating his metatheory for psychoanalysis, Bion, like Freud before him, had to confront the tenets of science as deter-

DOI: 10.4324/9781003348665-33

mined by the scientific establishment. Freud, it seems, never stopped in his attempts to win formal approval from science—confirmation that psychoanalysis *was* a science. Bion, the intrepid tank commander, took a different direction and attacked science's flank. "Science", he claimed, was appropriate only for *inanimate objects*. The "science" that is apposite for psychoanalysis is a "my*stical science*", a science of emotions that are infinite and consequently complex and non-linear in nature. In short, he seems to have been the first psychoanalyst to seize upon the idea of *complexity theory*, the "science" that studies non-linear phenomena. Using his now famous technique of reversible perspectives, he asserted that "science" (meaning the linear science of inanimate objects) was myth, and myth was science. I doubt that anyone else could have reversed fields so successfully against so formidable an establishment.[1]

Bion, the polymath and autodidact, summoned a significant portion of the wisdom of the Western—and perhaps even Eastern—World, infused it into psychoanalytic thinking, and rendered psychoanalysis a pragmatic practicing philosophy about the achievement and experience of intimacy and self-transcendence. Whatever else, he formulated the phenomenon of intimacy (with oneself as well as between self and other) as it had never been portrayed before. In retrospect it would seem that Bion's ideas would have been better served if his first major book had been entitled *Learning from Experience by Experiencing and Becoming*.

Another major theme that runs through the entirety of Bion's work is the practical philosophical notion of the consummate importance for the infant—and for his grown-up descendant, the adult—to develop the grace of being able to tolerate frustration stoically and meaningfully, with faith as his support, enabling him, in turn, to access his infinite potential for learning inwardly and outwardly from experience. Psychoanalysis does not heal the analysand. It prepares him to tolerate suffering emotional pain (passion, L, H, K), thereby letting personal *and* cosmic *meaning* emerge and allow the analysand to evolve and transcend himself at any given moment. A Kleinian koan would be: "We become what we do (in phantasy) to our objects." A Bionian koan would be: "We become what we agree to suffer."

While Bion has written a great deal about "container ↔ contained", "maternal reverie", "α-function", "contact-barrier", the Grid, "caesura", "transformations", I conclude (for the moment) that all the above belong to the "service organizations" that either subtend or actually constitute dreaming: that is, that α-function is a model for a process in which α-elements are produced for dreaming, which, in turn, generates dreams, phantasies, and personal myths, all of which stabilize the unconscious *and* conscious personalities. Dreaming is, in turn, organized and directed by the constraints of collective myths. According to Bion, as analysts, we must *dream* our emotions and those of our patients as our analytic task. Psychopathology thus ultimately devolves to being the result of incomplete or unsuccessful dreaming (containment) (by day and/or by night). I hasten to add *Faith* as another of Bion's most important contributions. Thus, *Faith, Dreaming*, and *Emotional Truth* (O) constitute the Bionian trinity.

Some Bion scholars may differ from these views. It has taken me years of perusing Bion's works and years of analysis with him to come to the conclusions presented here—and they still are tentative in my mind. This is one of the rewards and joys of "dreaming"—that is, absorbing and transforming—Bion's works and maintaining the personal faith, not that I would *understand* Bion and his works, but that I would *become* as much of the wisdom, O, of his works as my mind can possibly progressively accommodate.

Thus far I have distilled the quintessence of Bion's work in terms of dreaming, thinking, and becoming in the context of emotional truth and faith. To those we must surely add his gift for *shifting perspectives* and his penchant for *binocular vision*, both of which allowed him with ever-growing success to *"dare to disturb the universe"* of psychoanalytic ideas and beyond.

Of all his concepts, however, I turn to "wild thoughts"[2] (imagination) and their origin, the transcendental unconscious, the godhead (godhood) as his most important legacies. There his whimsy overturns the "topless towers" of psychoanalytic medievalism. Psychoanalysis will be radically different because of Bion's whimsy, daring, and genius. To mix metaphors, he was the latter-day Prometheus who brought the messiah message to psychoanalysis and ushered in its Renaissance!

Some other stray thoughts

As I now enter into the twilight of this book, I experience a mad rush of would-be epiphanies into my mind in the afterglow of this long writing adventure—seeking to be born and have life—before it is too late. Let me discursively give birth to some of them and place others in a thought-nursery for future consideration.

"Vixere fortes ante Agamemnona multi. . . ."

[Horace Odes, Bk. IV, 9.]

Bion alluded to this Horatian ode from time to time, principally in reference to the fate of anonymity of fetal memories. I think it may have another, more personal meaning for Bion—perhaps his concern for the anonymity of his ideas. I wish he could now see that his concepts have become the most defining ideas of our age in psychoanalysis and beyond: he has less chance than anyone else in psychoanalysis to be forgotten.

At the beginning of this work I likened Bion to the Titan Prometheus, the god who stole fire from heaven and gave it to mankind, following which there was a rage in heaven. I also suggested that he was a latter-day Socrates, a man who was dogmatic about what he did not know and who thought of himself only as the midwife of truth for whoever came to him for wisdom. When I latterly came across the theme of entelechy, I thought of how much Bion, the encyclopaedic autodidact and polymath, reminded me of Aristotle. Then, when I discovered the concept of conatus, I immediately thought of Spinoza. Spinoza then reminded me of Galileo, who also reminds me of Bion. Freud is yet another such example. All the above-mentioned giants, with the exception of Aristotle, suffered enormously for daring to disturb their respective universes, but we, their latter-day beneficiaries, are endlessly grateful.

Some variations of mine on themes by Bion

As I began to put the finishing touches on this long endeavour, which took place during the beginning of hostilities in the Middle East, I became occupied with reminiscences of an early visit there. I remembered a dinner party in Jerusalem; I sat next to Professor Chaim Tadmor, then the world's ranking authority on ancient Assyria during the days of Assurbanipal and Tiglath Pileser. I casually mentioned to him that I was just completing a paper, "Who was the Dreamer Who Dreams the Dream and Who is the Dreamer Who Understands It". Tadmor's response was pivoting. He related that the Assyrian gods were thought by ancient Assyrians to communicate with each other through human dreams. Dreams were held to be sacred: they were signifiers of divine intercourse, and it was considered blasphemy for any mortal to attend to them. They were often transcribed, perhaps dissociatively, by scribes, and placed in sacred jars for worship.

As I now began to recount this moment, I had a sudden epiphany, a "wild thought", an imaginative conjecture, which Bion personally taught me always to respect. In my reverie I thought of down-grading Freud's (and Klein's) life and death instincts, reconfiguring them, and subordinating them to entelechy and conatus (conation). Entelechy, you recall, is the activation of one's total inherent potential. It includes the life force, the sexual drives, and more—that is, all that you can be. Conatus is the principle of self-organization and self-regulation and functions as defences and resistances when necessary for adaptation and survival. The death instinct reports to *it*, not the other way around. I thought this alteration in theory was necessary for Bion's metatheory because his panoramic protocol fails to consider (or at least to emphasize) the vital forces impinging on one's emotional frontier. He did reroute and reconfigure the drives, in part, to L, H, and K emotional linkages, but he did not reckon with the economic (force) aspects. I think that entelechy and conatus do.

Now for the epiphany: "Gods speaking to one another through human dreams!" Now I understand better than ever why Bion was so taken with religious and mystic metaphors. Their language is closer to what psychoanalytic patients experience, once we do away with the superficiality of their politics and get beyond the need to idealize a deity and thereby surrender the mind. When Bion conceived of "godhead", for which I substitute "godhood", I don't think he realized that he was fundamentally altering our concept, not only of the unconscious, but also of the deity in all religions. Bion is transforming the positivistic–mechanistic drive unconscious into a numinous, mystical unconscious.

In short, Bion is telling us that the *deity, like the unconscious, is incomplete, not omnipotent, only infinite!* The deity needs man for it to become incarnated and realized—just as the unconscious needs consciousness to become known, to complete its mission. This we have learned from Bion. What I am now adding, thanks to Chaim Tadmor, is that entelechy and conatus comprise one aspect, an ever-surging aspect of O, and must meet up communicatively with the *transcendental analytic* (Kant, 1797), the other arm of O, which includes Plato's Ideal Forms (always in a state of flux, of "becoming") and Kant's noumena (things-in-themselves) and primary, secondary categories, and "empty thoughts". The third part of the numinous trinity is comprised of sensory stimuli from the outer and inner worlds.

Now here is the protocol: As entelechy, along with conatus as its regulator, surges relentlessly as our life trajectory, we are mandated to adjust to it and do its bidding by accepting our growing and developing selves—that is, keep our rendezvous with our destiny while at the same time accepting and dealing with our fate, destiny's default. As we accept and process (dreaming, α-function) our continuing experiences (fulfilling our *Dasein*) we become "enlivened"—that is, we become an ideal bridge or channel for one aspect of O, the Forms and noumena, being met by another aspect of O, conatus and entelechy. Both are aspects of "godhead" ("godhood"), and godhood is completed again as its two disparate aspects enter in the cycle of parting and return. Their catalyst are the impinging sensory stimuli. In short, man's destiny is to evolve by becoming transformed from the transcendental to the transcendent—as they pursue their destiny and suffer their fate.

Is there transference between them? They are also analogues to the sexual communication of one's parents, just as the birth and life of the infant ratifies and completes the parental intercourse, almost as if the infant/child constituted an affidavit for the parents, who now have achieved their task of entelechy. Do they constitute the true trinity? The other trinity is that between entelechy/conatus, the transcendental analytic, and the sense impressions of emotional significance.

I close by repeating a statement by Joan and Neville Symington (1996) that I cited earlier:

> Psychoanalysis seen through Bion's eyes is a radical departure from all conceptualizations which preceded him. We have not the slightest hesitation in saying that he is the deepest thinker within psychoanalysis—and this statement does not exclude Freud. [Symington & Symington, 1996, p. xii]

NOTES

1. The recent attacks against evolution by the Religious Right in the United States have come perilously close.

2. As the reader now knows, I consider "wild thoughts" to be "wild" only to our mortal conscious self. In their own domain, as conceived by shifting perspectives, the wild thoughts are not wild. I believe they are always being "thought" by the Thinker of the thoughts without a thinker, godhood, one of whose forms might be the Muses.

W. R. BION BIBLIOGRAPHY

Harry Karnac

Part 1: List of volumes

WRB 1   *Experiences in Groups and Other Papers*. London: Tavistock
Publications and New York: Routledge 1961
     reprinted Hove: Brunner-Routledge 2001

WRB 2   *Learning from Experience*. London: William Heinemann Medical
Books 1962
     reprinted in *Seven Servants* with WRB3, WRB4, & WRB6
     New York: Aronson 1977
     reprinted London: Karnac 1984

WRB 3   *Elements of Psycho-Analysis*. London: William Heinemann Medical
Books 1963
     reprinted in *Seven Servants* with WRB2, WRB4, & WRB6
     New York: Aronson 1977
     reprinted London: Karnac 1984

WRB 4   *Transformations*. London: William Heinemann Medical Books 1965
     reprinted in *Seven Servants* with WRB2, WRB3, & WRB6
     New York: Aronson 1977
     reprinted London: Karnac 1984

WRB 5   *Second Thoughts: Selected Papers on Psycho-Analysis*. London: William
Heinemann Medical Books 1967
     reprinted London: Karnac 1984

WRB 6   *Attention and Interpretation*. London: Tavistock Publications 1970
     reprinted in *Seven Servants* with WRB2, WRB3, & WRB4
     New York: Aronson 1977
     reprinted London: Karnac 1984

WRB 7   *Bion's Brazilian Lectures 1—São Paulo.* Rio de Janeiro: Imago Editora
         1973
                  reprinted in *Brazilian Lectures* (revised & corrected ed.) with
                  WRB 8 in one volume London: Karnac 1990

WRB 8   *Bion's Brazilian Lectures 2—Rio de Janeiro/São Paulo.* Rio de Janeiro:
         Imago Editora 1974
                  reprinted in *Brazilian Lectures* (revised & corrected ed.) with
                  WRB 7 in one volume London: Karnac 1990

WRB 9   *A Memoir of the Future, Book 1: The Dream.* Rio de Janeiro: Imago
         Editora 1975
                  reprinted in *A Memoir of the Future* (revised & corrected
                  edition) with WRB 10, WRB 13, & WRB 15 in one volume
                  London: Karnac 1991

WRB 10   *A Memoir of the Future, Book 2: The Past Presented.* Rio de Janeiro:
         Imago Editora 1977
                  reprinted in *A Memoir of the Future* (revised & corrected
                  edition) with WRB 9, WRB 13, & WRB 15 in one volume
                  London: Karnac 1991

WRB 11   *Two Papers: The Grid and Caesura.* Rio de Janeiro: Imago Editora 1977
                  reprinted (revised and corrected edition) London: Karnac
                  1989

WRB 12   *Four Discussions with W.R. Bion.* Perthshire: Clunie Press 1978
                  reprinted in *Clinical Seminars and Other Works* with WRB 18 in
                  one volume (edited by Francesca Bion) London: Karnac 2000

WRB 13   *A Memoir of the Future, Book 3: The Dawn of Oblivion* Rio de Janeiro:
         Imago Editora 1977
                  reprinted in *A Memoir of the Future* (revised & corrected
                  edition) with WRB 9, WRB 10, & WRB 15 in one volume
                  London: Karnac 1991

WRB 14   *Bion in New York and São Paulo.* Perthshire: Clunie Press 1980

WRB 15   *A Key to A Memoir of the Future.* Rio de Janeiro: Imago Editora 1977
                  reprinted in *A Memoir of the Future* (revised & corrected
                  edition) with WRB 9, WRB 10, & WRB 13 in one volume
                  London: Karnac 1991

WRB 16   *The Long Weekend: 1897–1919 (Part of a Life)* (edited by Francesca
         Bion) Abingdon: Fleetwood Press 1982
                  reprinted London: Free Association Books 1986
                  reprinted London: Karnac 1991

WRB 17   *All My Sins Remembered: Another Part of a Life* and *The Other Side
         of Genius: Family Letters* (edited by Francesca Bion). Abingdon:
         Fleetwood Press 1985
                  reprinted London: Karnac 1991

WRB 18   *Clinical Seminars and Four Papers* Abingdon: Fleetwood Press 1987
                  reprinted in *Clinical Seminars and Other Works* with WRB 12 in
                  one volume (edited by Francesca Bion) London: Karnac 2000

WRB 19   *Cogitations* (edited by Francesca Bion). London: Karnac 1992
        new extended edition London: Karnac 1994

WRB 20   *Taming Wild Thoughts* (edited by Francesca Bion). London: Karnac
        1997

WRB 21   *War Memoirs 1917–1919* (edited by Francesca Bion). London: Karnac
        1997

WRB 22   *Clinical Seminars and Other Works* (edited by Francesca Bion).
        London: Karnac 2000
                [single volume edition containing *Four Discussions with W. R.*
                Bion (WRB 12) and *Clinical Seminars and Four Papers (WRB 18)*]

WRB 23   *The Italian Seminars* (edited by Francesca Bion and transl. from the
        Italian by Philip Slotkin). London: Karnac 2005
                [earlier edition *Seminari Italiani: Testo Completo dei Seminari*
                tenuti da W. R. Bion a Roma. Edizioni Borla 1985]

WRB 24   *The Tavistock Seminars* (edited by Francesca Bion). London: Karnac
        2005

Part 2: Chronological

1940   War of Nerves, The
        in *The Neuroses in War*, ed. Miller & Crichton-
        Miller (pp 180–200). London: Macmillan 1940

1943   Intra-Group Tensions in Therapy (with Rickman, J.)   WRB 1: 11–26
        Lancet 2: 678/781—Nov. 27

1946   Northfield Experiment [The] (with Bridger, H. and
        Main, T.)
        Bulletin of the Menninger Clinic 10: 71–76

1946b Leaderless Group Project
        Bulletin of the Menninger Clinic 10: 77–81

1948a Psychiatry in a Time of Crisis
        British Journal of Medical Psychology XXI: 81–89

1948b Experiences in Groups I   WRB 1: 29–40
        Human Relations I: 314–320

1948c Experiences in Groups II   WRB 1: 41–58
        Human Relations I: 487–496

1948d Untitled paper read at the International Congress on
        Mental Health, London 1948.
        In Vol. III, *Proceedings of the International*
        Conference on Medical Psychotherapy: 106–109.
        London: H. K. Lewis & New York: Columbia
        University Press 1948

1949a Experiences in Groups III   WRB 1: 59–75
        Human Relations 2: 13–22

1949b   Experiences in Groups IV   WRB 1: 77–91
        Human Relations 2: 295–303

1950a   Experiences in Groups V   WRB 1: 93–114
        Human Relations 3: 3–14

1950b   Experiences in Groups VI   WRB 1: 115–126
        Human Relations 3: 395–402

1950c   Imaginary Twin, The   WRB 5: 3–22
        read to British Psychoanalytic Society, Nov. 1

1951   Experiences in Groups VII   WRB 1: 127–137
        Human Relations 4: 221–227

1952   Group Dynamics: A Review.   WRB 1: 141–191
        International Journal of Psychoanalysis 33: 235–
        247. Also in Klein, M. et al. (eds), *New
        Directions in Psychoanalysis*: 440–477. London:
        Tavistock Publications 1955

1954   Notes on the Theory of Schizophrenia   WRB 5: 23–35
        International Journal of Psychoanalysis 35:
        113–118

1955   Language and the Schizophrenic
        in Klein, M. et al. (eds), *New Directions in
        Psychoanalysis*: 200–239. London: Tavistock
        Publications 1955

1956   Development of Schizophrenic Thought, The   WRB 5: 36–42
        International Journal of Psychoanalysis 37:
        344–346

1957a   Differentiation of the Psychotic from the Non- WRB 5: 43–64
        Psychotic Personalities, The
        International Journal of Psychoanalysis 38:
        266–275

1957b   On Arrogance   WRB 5: 86–92
        International Journal of Psychoanalysis 39:
        144–146

1958   On Hallucination   WRB 5: 65–85
        International Journal of Psychoanalysis 39:
        341–349

1959   Attacks on Linking   WRB 5: 93–109
        International Journal of Psychoanalysis 40:
        308–315

1961   Melanie Klein—Obituary (with Herbert Rosenfeld
        and Hanna Segal)
        International Journal of Psychoanalysis 42: 4–8

1962   Psychoanalytic Study of Thinking, The   WRB 5: 110–119
       International Journal of Psychoanalysis 43:
       306–310 (published as "A Theory of
       Thinking")

1963   The Grid   WRB 20:. 6–21

1966a Catastrophic Change
       Bulletin of the British Psychoanalytic Society #5

1966b *Medical Orthodoxy and the Future of Psycho-Analysis,*
       K. Eissler. New York, I.U.P. 1965 (review)
       International Journal of Psychoanalysis 47:
       575–579

1966c *Sexual Behavior and the Law,* ed. R. Slovenko.
       Springfield, Thomas 1964 (review)
       International Journal of Psychoanalysis 47:
       579–581

1967   Notes on Memory and Desire
       Psychoanalytic Forum 11/3: 271–280. Reprinted
       in *Melanie Klein Today Vol.2—Mainly Practice:*
       17–21, ed. E. Bott Spillius. London: Routledge
       1988

1976a Evidence   WRB 18: 313–320
       Bulletin of the British Psychoanalytic Society 1976

1976b Interview with A. G. Banet Jr., Los Angeles 1976   WRB 24: 97–114
       Group and Organisation Studies 1 (3): 268–285

1977a Quotation from Freud (On a)   WRB 18: 306–311
       in *Borderline Personality Disorders,* ed. P.
       Hartocollis. New York: I.U.P.

1977b Emotional Turbulence   WRB 18: 295- 305
       in *Borderline Personality Disorders,* ed. P.
       Hartocollis. New York: I.U.P.

1977c *Seven Servants* (with an introduction by W.R. Bion)
       containing *Elements of Psycho-Analysis Learning
       from Experience, Transformations, Attention and
       Interpretation*
       New York: Aronson

1978   Seminar held in Paris, July 10th 1978 (unpublished in
       English)
       published in French, *Revue Psychotherapie
       Psychanalytique de Groupe* 1986

1979   Making the Best of a Bad Job   WRB 18: 321–331
       Bulletin of the British Psychoanalytic Society

Part 3: *Alphabetical*

1959   Attacks on Linking   WRB 5: 93–109
        International Journal of Psychoanalysis 40: 308–315

1966a   Catastrophic Change
        Bulletin of the British Psychoanalytic Society #5

1956   Development of Schizophrenic Thought, The   WRB 5: 36–42
        International Journal of Psychoanalysis 37: 344–346

1957a   Differentiation of the Psychotic from the Non-   WRB 5: 43–64
        Psychotic Personalities, The
        International Journal of Psychoanalysis 38: 266–275

1977b   Emotional Turbulence   WRB 18: 295–305
        in *Borderline Personality Disorders* ed. P.
        Hartocollis. New York: I.U.P.

1976a   Evidence   WRB 18: 313–320
        Bulletin of the British Psychoanalytic Society 1976

1948b   Experiences in Groups I   WRB 1: 29–40
        Human Relations I: 314–320

1948c   Experiences in Groups II   WRB 1: 41–58
        Human Relations I: 487–496

1949a   Experiences in Groups III   WRB 1: 59–75
        Human Relations 2: 13–22

1949b   Experiences in Groups IV   WRB 1: 77–91
        Human Relations 2: 295–303

1950a   Experiences in Groups V   WRB 1: 93–114
        Human Relations 3: 3–14

1950b   Experiences in Groups VI   WRB 1: 115–126
        Human Relations 3: 395–402

1951   Experiences in Groups VII   WRB 1: 127–137
        Human Relations 4: 221–227

1963   The Grid   WRB 20:. 6–21

1952   Group Dynamics: A Review.   WRB 1: 141–191
        International Journal of Psychoanalysis 33: 235–
        247. Also in Klein, M. et al. (eds), *New Directions
        in Psychoanalysis:* 440–477. London: Tavistock
        Publications 1955

1950c   Imaginary Twin, The   WRB 5: 3–22
        read to British Psychoanalytic Society, Nov. 1

1976b   Interview with A. G. Banet Jr., Los Angeles 1976   WRB 24: 97–114
        Group and Organisation Studies 1 (3): 268–285

1943   Intra-Group Tensions in Therapy (with Rickman, J.)   WRB 1: 11–26
        Lancet 2: 678/781—Nov. 27

1955   Language and the Schizophrenic
        in Klein, M. et al. (eds), *New Directions in
        Psychoanalysis*: 200–239. London: Tavistock
        Publications 1955

1946b   Leaderless Group Project
        Bulletin of the Menninger Clinic 10: 77–81

1979   Making the Best of a Bad Job   WRB 18: 321–331
        Bulletin of the British Psychoanalytic Society

1966b   *Medical Orthodoxy and the Future of Psycho-Analysis*,
        K. Eissler. New York, I.U.P. 1965 (review)
        International Journal of Psychoanalysis 47: 575–579

1961   Melanie Klein—Obituary (with Herbert Rosenfeld
        and Hanna Segal)
        International Journal of Psychoanalysis 42: 4–8

1946   Northfield Experiment [The] (with Bridger, H., and
        Main, T.)
        Bulletin of the Menninger Clinic 10: 71–76

1967   Notes on Memory and Desire
        Psychoanalytic Forum 11/3: 271–280. Reprinted in
        Melanie Klein Today Vol.2—Mainly Practice: 17–21,
        ed. E. Bott Spillius. London: Routledge 1988

1954   Notes on the Theory of Schizophrenia   WRB 5: 23–35
        International Journal of Psychoanalysis 35: 113–118

1957b   On Arrogance   WRB 5: 86–92
        International Journal of Psychoanalysis 39: 144–146

1958   On Hallucination   WRB 5: 65–85
        International Journal of Psychoanalysis 39: 341–349

1948a   Psychiatry in a Time of Crisis
        British Journal of Medical Psychology XXI: 81–89

1962   Psychoanalytic Study of Thinking, The   WRB 5: 110–119
        International Journal of Psychoanalysis 43: 306–310
        (published as "A Theory of Thinking")

1977a   Quotation from Freud (On a)   WRB 18: 306–311
        in *Borderline Personality Disorders*, ed. P.
        Hartocollis. New York: I.U.P.

1978   Seminar held in Paris, July 10th 1978 (unpublished
        in English)
        published in French, *Revue Psychotherapie
        Psychanalytique de Groupe* 1986

1977c   *Seven Servants* (with an introduction by W.R. Bion)
containing *Elements of Psycho-Analysis, Learning
from Experience, Transformations, Attention and
Interpretation*
New York: Aronson

1966c   *Sexual Behavior and the Law*, ed. R. Slovenko.
Springfield, Thomas 1964 (review)
International Journal of Psychoanalysis 47:
579–581

1948d   Untitled paper read at the International Congress
on Mental Health, London 1948.
In Vol. III, *Proceedings of the International
Conference on Medical Psychotherapy:* 106–109.
London: H. K. Lewis & New York: Columbia
University Press 1948

1940   War of Nerves, The
in *The Neuroses in War,* ed. Miller & Crichton-
Miller (pp 180–200). London: Macmillan 1940

Aisenstein, M. (2006). The indissociable unity of psyche and soma: A view from the Paris Psychoanalytic School. *International Journal of Psychoanalysis, 87* (3): 667–680.

Apprey, M. (1987). Projective identification and maternal misconception in disturbed mothers. *British Journal of Psychotherapy, 4* (1): 5–22.

Arnold, M. (1867). "Dover Beach." In: *New Poems*. London: Dover Publications, 1994.

Bandera, A. (2005). "Hysteria and the 'Transformation Spectrum'." Paper presented at the Scientific Meeting of the Northern California Society for Psychoanalytic Psychotherapy, 11 June.

Banet, A. G. (1976). Interview [of Bion] by Anthony G. Banet, Jr., Los Angeles, 3 April. In: *Wilfred R. Bion: The Tavistock Seminars* (pp. 97–114). London: Karnac, 2005.

Beebe, B., & Lachman, F. M. (1988). Mother–infant mutual influence and precursor of psychic structure. In: A. Goldberg (Ed.), *Progress in Self Psychology, Vol. 3* (pp. 3–25). Hillsdale, NJ: Analytic Press.

Billow, R. (2003). *Relational Group Psychotherapy: From Basic Assumption to Passion*. London/New York: Jessica Kingsley.

Bion, F. (1980). Preface. In: W. R. Bion, *Bion in New York and São Paulo*, ed. F. Bion. Strath Tay: Clunie Press.

Bion, W. R. (1950). The imaginary twin. In: *Second Thoughts: Selected Papers on Psychoanalysis* (pp. 3–22). London: Heinemann, 1967.

341

Bion, W. R. (1954). Notes on the theory of schizophrenia. In: *Second Thoughts: Selected Papers on Psychoanalysis* (pp. 23–35). London: Heinemann, 1967.

Bion, W. R. (1956). Development of schizophrenic thought. In: *Second Thoughts: Selected Papers on Psychoanalysis* (pp. 36–42). London: Heinemann, 1967

Bion, W. R. (1957a). On arrogance. In: *Second Thoughts: Selected Papers on Psychoanalysis* (pp. 86–92). London: Heinemann, 1967.

Bion, W. R. (1957b). Differentiation of the psychotic from the non-psychotic personalities. In: *Second Thoughts: Selected Papers on Psychoanalysis* (pp. 43–64). London: Heinemann, 1967.

Bion, W. R. (1958). On hallucination. In: *Second Thoughts: Selected Papers on Psychoanalysis* (pp. 65–85). London: Heinemann, 1967.

Bion, W. R. (1959). Attacks on linking. In: *Second Thoughts: Selected Papers on Psychoanalysis* (pp. 93–109). London: Heinemann, 1967.

Bion, W. R. (1961). *Experiences in Groups*. London: Tavistock.

Bion, W. R. (1962a). A theory of thinking. In: *Second Thoughts: Selected Papers on Psychoanalysis* (pp. 110–119). London: Heinemann, 1967.

Bion, W. R. (1962b). *Learning from Experience*. London: Heinemann. (Reprinted London: Karnac, 1984.)

Bion, W. R. (1963). *Elements of Psycho-Analysis*. London: Heinemann. (Reprinted London: Karnac, 1984.)

Bion, W. R. (1965). *Transformations*. London: Heinemann. (Reprinted London: Karnac, 1984.)

Bion, W. R. (1967a). Commentary. In: *Second Thoughts: Selected Papers on Psychoanalysis* (pp. 120–166). London: Heinemann.

Bion, W. R. (1967b). Notes on memory and desire. In: *Cogitations* (pp. 380–385). London: Karnac.

Bion, W. R. (1967c). *Second Thoughts: Selected Papers on Psychoanalysis*. London: Heinemann. (Reprinted London: Karnac, 1984.)

Bion, W. R. (1970). *Attention and Interpretation*. London: Tavistock. (Reprinted London: Karnac, 1984.)

Bion, W. R. (1973). *Bion's Brazilian Lectures 1*. Rio de Janeiro: Imago Editora. (Also in: *Brazilian Lectures: 1973 Sao Paulo; 1974 Rio de Janeiro/Sao Paulo*. London: Karnac, 1990.)

Bion, W. R. (1974). *Bion's Brazilian Lectures 2*. Rio de Janeiro: Imago Editora. (Also in: *Brazilian Lectures: 1973 Sao Paulo; 1974 Rio de Janeiro/Sao Paulo*. London: Karnac, 1990.)

Bion, W. R. (1975). *A Memoir of the Future, Book I: The Dream*. Rio de Janeiro: Imago Editora. (Also in: *A Memoir of the Future, Books 1–3*. London: Karnac, 1991).

Bion, W. R. (1976). Evidence. In: *Clinical Seminars and Four Papers*. Oxford: Fleetwood Press, 1987.

Bion, W. R. (1977a). *Two Papers: The Grid and Caesura*, ed. J. Salomao. Rio de Janeiro: Imago Editora. (Revised edition London: Karnac, 1989.)

Bion, W. R. (1977b). *A Memoir of the Future, Book II: The Past Presented*. Brazil: Imago Editora. (Also in: *A Memoir of the Future, Books 1–3*. London: Karnac, 1991).

Bion, W. R. (1977c). *Seven Servants*. New York: Jason Aronson.

Bion, W. R. (1979). *A Memoir of the Future, Book III: The Dawn of Oblivion*. Perthshire: Clunie Press. (Also in: *A Memoir of the Future, Books 1–3*. London: Karnac, 1991.)

Bion, W. R. (1980). *Bion in New York and São Paulo*, ed. F. Bion. Strath Tay: Clunie Press.

Bion, W. R. (1981). *A Key to A Memoir of the Future*, ed. F. Bion. Strath Tay: Clunie Press. (Also in: *A Memoir of the Future, Books 1–3*. London: Karnac, 1991.)

Bion, W. R. (1982). *The Long Week-End 1897–1919: Part of a Life*. Oxford: Fleetwood Press.

Bion, W. R. (1985). *All My Sins Remembered and The Other Side of Genius*. Abingdon: Fleetwood Press.

Bion, W. R. (1987). Making the best of a bad job. In: *Clinical Seminars and Four Papers* (pp. 247–257). Abingdon: Fleetwood Press. (Reprinted London: Karnac, 2000.)

Bion, W. R. (1991). *A Memoir of the Future*. London: Karnac.

Bion, W. R. (1992). *Cogitations*. London: Karnac.

Bion, W. R. (1997). *Taming Wild Thoughts*, ed. F. Bion. London: Karnac.

Bion, W. R. (2005a). *The Italian Seminars*. London: Karnac.

Bion, W. R. (2005b). *The Tavistock Seminars*. London: Karnac.

Blakeslee, S. (2000). Experts explore deep sleep and the making of memory. *New York Times: Science Times*, Tuesday, 14 November, p. D2.

Bléandonu, G. (1993). *Wilfred R. Bion: His Life and Works. 1897–1979*, trans. C. Pajaczkowska. London: Free Association Books, 1996.

Bloom, H. (1983). *Kabbalah and Criticism*. New York: Continuum.

Bohm, D. (1980). *Wholeness and the Implicate Order*. London/Boston, MA: Routledge & Kegan Paul.

Bollas, C. (1987). *The Shadow of the Object: Psychoanalysis of the Unthought and Known*. New York: International Universities Press.

Borges J. L. (1998). *Collected Fictions: Jorge Luis Borges*. New York: Viking.

Bowlby, J. (1969). *Attachment and Loss, Vol. I: Attachment*. New York: Basic Books.

Bråten, S. (1998). Infant learning by altero-centric participation: The reverse of egocentric observation in autism. In S. Bråten (Ed), *Intersubjective Communication and Emotion in Early Ontogeny* (pp. 105–124). Cambridge: Cambridge University Press.

Britton, R. (1998). *Belief and Imagination: Explorations in Psychoanalysis.* London: Routledge.

Britton, R. (2006). "The Pleasure Principle, the Reality Principle and the Uncertainty Principle." Unpublished manuscript.

Brown, L. (2005). The cognitive effects of trauma: Reversal of alpha-function and the formation of a beta-screen. *Psychoanalytic Quarterly, 74:* 397–420.

Brown, L. (2006). Julie's Museum: The evolution of thinking, dreaming and historicization in the treatment of traumatized patients. *International Journal of Psychoanalysis, 87:* 1569–1585.

Brunschwig, J., & Lloyd, G. (2000). *Greek Thought: A Guide to Classical Knowledge.* Cambridge, MA: Harvard University Press.

Carvalho, R. (2005). Translator's introduction to Matte Blanco's "Four antimonies of the death instinct". *International Journal of Psychoanalysis, 86:* 1463–1464.

Chomsky, N. (1957). *Syntactic Structures.* The Hague: Mouton.

Chomsky, N. (1968). *Language and Mind.* New York: Harcourt Brace and World.

Chuster, A., & Conte, J. (2003). The negative grid. In: *W. R. Bion: Novas leituras, Vol. 2: A psicanályse dos principos ético-estéticos à clinica.* Rio de Janeiro: Companhia de Freud.

Chuster, A., & Frankiel, R. W. (2003). The clinical value of the ideas of Wilfred Bion. *International Journal of Psychoanalysis, 83:* 463–467.

Couzin, I. D., & Krause, J. (2003). Self-organization and collective behaviour in vertebrates. *Advances in the Study of Behaviour, 21:* 1–75.

Damasio, A. (1999). *The Feeling of What Happens: Body Emotion in the Making of Consciousness.* New York: Harcourt Brace.

Damasio, A. (2003). *Looking for Spinoza: Joy, Sorrow, and the Feeling Brain.* New York: Harcourt.

de Bianchedi, E. T. (1993). Lies and falsities. *Journal of Melanie Klein and Object Relations, 11:* 30–46.

de Bianchedi, E. T. (1997). From objects to links: Discovering relatedness. *Journal of Melanie Klein and Object Relations, 15:* 227–234.

de Bianchedi, E. T. (2004). "Evolution in and of Bion." Lecture presented at the Fourth Bion Conference, São Paulo, 14 July.

de Bianchedi, E. T. (2005). Whose Bion? Who is Bion? *International Journal of Psychoanalysis, 56:* 1529–1534.

de Bianchedi, E., Bregazzi, C., Crespo, C., Grillo de Rimoldi, E., Grimblat de Notrica, S., Saffories, D., Szpunberg de Bernztein, A., Werba, A., & Zamkow, R. (2000). The various faces of lies. In: *W. R. Bion: Between Past and Future*, ed. P. Bion Talamo, F. Borgogno, & S. A. Merciai. London: Karnac.

Decety, J., & Chaminade, T. (2003). Neural correlates of feeling sympathy. *Neuropsychologia, 41*: 127–138.

Dimock, G. (1989). *The Unity of the Odyssey.* Amherst, MA: University of Massachusetts Press.

Dodds, E. R. (1965). *The Greeks and the Irrational.* Cambridge: Cambridge University Press.

Edelman, G. (2004). *Wider than the Sky: The Phenomenal Gift of Consciousness.* New Haven, CT/London: Yale University Press.

Ehrenzweig, A. (1967). *The Hidden Order of Art.* Berkeley, CA/London: University of California Press.

Eigen, M. (1985). Toward Bion's starting point between catastrophe and faith. *International Journal of Psychoanalysis, 66*: 321–330.

Eigen, M. (1998). *The Psychoanalytic Mystic.* Binghamton, NY: ESF Publications.

Eigen, M. (2005). *Emotional Storms.* Middletown, CT: Wesleyan University Press.

Fagles, R. (1991). *Homer's "The Iliad."* New York: Penguin Books.

Fairbairn, W. R. D. (1940). Schizoid factors and personality. In: *Psychoanalytic Studies of the Personality* (pp. 3–27). London: Tavistock, 1952.

Fairbairn, W. R. D. (1943). The repression and the return of bad objects (with special reference to the "war neuroses."). In: *Psychoanalytic Studies of the Personality* (pp. 59–81). London: Tavistock, 1952.

Federn, P. (1949). The ego in schizophrenia. In: *Ego Psychology and the Psychoses* (pp. 227–240), ed. E. Weiss. New York: Basic Books, 1952.

Federn, P. (1952). The psychoanalysis of psychoses. In: *Ego Psychology and the Psychoses* (pp. 117–165), ed. E. Weiss. New York: Basic Books.

Ferro, A. (1999). *Psychoanalysis as Therapy and Storytelling.* London/New York: Routledge.

Ferro, A. (2002a). *In the Analyst's Consulting Room*, trans. P. Slotkin. Hove/New York: Brunner-Routledge.

Ferro, A. (2002b). *Seeds of Illness, Seeds of Recovery: The Genesis of Suffering and the Role of Psychoanalysis.* Hove/New York: Brunner-Routledge, 2005.

Ferro, A. (2005). Bion: Theoretical and clinical observations. *International Journal of Psychoanalysis, 86*: 1535–1542.

Ferro, A. (2006). Clinical implications of Bion's thought. *International Journal of Psychoanalysis, 87*: 989–1003.

Fitch, W. T. (2005). Dancing to Darwin's tune: Review of Steve Mithen's *The Singing Neanderthal: The Origins of Music, Language, Mind and Body* [Weidenfeld & Nicholson, 2005]. *Nature, 438* (17): 287.

Fliess, R. (1942). The metapsychology of the analyst. *Psychoanalytic Quarterly, 11*: 211–227.

Fonagy, P., & Target, M. (1996). Playing with reality: Theory of mind and the normal development of psychic reality. *International Journal of Psychoanalysis, 77*: 217–233.

Fonagy, P., & Target, M. (2000). Playing with reality III: The persistence of dual psychic reality in borderline patients. *International Journal of Psychoanalysis, 81*: 853–874.

Fox, M. (1981). Meister Eckhart on the fourfold path of creation. In: M. Fox (Ed.), *Western Spirituality: Historical Roots, Ecumenical Roots* (pp. 215–248). Santa Fe, NM: Bear & Co.

Frazer, J. (1992). *The Golden Bough*. New York: Macmillan.

Freud, A. (1936). *The Ego and the Mechanisms of Defense*. New York: International Universities Press.

Freud, S. (1895d) (with Breuer, J.). *Studies on Hysteria. Standard Edition*, 2: 1–309. London: Hogarth Press, 1955.

Freud, S. (1896b). Further remarks on the neuro-psychoses of defence. *Standard Edition*, 3: 159–185. London: Hogarth Press, 1962.

Freud, S. (1897a–1950 [1892–1899]). Letter 61. Extracts from the Fliess papers. *Standard Edition*, 1: 247–248. London: Hogarth Press, 1966.

Freud, S. (1897b). Draft L: [Notes 1]. Extracts from the Fliess papers. *Standard Edition*, 1: 247–248. London: Hogarth Press, 1966.

Freud, S. (1900a). *The Interpretation of Dreams. Standard Edition*, 4/5. London: Hogarth Press, 1958.

Freud, S. (1905d). *Three Essays on the Theory of Sexuality. Standard Edition*, 7: 125–245. London: Hogarth Press, 1953.

Freud, S. (1910i). The psycho-analytic view of psychogenic disturbance of vision. *Standard Edition*, 11: 209–218. London: Hogarth Press, 1957.

Freud, S. (1911b). Formulations on the two principles of mental functioning. *Standard Edition*, 12: 213–226. London: Hogarth Press, 1958.

Freud, S. (1912e). Recommendations to physicians practising psycho-analysis. *Standard Edition*, 12: 109–120. London: Hogarth Press, 1958.

Freud, S. (1914d). On the history of the psycho-analytic movement. *Standard Edition*, 14:3 –66. London: Hogarth Press, 1957.

Freud, S. (1915c). Instincts and their vicissitudes. *Standard Edition*, 14: 109–140. London: Hogarth Press, 1957.

Freud, S. (1915d). Repression. *Standard Edition*, 14: 141–158. London: Hogarth Press, 1957.

Freud, S. (1915e). The unconscious. *Standard Edition* 14: 159–215. London: Hogarth Press, 1957.

Freud, S. (1917e [1915]). Mourning and melancholia. *Standard Edition*, 14: 237–260. London: Hogarth Press, 1957.

Freud, S. (1920g). *Beyond the Pleasure Principle. Standard Edition*, 18: 3–66. London: Hogarth Press, 1955

Freud, S. (1921c). *Group Psychology and the Analysis of the Ego. Standard Edition*, 18: 67–144. London: Hogarth Press, 1955.

Freud, S. (1924d). The dissolution of the Oedipus complex. *Standard Edition*, 19: 173–182. London: Hogarth Press, 1961.

Freud, S. (1926d). *Inhibitions, Symptoms and Anxiety. Standard Edition*, 20: 77–178. London: Hogarth Press, 1959.

Freud, S. (1950 [1895]). Project for a scientific psychology. *Standard Edition*, 1: 281–397. London: Hogarth Press, 1966.

Freud, S., & Andreas-Salomé, L. (1966). Letter dated "25.5.16." In: *Letters* (p. 45), ed. E. Pfeiffer, trans. W. Robson-Scott & E. Robson-Scott. London: Hogarth Press, 1972.

Gais, S., Plihal, W., Wagner, U., & Born, J. (2000). Early sleep triggers memory for early visual discrimination skills. *Nature Neuroscience, 3*: 1335–1339.

Gallese, V. (2001). The "shared manifold" hypothesis: From mirror neurons to empathy. *Journal of Consciousness Studies, 8*: 33–50.

Gallese, V., & Goldman, A. (1998). Mirror neurons and the simulation theory of mind reading. *Trends in Cognitive Science, 2*: 493–501.

Ghazanfar, A. A., & Logothetis, N. K. (2003). Facial expressions linked to monkey calls. *Nature, 423*: 937–938.

Gleik, J. (1987). *Chaos: Making a New Science.* New York: Viking Press.

Godbout, C. (2004). Reflections on Bion's "elements of psychoanalysis". *International Journal of Psychoanalysis, 85*: 1123–1136.

Gordon, J. (1994). Bion's post-*Experiences in Groups* thinking on groups: A clinical example of –K. In: V. L. Schermer & M. Pines (Eds.), *Ring of Fire: Primitive Affects and Object Relations in Group Psychotherapy* (pp. 107–127). London: Jessica Kingsley.

Greatrex T. (2002). Projective identification: How does it work? *Neuro-Psychoanalysis, 4*: 187–197.

Green, J. (1947). *If I Were You . . .*, trans. J. H. F. McEwen. London: Eyre & Spottiswoode, 1950.

Greenberg, J. (2005). Conflict in the middle voice. *Psychoanalytic Quarterly, 74*: 105–120.

Grinberg, L. (1979). Countertransference and projective counter-identification. *Contemporary Psychoanalysis, 15*: 226–247.

Grinberg, L., Sor, D., & de Bianchedi, E. T. (1977). *Introduction to the Work of Bion*. New York: Jason Aronson.

Grinberg, L., Sor, D., & de Bianchedi, E. T. (1993). *New Introduction to the Work of Bion*. Northvale, NJ: Jason Aronson.

Grotstein, J. (1978). Inner space: Its dimensions and its coordinates. *International Journal of Psychoanalysis, 59*: 55–61.

Grotstein, J. (1979). Demoniacal possession, splitting, and the torment of joy. *Contemporary Psychoanalysis, 15*: 407–453.

Grotstein, J. (1981a). *Splitting and Projective Identification*. New York: Jason Aronson.

Grotstein, J. (1981b). Bion the man, the psychoanalyst, and the mystic: A perspective on his life and work. In: J. S. Grotstein (Ed.), *Do I Dare Disturb the Universe? A Memorial to Wilfred R. Bion* (pp. 1–36). Beverly Hills, CA: Caesura Press.

Grotstein, J. (1981c). Who is the dreamer who dreams the dream and who is the dreamer who understands it? (Revised). In: J. S. Grotstein (Ed.), *Do I Dare Disturb the Universe? A Memorial to Wilfred R. Bion* (pp. 357–416). Beverly Hills, CA: Caesura Press.

Grotstein, J. (Ed.) (1981d). *Do I Dare Disturb the Universe? A Memorial to Wilfred R. Bion*. Beverly Hills, CA: Caesura Press.

Grotstein, J. (1985). W. R. Bion: A voyage into the deep and formless infinite. In: J. Reppen (Ed.), *Beyond Freud* (pp. 297–314). Hillsdale, NJ: Analytic Press.

Grotstein, J. (1986). The dual-track: A contribution toward a neurobehavioral model of cerebral processing. *Psychiatric Clinics of North America, 9* (2): 353–366.

Grotstein, J. (1987). Making the best of a bad deal: On Harold Boris' "Bion Revisited". *Contemporary Psychoanalysis, 23* (1): 60–76.

Grotstein, J. (1993a). Towards the concept of the transcendent position: Reflections on some of "the unborns" in Bion's *Cogitations. Journal of Melanie Klein and Object Relations, 11* (2): 55–73. [Special Issue: "Understanding the Work of Wilfred Bion".]

Grotstein, J. (1993b). Editorial. *The Journal of Melanie Klein and Object Relations, 11* (2): 1–2. [Special Issue: "Understanding the Work of Wilfred Bion".]

Grotstein, J. (1995). A reassessment of the couch in psychoanalysis. *Psychoanalytic Inquiry, 15*: 396–405. [Special issue: "The Relevance of the Couch in Contemporary Psychoanalysis."]

Grotstein, J. (1996a). Bion's transformation in "O", Lacan's "thing-in-itself," and Kant's "Real": Towards the concept of the transcendent position. *Journal of Melanie Klein and Object Relations, 14* (2): 109–141.

Grotstein, J. (1996b). The significance of Bion's concepts of P-S→D and transformations in "O": A reconsideration of the relationship between the paranoid–schizoid and depressive positions—and beyond. In: K. Hall & B. Burgoyne (Eds.), *Schemas and Models in Psychoanalysis*. London: Rebus Press.

Grotstein, J. (1997a). Bion: The pariah of "O". *British Journal of Psychotherapy, 14* (1): 77–90.

Grotstein, J. (1997b). "Fearful symmetry" and the calipers of the infinite geometer: Matte-Blanco's legacy to our conception of the unconscious. *The Journal of Melanie Klein and Object Relations, 15* (4): 631–646. [Special Issue on Matte Blanco.]

Grotstein, J. (1997c). Integrating one-person and two-person psychologies: Autochthony and alterity in counterpoint. *Psychoanalytic Quarterly, 66*: 403–430.

Grotstein, J. (1997d). Mens sane in corpore sano: The mind and body as an "odd couple" and as an oddly coupled unity. *Psychoanalytic Inquiry, 17* (2): 204–222.

Grotstein, J. (1998). The numinous and immanent nature of the psychoanalytic subject. *Journal of Analytical Psychology, 43*: 41–68.

Grotstein, J. (1999a). Bion's "transformations in O and the concept of the transcendent position". In: P. Bion, F. Borgogno, & S. A. Merciai (Eds.), *W. R. Bion: Between Past and Future*. London: Karnac.

Grotstein, J. (1999b). The significance of Bion's concepts of PS↔D and transformations in "O": A reconsideration of the relationship between Klein's "positions". In: K. Hall & O. Rathbone (Eds.), *Psychoanalytic Schemas and Models and Their Graphic Representations*. London: Rebus Press.

Grotstein, J. (2000a). *Who Is the Dreamer Who Dreams the Dream? A Study of Psychic Presences*. Hillsdale, NJ: Analytic Press.

Grotstein, J. (2000b). The relationship between Bollas's "unthought known" and Bion's "thoughts without a thinker" and "memoirs of the future". In: J. Scalia & L. Mitchell (Eds.), *The Vitality of Objects: Exploring the Work of Christopher Bollas*. Middletown, CT: Wesleyan University Press.

Grotstein, J. (2000c). Notes on Bion's "Memory and Desire." *Journal of the American Academy of Psychoanalysis, 28* (4): 687–694.

Grotstein, J. (2001a). Bion on free associations. *Revista di Psicoanalisi*: 365–373. [Special Issue: "Free Association and Free-Floating Discourse."]

Grotstein, J. (2001b). Commentary on "Bion's: A Tool for Transformation" by Marilyn Charles. *Journal of the American Academy of Psychoanalysis, 30*: (3): 447–450.

Grotstein, J. (2002). "We are such stuff as dreams are made on": Annotations on dreams and dreaming in Bion's works. In: C. Neri, M. Pines, & R. Friedman (Eds.), *Dreams in Group Psychotherapy: Theory and Technique* (pp. 110–145). London/Philadelphia: Jessica Kingsley.

Grotstein, J. (2003). Introduction: Early Bion. In: R. M. Lipgar & M. Pines (Eds.), *Building on Bion: Origins and Context of Bion's Contributions to Theory and Practice*. London/Philadelphia: Jessica Kingsley.

Grotstein, J. (2004a). "The Light Militia of the Lower Sky": The deeper nature of dreaming and phantasying. *Psychoanalytic Dialogues, 14* (1): 99–118.

Grotstein, J. (2004b). "The seventh servant": The implications of a truth drive in Bion's theory of O. *International Journal of Psychoanalysis, 85*: 1081–1101.

Grotstein, J. (2005). "Projective *trans*identification: An extension of the concept of projective identification. *International Journal of Psychoanalysis, 86*: 1051–1069.

Grotstein, J. (2006a). Foreword. In: A. Casement & D. Tacey (Eds.), *The Idea of the Numinous: Contemporary Jungian and Psychoanalytic Perspectives* (pp: xi–xv). Hove: Routledge.

Grotstein, J. (2006b). On: "Whose Bion?" [Letter to the Editors]. *International Journal of Psychoanalysis, 87* (2): 577–579.

Grotstein, J. (2009). *"But at the Same Time and on Another Level . . .": Psychoanalytic Technique in the Kleinian/Bionian Mode. A Beginning.* New York: Other Press.

Grotstein, J. (unpublished-a). Notes on unconscious phantasies from the Kleinian/Bionian perspective. *Psychoanalytic Inquiry.*

Grotstein, J. (unpublished-b). The voice from the crypt: The negative therapeutic reaction and the longing for the infancy that never was. *Contemporary Psychoanalysis.*

Hampshire, S. (2005). *Spinoza and Spinozism.* Oxford: Oxford University Press.

Hargreaves, E., & Varchevker, A. (Eds.) (2004). *In Pursuit of Psychic Change: The Betty Joseph Workshop.* Hove/New York: Brunner-Routledge.

Hartmann, H. (1939). *Ego Psychology and the Problem of Adaptation.* New York: International Universities Press, 1958.

Heidegger, M. (1927). *Being and Time,* trans. J. Macquarrie & E. Robinson. San Francisco: HarperCollins, 1962.

Heidegger, M. (1968). *What Is Called Thinking?,* trans. F. Wieck & G. Gray. New York: Harper & Row.

Heimann, P. (1950). On counter-transference. *International Journal of Psychoanalysis, 31*: 81–84.

Heimann, P. (1960). Countertransference. *British Journal of Medical Psychology, 33*: 9–15.

Heisenberg, W. (1958). *Physics and Philosophy*. New York: Harper & Brothers.

Helm, F. (2004). "Conscious, Unconscious and Non-conscious Communication." Unpublished manuscript.

Hoffman, I. Z. (1992). Some practical implications of a social constructivist view of the psychoanalytic situation. *Psychoanalytic Dialogues, 2*: 287–304.

Hoffman, I. Z. (1994). Dialectical thinking and therapeutic action in the psychoanalytic process. *Psychoanalytic Quarterly, 63*: 187–213.

Humphrey, N. (2006). *Seeing Red: A Study in Consciousness*. Cambridge, MA: Harvard University Press.

Isaacs, S. (1952). The nature and function of phantasy. In: M. Klein, P. Heimann, S. Isaacs, & J. Riviere (Eds.), *Developments in Psycho-Analysis* (pp. 67–121). London: Hogarth Press.

Jacobson, E. (1964). *The Self and the Object World*. New York: International Universities Press.

James, W. (1890). *The Principles of Psychology*. Cambridge, MA: Harvard University Press, 1981.

Joseph, B. (1989). *Psychic Equilibrium and Psychic Change*. London: Routledge

Jowett, B. (1892). *The Dialogues of Plato, Vols. 1 & 2*. London: MacMillan.

Joyce, J. (1916). *Portrait of the Artist as a Young Man*. New York: Penguin Classics, 2003.

Jung, C. G. (1916). The transcendent function. In: *The Collected Works of C. G. Jung, Vol. 8* (2nd edition), trans. R. F. C. Hull. Princeton, NJ: Princeton University Press, 1972, pp. 67–91.

Jung, C. G. (1967). *Psychology and Alchemy. The Collected Works of C. G. Jung, Vol. 12* (2nd edition), trans. G. Adler & R. F. C. Hull. Princeton, NJ: Princeton University Press, 1968.

Kant, I. (1783). *Prolegomena zu einer jeden kuenftigen Metaphysik*. Riga: Hartknoch.

Kant, I. (1787). *Critique of Pure Reason* (revised edition), trans. N. Kemp Smith. New York: St. Martin's Press, 1965.

Kauffman, S. (1993). *The Origin of Order: Self-Organization and Selection in Evolution*. New York: Oxford University Press.

Kauffman, S. (1995). *At Home in the Universe: The Search for the Laws of Self-Organization and Complexity*. New York/Oxford: Oxford University Press.

Keats, J. (1817). Letter to George and Thomas Keats, 21 December 1817.

In: *Letters* (4th edition), ed. M. B. Forman. Oxford: Oxford University Press, 1952.

Kernberg, O. (1987). Projection and projective identification: Developmental and clinical aspects. In: J. Sandler (Ed.), *Projection, Identification, and Projective Identification* (pp. 93–116). Madison, CT: International Universities Press, 1987.

Kitayama, O. (1998). Transience: Its beauty and its danger. *International Journal of Psychoanalysis, 79*: 937–954.

Klein, M. (1921). The development of a child. In: *Contributions to Psycho-Analysis, 1921–1945* (pp. 13–67). London: Hogarth Press, 1950.

Klein, M. (1928). Early stages of the Oedipus conflict. In: *Contributions to Psycho-Analysis, 1921–1945* (pp. 202–214). London: Hogarth Press, 1950.

Klein, M. (1929). Personification in the play of children. In: *Contributions to Psycho-Analysis, 1921–1945* (pp. 215–226). London: Hogarth Press, 1950.

Klein, M. (1930). The importance of symbol formation in the development of the ego. *International Journal of Psychoanalysis, 11*: 24–39.

Klein, M. (1933). The early development of conscience in the child. In: *Contributions to Psycho-Analysis, 1921–1945* (pp. 267–277). London: Hogarth Press, 1950.

Klein, M. (1935). A contribution to the psychogenesis of manic-depressive states. In: *Contributions to Psycho-Analysis, 1921–1945* (pp. 282–310). London: Hogarth Press, 1950.

Klein, M. (1940). Mourning and its relation to manic-depressive states. In: *Contributions to Psycho-Analysis, 1921–1945* (pp. 311–338). London: Hogarth Press, 1950.

Klein, M. (1946). Notes on some schizoid mechanisms. In: M. Klein, P. Heimann, S. Isaacs, & J. Riviere (Eds.), *Developments in Psycho-Analysis* (pp. 292–320). London: Hogarth Press, 1952.

Klein, M. (1955). On identification. In: M. Klein, P. Heimann, S. Isaacs, & R. Money-Kyrle (Eds.), *New Directions in Psycho-Analysis* (pp. 309–345). London: Hogarth Press.

Klein, M. (1960). *Narrative of a Child Analysis*. New York: Basic Books.

Kohut, H. (1971). *The Analysis of the Self: A Systematic Approach to the Psychoanalytic Treatment of Narcissistic Personality Disorders*. New York: International Universities Press.

Korbivcher, C. (1999). Mente primitiva e pensamento. *Revista Brasileira de Psicanálise, 33* (4): 687–707.

Korbivcher, C. (2001). A teoria das transformações e os estados autisticos. Transformações autisticas. Uma proposta. *Revista Brasileira de Psicanálise, 35* (4): 935–958.

Korbivcher, C. (2005a). "The Analyst's Mind and Autistic Transformations." Paper presented at the Annual Francis Tustin Memorial Lectureship, Los Angeles, November 5.

Korbivcher, C. (2005b). The theory of transformations and autistic states. *International Journal of Psychoanalysis, 86*: 1595–1610.

Kristeva, J. (1989). *Black Sun: Depression and Melancholia.* New York: Columbia University Press.

Lacan, J. (1966). *Écrits: 1949–1960*, trans. A. Sheridan. New York: W. W. Norton, 1977.

Lawlor, R. (1982). *Sacred Geometry: Philosophy and Practice.* Crestone, CO: Thames & Hudson.

Lebow, R. (2003). *The Tragic Vision of Politics: Ethics, Interests and Orders.* Cambridge: Cambridge University Press.

Lévi-Strauss, C. (1958). *Structural Anthropology*, trans. C. Jacobson & B. Grundfest. Harmondsworth: Penguin, 1968.

Lévi-Strauss, C. (1970). *The Elementary Structures of Kinship.* London: Tavistock.

Llinàs, R. (2001). *I of the Vortex: From Neurons to Self.* Cambridge, MA/London: MIT Press.

López-Corvo, R. (2003). *The Dictionary of the Work of W. R. Bion.* London: Karnac.

López-Corvo, R. (2006a). *Wild Thoughts Searching for a Thinker.* London: Karnac.

López-Corvo, R. (2006b). The forgotten self: With the use of Bion's theory of negative links. *Psychoanalytic Review, 93*: 363–377.

Maquet, P. (2000). Sleep on it. *Nature Neuroscience, 3*: 1235–1236.

Mason, A. (1981). The suffocating super-ego: Psychotic break and claustrophobia. In: J. S. Grotstein (Ed.), *Do I Dare Disturb the Universe? A Memorial to Wilfred R. Bion.* Beverly Hills, CA: Caesura Press.

Mason, A. (1994). A psychoanalyst looks at a hypnotist: A study of folie à deux. *Psychoanalytic Quarterly, 63* (4): 641–679.

Mason, A. (2000). Bion and binocular vision. *International Journal of Psychoanalysis, 81*: 983–989.

Massidda, G. B. (1999). Shall we ever know the whole truth about projective identification? [Letter to the Editor.] *International Journal of Psychoanalysis, 80*: 365–367.

Matte Blanco, I. (1975). *The Unconscious as Infinite Sets.* London: Duckworth.

Matte Blanco, I. (1981). Reflecting with Bion. In: J. S. Grotstein (Ed.), *Do I Dare Disturb the Universe? A Memorial to Wilfred R. Bion* (pp. 489–528). Beverly Hills, CA: Caesura Press.

Matte Blanco, I. (1988). *Thinking, Feeling, and Being: Clinical Reflections on the Fundamental Antinomy of Human Beings*. London/New York: Routledge.

Matte Blanco, I. (2005). The four antinomies of the death instinct [trans. R. Carvalho]. *International Journal of Psychoanalysis, 86*: 1463–1476.

Mattos, J. A. J. de (1997). "Transference and Counter-transference as Transience." Paper presented at the International Centennial Conference on the Work of W. R. Bion, Turin, Italy, 16 July.

Maturana, H. R., & Varela, F. J. (1972). *Autopoiesis and Cognition: The Realization of the Living*. Boston/London: Reidel.

Maugham, W. S. (1945). *The Razor's Edge*. London: Penguin Classics, 1992.

McGinn, B. (1994). *The Foundations of Mysticism: Origins to the Fifth Century*. New York: Crossroad Publishing.

McGinn, B. (1996). *The Growth of Mysticism*. New York: Crossroad Publishing.

Meares, R. (2000). Priming and projective identification. *Bulletin of the Menninger Clinic, 64*: 1–15.

Meltzer, D. W. (1966). The relation of anal masturbation to projective identification. *International Journal of Psychoanalysis, 47*: 335–342.

Meltzer, D. W. (1978). *The Kleinian Development, Part III: The Clinical Significance of the Work of Bion*. Strath Tay: Clunie Press.

Meltzer, D. W. (1980). "The diameter of the circle" in Wilfred Bion's work. In: *Sincerity and Other Works: Collected Papers of Donald Meltzer* (pp. 469–474), ed. A. Hahn. London: Karnac, 1994.

Meltzer, D. W. (1985). Three lectures on W. R. Bion's *A Memoir of the Future* [with Meg Harris Williams]. In: *Sincerity and Other Works: Collected Papers of Donald Meltzer* (pp. 520–550), ed. A. Hahn. London: Karnac, 1994.

Meltzer, D. W. (1986). *Studies in Extended Metapsychology: Clinical Applications of Bion's Ideas*. Strath Tay: Clunie Press.

Meltzer, D. W. (1992). *The Claustrum: An Investigation of Claustrophobic Phenomena*. Strath Tay: Clunie Press.

Meltzer, D. W. (2000). A review of my writings. In: M. Cohen & A. Hahn (Eds.), *Exploring the Work of Donald Meltzer: A Festschrift* (pp. 1–11). London: Karnac.

Modell, A. H. (1980). Affects and their non-communication. *International Journal of Psychoanalysis, 61*: 259–267.

Money-Kyrle, R. (1956). Normal concepts of counter-transference and some of its deviations. *International Journal of Psychoanalysis, 37*: 360–366.

Money-Kyrle, R. (1968). Cognitive development. In: *The Collected Papers of Roger Money-Kyrle* (pp. 416–433), ed. D. Meltzer & E. O'Shaughnessy. Strath Tay: Clunie Press, 1978.

Moore, B., & Fine, B. (Eds.) (1990). *Psychoanalytic Terms and Concepts.* New Haven, CT: Yale University Press.

Muir, R. (1995). Transpersonal processes: A bridge between object relations and attachment theory in normal and psychopathological development. *British Journal of Medical Psychology, 68*: 243–257.

Nietzsche, F. (1883). *Thus Spake Zarathustra*, trans. W. Kaufman. London: Penguin Books, 1961.

Norman, J. (2004). Transformations of early infantile experiences: A 6-month-old in psychoanalysis. *International Journal of Psychoanalysis, 85*: 1103–1122.

Novick, J., & Kelly, K. (1970). Projection and externalization. *Psychoanalytic Study of the Child, 25*: 69–98.

Ogden, T. (1982). *Projective Identification and Psychotherapeutic Technique.* New York/London: Jason Aronson.

Ogden, T. (1994a). The analytic third: Working with intersubjective clinical facts. *International Journal of Psychoanalysis, 75*: 3–20.

Ogden, T. (1994b). The concept of interpretive action. *Psychoanalytic Quarterly, 63*: 219–245.

Ogden, T. (1997). *Reverie and Interpretation: Sensing Something Human.* Northvale, NJ/London: Jason Aronson.

Ogden, T. (2001). *Conversations at the Frontier of Dreaming.* Northvale, NJ/London: Jason Aronson.

Ogden, T. (2003). On not being able to dream. *International Journal of Psychoanalysis, 84*: 17–30.

Ogden, T. (2004a). On holding and containing, being and dreaming. *International Journal of Psychoanalysis, 86*: 1349–1364.

Ogden, T. (2004b). An introduction to the reading of Bion. *International Journal of Psychoanalysis, 85*: 285–300.

Ogden, T. (2007a). Elements of analytic style: Bion's clinical seminars. *International Journal of Psychoanalysis, 88*: 1185–1200.

Ogden, T. (2007b). On talking-as-dreaming. *International Journal of Psychoanalysis, 88* (2): 575–590.

O'Shaughnessy, E. (2005). Whose Bion? *International Journal of Psychoanalysis, 86*: 1523–1528.

Peirce, C. S. (1931). *Collected Papers* (8 vols.), ed. C. Hartshore & P. Weiss. Cambridge, MA: Harvard University Press.

Peradotto, J. (1990). *Man in the Middle Voice: Name and Narration in "The Odyssey."* Princeton, NJ: Princeton University Press.

Piaget, J. (1926). *The Child's Conception of the World*, trans. J. Tomlinson & A. Tomlinson. Totowa, NJ: Littlefield, Adams, 1969.

Plato (1892). *The Dialogues of Plato, Vols. 1 & 2*, trans. B. Jowett. New York: Random House, 1937.

Poincaré, H. (1963). *Science and Method*. New York: Dover Publications.

Racker, H. (1968). *Transference and Countertransference*. London: Hogarth Press.

Rather, L. (2005). "'Saturated-O' and 'Unsaturated-O' Experience: A Contribution to Bion's Theory of Transformations." Paper presented at the Hysteria and the Transformation Spectrum Conference, Scientific Meeting of the Northern California Society for Psychoanalytic Psychology, San Francisco, 11 June.

Rezende, A. (2004). "The Experience of Truth in Clinical Psychoanalysis." Paper presented at Bion 2004 Conference, sponsored by the Sociedade Brasileira de Psicanálise de São Paulo, São Paulo, 17 July.

Ricoeur, P. (1970). *Freud and Philosophy: An Essay on Interpretation*, trans. D. Savage. New Haven, CT: Yale University Press.

Rosenfeld, H. (1965). *Psychotic States*. New York: International Universities Press

Rosenfeld, H. (1971). Contribution to the psychopathology of psychotic states: The importance of projective identification in the ego structure and the object relations of the psychotic patient. In: *Problems of Psychosis* (pp. 115–128), ed. P. Doucet & C. Laurin. Amsterdam: Excerpta Medica.

Salomonsson, B. (2007). "Talk to me baby, tell me what's the matter now": Semiotic and developmental perspectives on communication in psychoanalytic infant treatment. *International Journal of Psychoanalysis, 88*: 127–146.

Sandler, J. (1976). Countertransference and role responsiveness. *International Review of Psychoanalysis, 3*: 43–47.

Sandler, P. (1999). Um desenvolvimento e aplicação clinica do instrumento de Bion, o Grid. *Revista Brasileira de Psicanálise, 33* (1): 13–38.

Sandler, P. (2005). *The Language of Bion*. London: Karnac.

Sandler, P. (2006a). The origin of Bion's work. *International Journal of Psychoanalysis, 87*: 179–201.

Sandler, P. (2006b). "The Three-Dimensional Grid." Unpublished manuscript.

Schermer, M. (2003). The demon of determinism: Discussion of Daniel Dennet's, *Freedom Evolves*. *Science, 300*: 56–57.

Schermer, V. (2003). "O": Bion and epistemology. In: R. Lipgar & M. Pines (Eds.), *Building on Bion, II: Roots*. London: Jessica Kingsley.

Schneider, J. (2005). Experiences in K and –K. *International Journal of Psychoanalysis, 86*: 825–839.

Schore, A. (2003a). *Affect Dysregulation and Disorders of the Self*. New York: W. W. Norton.

Schore, A. (2003b). *Affect Dysregulation and Repair of the Self*. New York: W. W. Norton.

Schreber, D. P. (1903). *Memoirs of My Mental Illness*, ed & trans. I. Macalpine & R. Hunter. London: William Dawson & Sons, 1955.

Schwalbe, M. L. (1991). The autogenesis of the self. *Journal for the Theory of Social Behaviour, 21* (3): 269–295.

Segal, H. (1957). Notes on symbol formation. *International Journal of Psychoanalysis, 38*: 391–397.

Segal, H. (1981). Notes on symbol formation. In: *The Work of Hanna Segal: A Kleinian Approach to Clinical Practice* (pp. 49–68). New York/London: Jason Aronson.

Seligman, S. (1993). Integrating Kleinian theory and intersubjective infant research observing projective identification. *Psychoanalytic Dialogues, 9*: 129–159.

Seligman, S. (1994). Applying psychoanalysis in an unconventional context. *Psychoanalytic Study of the Child, 49*: 481–510.

Sells, M. A. (1994). *Mystical Language of Unsaying*. Chicago: University of Chicago Press.

Sodré, I. (2004). Who's who? Notes on pathological identifications, In: *In Pursuit of Psychic Change: The Betty Joseph Workshop* (pp. 53–64), ed. E. Hargreaves & A. Varchevker. Hove/New York: Brunner-Routledge.

Sor, D., & Senet de Gazzano, M. R. (1988). *Cambio catastrófico* [Catastrophic Change]. Buenos Aires: Kargieman.

Sor, D., & Senet de Gazzano, M. R. (1993). *Fanatismo* [Fanaticism]. Buenos Aires: Ananké.

Spillius, E. B. (1988). General introduction. In: *Melanie Klein Today: Developments in Theory and Practice, Vol. 1: Mainly Theory* (pp. 1–7), ed. E. Spillius. London/New York: Routledge.

Spillius, E. B. (1992). Clinical experiences of projective identification. In: *Clinical Lectures on Klein and Bion* (pp. 59–73), ed. R. Anderson. London/New York: Routledge.

Spillius, E. B. (2001). Freud and Klein on the concept of phantasy. *International Journal of Psychoanalysis, 82*: 361–373.

Stanislavski, C. (1936). *An Actor Prepares*, trans. E. Reynolds Hapgood. New York: Routledge, 1989.

Steiner, J. (1993). *Psychic Retreats: Pathological Organizations in Psychotic, Neurotic and Borderline Patients*. London: Routledge.

Steiner, R. (1999). Who influenced whom? And how? [Letter to the Editor]. *International Journal of Psychoanalysis, 80*: 369–376.

Stern, D. (2004). *The Present Moment in Psychotherapy and Everyday Life*. New York: W. W. Norton.

Stickgold, R., James, L.-T., & Hobson, J. A. (2000). Visual discrimination learning requires sleep after training. *Nature Neuroscience, 3*: 1237–1238.

Stitzman, L. (2004). At-one-ment, intuition, and "suchness". *International Journal of Psychoanalysis, 85*: 1137–1155.

Sullivan, B. (2007). "The Nature of Psychological Growth: Parallels between Bion and Jung." Unpublished manuscript.

Sutherland, J. D. (1985). Bion revisited: Group dynamics and group psychotherapy. In: *Bion and Group Psychotherapy*, ed. M. Pines. London: Kegan Paul.

Sutherland, J. D. (1994). Bion's group dynamics. In: *The Autonomous Self: The Work of Jon D. Sutherland*, ed. J. S. Scharff. Northvale, NJ: Jason Aronson.

Symington, J. D., & Symington, N. (1996). *The Clinical Thinking of Wilfred Bion*. London/New York: Routledge.

Target, M., & Fonagy, P. (1996). Playing with reality II: The development of psychic reality from a theoretical perspective. *International Journal of Pyschoanalysis, 77*: 459–479.

Tausk, V. (1919). On the origin of the "influencing machine" in schizophrenia. *Psychoanalytic Quarterly, 2*: 519–556.

Trevarthen, C. (1999). Musicality and the intrinsic motive pulse: Evidence from human pychobiology and infant communication. *Musicae Scientiae*: 157–213. [Special Issue: "Rhythms, Musical Narrative, and Origins of Human Communication."]

Tucker, W., & Tucker, K. (1988). *The Dark Matter: Contemporary Science's Quest for the Mass Hidden in the Our Universe*. New York: William Morrow.

Tustin, F. (1981). *Autistic States in Children*. London: Routledge & Kegan Paul.

Tustin, F. (1986). *Autistic Barriers in Neurotic Patients*. New Haven, CT: Yale University Press.

Tustin, F. (1990). *The Protective Shell in Children and Adults*. London: Karnac.

Vasta, R. (2006). "The Negative." Unpublished manuscript.

Vernant, J.-P. (1990). The historical moment of tragedy in Greece: Some of the social and psychological conditions. In: *Myth and Tragedy in Ancient Greece*, ed. J.-P. Vernant & P. Vidal-Niquet, trans. J. Lloyd. New York: Zone Books.

Wade, N. (2006). *New York Times: Science Times*, Tuesday, 25 July, p. D2.

Webb, R. E., & Sells, M. A. (1997). Lacan and Bion: Psychoanalysis and the mystical language of "unsaying". *Journal of Melanie Klein and Object Relations, 15*: 243–264.

Weisberg, J. (2006). Red in the head [Book review of *Seeing Red: A Study in Consciousness*]. *Nature, 441* (1 June).

Weiss, E. (1925). Der eine noch nicht beschriebene Phase der Entwicklung zur heterosexuellen Liebe. *International Zeitschrift für Psychoanalyse, 11*: 429–443.

Williams, C. (2006). *Heidegger, Bion, and Varela*. Unpublished book.

Williams, M. H. (1985). The tiger and "O": A reading of Bion's *Memoir of the Future*. *Free Associations, 1*: 33–56.

Winnicott, D. W. (1951). Transitional objects and transitional phenomena. In: *Collected Papers: Through Paediatrics to Psycho-Analysis* (pp. 229–242). London: Tavistock Publications; New York: Basic Books, 1958.

Winnicott, D. W. (1956). Primary maternal preoccupation. In: *Collected Papers: Through Paediatrics to Psycho-Analysis* (pp. 300–305). London: Tavistock Publications; New York: Basic Books, 1958.

Winnicott, D. W. (1960a). Ego distortion in terms of the true and false self. In: *The Maturational Processes and the Facilitating Environment* (pp. 140–152). London: Hogarth Press; New York: International Universities Press, 1965.

Winnicott, D. W. (1960b). The theory of the parent–infant relationship. In: *The Maturational Processes and the Facilitating Environment* (pp. 37–55). London: Hogarth Press; New York: International Universities Press, 1965.

Winnicott, D. W. (1963). Communicating and not communicating leading to a study of certain opposites. In: *The Maturational Processes and the Facilitating Environment* (pp. 37–55). London: Hogarth Press; New York: International Universities Press; 1965.

Winnicott, D. W. (1969). The use of an object. *International Journal of Psycho-analysis, 50*: 711–716.

Winnicott, D. W. (1971a). Creativity and its origins. In: *Playing and Reality* (pp. 65–85). London: Routledge; New York: Basic Books.

Winnicott, D. W. (1971b). Playing: A theoretical statement. In: *Playing and Reality* (pp. 38–52). London: Routledge; New York: Basic Books.

INDEX

Abraham, 56
Absolute Experience, 148
Absolute Space, 275
Absolute Time, 275
Absolute Truth, 68, 121, 138, 161, 214,
        261, 265, 266, 275, 281, 297, 303
    about Ultimate Reality:
    and curiosity, 20
    and dreaming, 94, 261, 265, 266
    and emotions, 62, 166
    O, 2, 41, 44, 97, 115, 148, 135, 136,
        156, 265, 270
    and psychoanalytic theory and
        practice, 80
    of raw Circumstance, 295–297, 300
    and transformation, 21, 55, 78, 136,
        139, 143–145
    transformation to tolerable truth
        (K), 40, 143–146, 156
    and the unconscious, 293–297
abstraction, Bion's use of, 111
adaptive editorial transformation, as
        function of dreaming, 281–288
aesthetic capacities, use of, 56, 218
aesthetics, 25, 218, 255
affect regulation, 209

aggressor, identification with, 154
Aisenstein, M., 61
aletheia, 128
alimentary canal model, 56, 153, 215
    of thinking, 272, 319
α-elements (*passim*):
    constellations of, 63, 263
    degraded, 67, 97
    for dreaming, 329
    and dream narratives, 80, 273
    as emotions, 44, 62, 204, 235, 236
    as free associations, 321
    inchoate, 272
    infant's rudimentary, 46, 92, 181,
        274
    mentalizable, 61, 68, 80, 86, 156, 161,
        166, 249, 261
    as models for thoughts and thinking,
        59, 138
    reinforcement of contact-barrier by,
        267, 277, 291, 293, 299, 300
    row B of the Grid, 245, 255
    transformation of β-elements into,
        40, 44, 50, 59, 62, 67, 122, 137, 156,
        157, 161, 217, 225, 261, 271, 291
    see also psychoanalytic element(s)

α-function (*passim*):
  analogue-model for dreaming, 46
  autochthonous, 157
  Bion's views, 45
  capacity for, 46, 321
    infant's, 45
    mother's, infant's introjection of, 45
  container's, 156
  day and night, 68, 164, 261, 279
  and dreaming, 45, 50, 59, 150, 215,
      217, 230, 236, 261–263, 288
    analogue-model, 46
    vs. primary and secondary
      processes, 79–81
  infant's, 122, 175
  mathematical roots of, 104
  mother's, 45, 50, 68, 89, 122, 138, 166,
      274, 292, 296
  in reverse, 71, 204, 206, 255, 295, 322
  rudimentary (inherited), 45
  transformation by, 136
α-megafunction, 271
altero-centred participation, 182
ambivalence, 210
American Psychoanalytic Association,
    32
analogic thinking, Bion's, 46
analyst (*passim*):
  abandoning memory and desire, 2,
      23, 27, 83, 86, 90, 107, 117, 200,
      204, 214, 225, 228, 237, 298, 317
    and containment, 165
    and projective identification, 185
    as protocol, 47–50
    and psychosis, 205, 210
  "of achievement", 44
  "becoming" the analysand/infant, 48
  as container, 291
  dreaming analytic session, 39, 86, 91,
      94, 165, 233, 263, 268, 273, 279
  faith in coherence, 85
  obligatory preconceptions, list of, 87,
      89, 95, 226
  patience, need for, 48, 85, 93, 110, 291
  reverie of, *see* reverie, analytic
analytic frame, 27, 188, 200, 269, 300
analytic resistance, 200
analytic technique:
  right-hemispheric, 82

sense, myth, passion, 82, 84, 91, 100,
    106, 113, 237, 248
Ananke [necessity or fate], 115, 130, 262,
    278
Andreas-Salomé, L., 1, 120, 304
animism, 179
annihilation, dread of, 202
Apprey, M., 188
archetypes, 135, 136
Aristotelian logic, 51, 79, 118, 271, 300
Aristotle, 86, 115, 127, 330
Arnold, M., 268
arrogance, and death instinct, 206–207
asymmetrical logic, 118
asymmetrical thinking, 80
asymmetry, principle of, 270–271
attachment, 41, 160, 166, 178, 181, 279
  concept of, 103, 155
autistic transformations, 229–230
autochthonous creativity, as function of
    dreaming, 268, 281–288
autochthony, 125, 144, 158, 281, 282
autogenesis, 159, 215
autopoiesis, 215
awe, capacity for, 211

balpha-element(s), 46, 272, 274
Bandera, A., 251, 272
Banet, A. G., 16
basic assumption(s), 191–193, 196
  groups, 63
"beam of intense darkness", 1, 84, 298
Beckett, S., 326
"become"/"becoming", 2, 17, 52–55, 63,
    107, 116, 123, 133, 183, 185, 186,
    205, 279, 291, 305–307, 317
  Platonic, 43
  thinking as, 50
Beebe, B., 278
Berkeley, G., 59, 316
β-elements (*passim*):
  analysand's projections, 48, 182, 183,
      184, 186, 231, 291
  and balpha-elements, 46
  conceptualization of, 59–63
  emotional sense impressions, 55
  infant's, 156, 157, 164, 166, 299
  inherent pre-conceptions, 62, 122
  invasion of dangerous, 216

pre-processed sensory stimuli, 46, 55
proto-emotions, 45, 156, 157, 166, 192, 204, 205, 208, 261, 263
proto-mental systems, 258
sense impression, 61
sensory impressions, 50
transformation of , 62, 80
    into α-elements, via α–function: see α-elements, transformation of β-elements into
unmentalized sensory impressions of emotional experience, 156
untransformed, 60, 67
see also psychoanalytic element(s)
β-screen, 60, 237
β-space, 63
Bianchedi, E. T. de, xi, xii, 5, 7, 12, 13, 134, 147–148, 226, 240, 273, 313
bi-logic, 79, 80, 118, 268, 270, 271
binary opposition, as model of dreaming, 265
binary-oppositional structure(s), 80, 91, 118, 246, 250, 270–272, 278, 282, 284, 297
binocular perspective, 269, 291
    as model of dreaming, 265
binocular thinking, 79, 95, 165
binocular vision, 6, 23, 24, 77, 78, 112, 113, 146, 200, 293–297, 308, 329
    breakdown of, 294–295
Binswanger, L., 325
Bion, F., xii, 11, 16, 19, 21, 26, 35, 231, 304
Bion, W. R. (passim):
    analogic thinking of, 46
    as analyst, 27–33, 102–108
    as bearer of the "messiah thought", 105
    conception of thinking, 47–48
    departure for US, 21
    discovery of O, 114–120
    epistemology of, 50–51
    and Freud:
        differences in dream theories, 39–40
        differing psychoanalytic aims, 38–39
    genius of, 18–21
    groups, work with, 190–196
    identification of with Socrates, 10, 11

and Klein:
    differing psychoanalytic aims, 38–39
    differing theories, 40–42
as Kleinian, 30, 42, 90, 95
"left-hemispheric", 86, 225
legacy of, 44–64, 91
and London Kleinians, 19, 34, 96, 105, 114, 156, 173, 200, 206, 215, 221, 228, 230
as mathematician, 102–108
metatheory, 65–81, 327, 331
    for psychoanalysis, 135–138
modifications and extension of Kleinian technique, 93–97
as mystic, 2–3, 102–108
ontological and phenomenological epistemology of, 54–56
as "pariah of O", 20–21
as person, 34–35
personal appearance of, 22, 35
personal relationship to O, 119–120
as Platonist, 73
as "post-post-Kleinian", 95–97
projective identification, extending of, 41
as Promethean, 1, 12, 20–23, 76, 137, 142, 277, 329, 330
psychoanalytic epistemology of, 291–292
psychosis, studies in, 197–212
pursuit of truth, 51
and religion, 74, 107, 128, 129, 137, 231
shift from positivism to ontology, epistemology, and phenomenology, 96–97
as Socrates' descendant, 10, 11, 12, 30, 34, 306, 307, 330
in South America, 22
study of groups, 41
style of writing and communicating, 11–18
supervision, attitude to, 12, 28
technical ideas (clinical vignette), 98–101
on technique, 82–97
theories, observational, 65
tools for exploration, 23–24
as transcendentalist, 37–38

Bion, W. R. (*continued*):
    transformational protocol, 122
    in United States, 21
    use of models vs. theories, 55–58
    use of plane (Euclidean) geometry,
        240–242
    vision of, 36–43
    war experiences of, 12, 19, 35, 119, 195
    works of, holographic nature of, 8,
        165
"bipolar man", 37
"bivalent logic", 79, 80, 118, 270, 271
bizarre objects, 206, 323
Blake, W., 325
Blanchot, M., 25
Bléandonu, G., xi, 5, 12, 51
Blomfield, O. H. D., 134
Bloom, H., 117
Bohr, N., 269
Borges, J. L., 9
Boss, M., 325
Bowlby, J., 103, 155
Bråten, S., 182
breast, 88, 95, 155, 187, 204, 209, 228, 253,
        316
    absent, 119, 122, 239, 321
    attack on, 171,
    bad, 208, 310, 321
    as container ↔ contained relation,
        160–164,
    good, 72, 208, 240, 310
        introjection of, 208
    /mother, 194, 316
    "no-breast", 103, 122, 163, 164, 194,
        208, 210, 239, 241, 242, 321
    role of, in Bion's metatheory, 65–70
    as twin, 198
British Psychoanalytic Institute, 102
Britton, R., 134, 141, 173, 262, 272, 282
Brown, L., 60, 154, 279, 286
Brunschwig, J., 84
"brute reality", 121
Buber, M., 105

caesura, 56, 96, 161, 197, 216, 250, 269,
        273, 274, 292, 300, 328
    of birth, and fetal mental life, 256–258
Cantor, G., 127
Carlyle, T., 129

Cartesian (cognitive) thinking, 51, 54,
        55, 292, 305
Carvalho, R., 270
castration anxiety, 195, 199, 201
catastrophic anxiety(ies), 142
catastrophic change, 3, 115, 258
censorship, as function of dreaming,
        281–288
cerebral hemispheres, harmony of
        functioning between, 25
Chaminade, T., 170, 185
chaos, 62, 74, 104, 115, 117, 118, 130, 136,
        262, 276, 318
    psychotic, 237
    theory, 58, 85, 211, 298
Chomsky, N., 45, 157, 166
Chuster, A., xii, 254
circles: *see* Euclidean geometry
claustrophobic anxiety, 179
claustrum, 173
clinical depressive illness (melancholia),
        131
co-construction and transformations,
        214
Coleridge, S. T., 140
communication(s):
    abnormal, 169
    between analysts, universal analogue
        language for, 15
    emotional, 9
    interpersonal, 209
        projective identification as, 49–50
    intersubjective, 188, 209
    pre-lexical, 9, 45
    projective identification as, 41
    prosodic lexical, 45
communicative projective identification,
        20, 22, 57, 67, 92
com-passion, 2
complementarity, 160, 293, 299
    binocular principle of, 270
conatus, 115–116, 120, 215, 278, 330–332
condensation, 260, 280, 287
consciousness, 6, 70, 140
    and the unconscious, 79, 156
    in binary opposition, 95
constant conjunction(s), 13, 21, 24, 104,
        224, 230, 232, 238, 240
    concept of, 251–252

and containment, 49
and curiosity, 141
and dreaming, 275, 283
and the Grid, 248, 251–252
Hume's concept of, 65–66
and interpreting, 291
meaning of, 221
and origins of thinking, 69
and selected fact, 48
and the transcendent position, 127
and transformations, 221, 230, 239,
    240
constructivism, 196, 215
    social, 159, 214
contact-barrier (*passim*):
    concept of, 78, 161
    and curiosity, 142
    and distinction between sleep and
        wakefulness, 103, 202, 236
    and dreaming, 50, 250, 269, 299–300
    function of, 49–51, 78, 161, 260, 265,
        321
    intactness of, analyst's faith in, 2, 186
    reinforcement of, by α-elements, 68,
        80, 136, 161, 267, 269, 271, 277,
        283, 291, 293, 299, 300
    relationship with container ↔
        contained, the Grid, and α-
        function, 49–51, 62, 122, 161
    selectively permeable, 50, 56–57, 94,
        165, 214, 272, 292
    and separation of consciousness and
        the unconscious, 57, 236, 258,
        261–265, 269, 308, 321
container(s):
    analyst as, 291
    and attachment, 154–155
        concept of, 41, 103
        relationships, categories of,
            160–161
        significance of, 163–165
    component functions of, 156–158
    and contained (*passim*):
        alternating, 159, 259, 324
        concept of, 151–167, 324
    good-enough, 162, 164
    infinite, 139
    –mother: *see* mother, container–
    negative, 21, 151–152, 153, 154, 156

persecutory, 153–154
positive, 151, 153, 156
container ↔ contained, 5, 49, 66, 67,
    84, 93, 103, 105, 116, 127, 132,
    151–168, 169, 173, 175, 202–204,
    212, 215, 262, 272, 283, 288, 310
    concept of, 20, 37, 41
    and dreaming, 297–299
    model, 94
containment, 23, 50, 103, 106, 138, 153,
    157–160, 164, 175, 192, 206–209,
    279, 284, 288, 292, 313, 327, 329
    failures of, 116
    secondary, 159
Conte, J., 254
Controversial Discussions (Melanie
    Klein and Anna Freud), 15, 251
counteridentification, projective, 181
countertransference, 22, 94, 101, 188,
    200, 202, 225, 294
    concept of, as analytic instrument, 165
    introjective, 181
    vs. reverie, 41, 212
    and transference, and projective
        identification, 185–186
Couzin, I. D., 188
curiosity, 14, 19, 88, 206, 207
    and arrogance, 141
    dangers of, 141–143
    deity's proscription against, 20, 21
    about truth, 139–146

Damasio, A., 120, 175, 182, 183, 215, 277
"*Dasein*", 123, 128, 332
day residue, 39
death instinct/drive, 39–42, 46, 96–97,
    114–121, 130, 136, 193, 203, 209,
    240, 298, 303–304, 313
    and arrogance, 206–207
    supraordinate position of, in Kleinian
        theory, 42, 52, 79, 96, 115, 121,
        135, 158, 295, 331
Decety, J., 170, 185
"definitory hypothesis", 32, 69, 70, 100,
    293
    Column 1 of the Grid, 74, 250, 283
delta-elements, 238
delusions, 201, 227, 282
Demiurge, 118

"dependency" group, 191
depressive anxiety(ies), 30, 115
depressive position, 89, 117, 128–133,
　　140, 158, 226, 293, 296, 297, 301,
　　302, 316
　ability to tolerate, 85
　Bion's reconceptualization of, 41, 79,
　　308–310
　depressive anxiety of, 115
　and dreaming, 270, 288
　and groups, 192
　infantile, 201
　and interpretation, 90
　and mystic, 3
　and paranoid–schizoid position:
　　Kleinian theory of, 47, 90, 121, 139,
　　　155, 308, 323, 324
　　relationship between, 30, 47, 95,
　　　165
　　transformation to, 86, 90, 307
　primitive, 324
　and psychosis, 197, 200–202, 210
　as "security", 41
　and selected fact, 58
　and "thinkers", 66
　and transcendent position, 97, 121
　transcending, 38
　see also paranoid–schizoid position
Derrida, J., 117
Descartes, R., 107
destructiveness, primary infantile, 21
Dilke, J., 109
Dimock, G., 143
displacement, 185, 223, 262, 287
　as function of dream-work, 260
dream(s)/dreaming (passim):
　and α-function, 45, 50, 59, 79, 80, 150,
　　215, 217, 230, 236, 261–263, 288
　　vs. primary and secondary
　　　processes, 79
　analytic, 39, 86, 91, 94, 165, 186, 233,
　　236, 263, 268, 273, 279
　autochthonous creativity of, 268
　Bion's theory of, vs.. Freud's, 39–40
　capacity to, 205, 321
　clinical vignette, 285–289
　Column 2 as, 249
　concept of, 68, 94, 164, 233, 259
　and contact-barrier, 50, 299–300

and container ↔ contained, 164–165,
　　297–299
　defective or inadequate, incomplete
　　or unsuccessful, and
　　psychopathology, 267, 268, 290,
　　295, 329
　demonstrating transcendence
　　(clinical vignette), 123–126
　as "editing function", 233
　"ensemble", 50, 68, 219, 233, 274
　exorcistic, 45
　Freud's theory, in service of pleasure
　　principle, 40
　functions of, 51, 80, 161, 202, 263,
　　274–288, 299, 327
　images, sensory, 40
　inability to, 92, 201, 236, 268
　interpretation, 111
　latent content of, 275
　meaning of, 267
　mother:
　　infant's experiences, 39
　　infant's projections, 45
　narratives, 80, 263
　night and day, 39, 68, 94, 164, 261, 269,
　　279
　as proto-language, 266
　and schizophrenia, 200–203
　theory, 259–289
　thinking, wakeful, 45, 83
　thoughts, 68, 69, 122, 136, 175, 261,
　　262, 271, 273
　　latent, 260
　unsuccessful:
　　and psychopathology, 280
　　or incomplete, as source of
　　　psychopathology, 266
　wakeful, 83, 91, 92
　　thinking, 152, 264, 268
　and wish-fulfilment, 293
　see also dream-work
"dreamer who dreams the dream", 77,
　126, 266, 268, 275, 330
dream-work, 86, 145, 146, 149, 249, 259–
　263, 269, 272, 275, 288, 291, 293
drives:
　importance of, 39
　shift from, to emotions and emotional
　　communication, 155–156

dying, fear of, 45, 46, 166, 209, 298, 324, 325

Eckhart, Meister, 26, 46, 53, 64, 105, 113, 127, 129, 137, 232
Edelman, G., 37
ego, splitting of, 203
Ehrenzweig, A., 56, 218, 277, 279–281, 294
Eigen, M., 3, 13
Einstein, A., 161, 231
Emerson, R. W., 124, 129
emotion(s):
    experience of, 2
    and personal truth, 10
    primal language of, Language of Achievement as, 15
    as template for thinking, 327
    as vehicular carriers of Truth, 44
emotional notation system, 312
Emotional Truth, 79, 87, 96, 101, 141, 156, 190, 219, 276, 281, 329
emotional turbulence, 3, 115, 131, 192, 258, 324
empathic resonance, 182, 186
empathy, 172, 173, 176, 177, 182, 183, 186
entelechy, 46, 115, 116, 120, 166, 209, 278, 297, 330, 331, 332
    ever-evolving, 46
entropy, 262, 323, 324, 325
envy, 10, 30, 38, 42, 49, 87, 88, 89, 95, 119, 226, 229, 236
    and greed, Kleinian theory of, 88
epistemology, 3, 50, 52, 54, 55, 57, 74, 96, 129, 143, 175, 207, 210, 212
    ontological, 2, 69, 103, 153, 200
    phenomenological, 153, 200
    psychoanalytic, Bion's, 291–292
epistemophilic instinct, 41
Eriugena, John Scotus, 129
Eternal Forms [Plato], 117, 135, 142, 210
Euclidean geometry, 72, 242
    Bion's use of, 240–242
Euclidean space, 70, 71
evolution(s), 5, 56, 67, 107, 261, 324
    of godhead, 67, 107
    of O, 116, 119, 211, 213, 261, 296, 302, 315

of self, 131–132, 209, 218–219
"excluded middle", law of, 51, 248
exhibitionism, 179
exorcism, 44, 48, 312
    as model for "becoming", 48–49
exorcistic dreaming, 45
experience, learning from, 143, 148, 213, 236
    clinical vignette, 144–145

Fagles, R., 143
Fairbairn, W. R. D., 116, 154, 297
Fairbairnian analysis, 39
Faith/faith (F), 2, 10, 105, 127, 233, 315, 316, 317, 318, 328, 329
    act of, 316, 317–318
    concept of, 141, 315–318
falsehoods, vs. Lies and lies, 147–150
falsification, 51, 249, 273, 275, 282, 313, 314
Fate, 61, 62
Ferguson, C. A., 24
Ferro, A., xi, xii, 7, 40, 56, 80, 91, 92, 95, 115, 266, 271, 272, 274
fetal memories, 330
fetal mental life, caesura with postnatal mental life, 256–258
fictionalization, 51, 273, 276, 282, 284, 297
"fight/flight" group, 191
Fitch, W. T., 266
Fliess, R., 185
"formless infinite", 63
Fox, M., 53
fragmentation, 205, 308, 323
Frankiel, R. W., 254
Frazer, J., 184, 187
free association(s), 27, 58, 66, 74, 75, 91, 94, 101, 127, 201, 219, 257, 260, 317, 320, 321
Freud, A., 15, 154, 174, 251
    Controversial Discussions, 15, 251
Freud, S. (passim):
    and Bion
        differing psychoanalytic aims, 38–39
        challenge of, 25
        original spirit of psychoanalysis in, 11

Freud, S. (*continued*):
    death instinct, concept of, 121
    dream:
        interpretation, 111
        theory of, differences with Bion, 39–40
    instinctual drives of, rerouted to emotions, 6
    "*Nachträglichkeit*", 214
    positivism of, 37, 41, 96–97, 114, 116, 200, 222
        and Bionian uncertainty, 44
    primary and secondary processes of Bion's erasure of distinction between, 6
    topographic and structural models of the psyche, 121
    twentieth-century science of, 3
    and the unconscious, 43, 66, 82, 134, 135, 168, 265, 277, 300
Freudian analysis, 39
frustration, 3, 66, 155, 194, 203, 205, 239,
    tolerance of, 10, 58, 69, 73, 85, 88, 122, 163, 164, 204, 208, 210, 223, 224, 316, 328
        lack of, 87, 89, 103, 206, 226, 228, 262, 295
function(s):
    mathematical, concept of, 104
    psychoanalytic, 235–237
    see also α-function

Galatzer-Levy, J., 24
Galileo, 330
Gallese, V., 307
gamma-elements, 238
"Garden of Eden" myth, 20, 21, 141, 143, 277
geometry, 72, 73, 222, 232, 240, 242, 253
    and emotions, 73
    use of plane (Euclidean) Bion's use of, 240–242
Gnostic Gospels, 129
Godbout, C., xii, 52, 108, 262
God of Essence, 137
godhead ("godhood", "godliness"), 21, 37, 42, 67, 102, 123, 231, 303, 331, 332
    and β-elements, 59, 62

and contact-barrier, 78, 142
and containment, 161, 165
and curiosity, opposition to, 143
and dreaming, 293
and homunculus, 53
and Ideal Form, 26, 43, 64
immanent, 122, 123, 137–138
and incarnation, 49, 52, 53, 107, 228
"Librarian Extra-Ordinaire" for the Library of the Ideal Forms, 54, 106
and O, 68, 106–107, 115, 117, 228, 231, 318
and psychosis, 209, 222
and quest for truth, 20, 139, 142
realization of, 122
and selected fact, 317, 318
as the "thinker", 76–78, 97, 108, 234
and wild thoughts, 329

godliness, 42, 53, 77, 106, 137
Goldman, A., 307
Gordon, J., 192, 193
Greatrex, T., 182
greed, 30, 38, 42, 87, 88, 89, 95, 119, 226
Green, J., 172
Greenberg, J., 3, 142, 183, 266
Grid, the, 6, 45, 49–50, 56, 67, 75, 88, 109, 165, 210, 217, 221, 272, 274, 279, 288, 291–292, 303, 324, 327, 328
    Column 1 (Definitory Hypothesis), 74, 248–250, 283, 293
    Column 2 (psi), 32, 51, 136, 234, 236, 238, 246, 248–255, 282–284, 293, 313
    concept of, 69, 243–255
    as form of transformation, 253–254
    tri-dimensional, 254
    use of, 245, 248
Grinberg, L., xi, 5, 12, 13, 181, 226
group(s):
    anxieties, primitive, 194
    basic assumption, 191, 196
    Bion's study of, 18, 41, 51, 190–196
    psychology, 4, 183, 190, 193–196
    resistance, 191
    work-, 191, 194–196, 258

H (hate), 67, 105

hallucination(s), 147, 201, 205–206, 226–228, 238, 278
hallucinosis, 295, 322
    transformations in, 222, 226–229, 258
Hampshire, S., 14
Hargreaves, E., 42, 94
Hartmann, H., 303, 304
hate, 6, 42, 67, 105, 179, 192, 193, 206, 229, 236, 287, 312, 314
Hegel, G. W. F., 49, 129, 135
Heidegger, M., 117, 123, 128, 129, 134, 143
Heimann, P., 41, 294
Heisenberg, W., 16, 161, 231
Helm, F., 182, 184
Hemingway, E., 316
Heraclitus, 4, 27, 105, 213, 306
"higher man/self ["Übermensch"], 2, 3, 38, 53
Hillel, Rabbi, 44
Hoffman, I. Z., 159, 214
holding:
    concept of, 162
    vs. containing, 162–163
    environment, 162, 298
Hooke's Law, 284
Horace, 330
Hume, D., 65, 66, 127, 251
Humphrey, N., 288
hypnosis, mutual, 185

I (Idea), 105, 237
Ibn'Arabi, M., 129
iconic signs, abstract, use of, 221–222
Ideal Forms, 12, 52–54, 59–67, 70, 106–108, 122, 231, 331
    and β-elements, 59, 258
    and dreaming, 265, 277, 278
    and emotional pain, 42
    and entelechy, 46
    godhead, 26, 43, 64, 137
    and the Grid, 254
    infinite self, 53
    infusion of the ego by, 38
    and O, 67, 115, 122, 143, 214, 331
    and pre-conceptions, 87, 122, 240, 317
    and transcendent position, 126
    transformation of, 53
    and unrepressed unconscious, 43, 74

idealization of Bion, 5, 10, 17, 22, 30, 331
idealizing selfobject function, 160
identification, 174
    partial, 185, 187
    role of, in projection, 173–174
    total, 185
    trial, 185
ideograph, 204
illusion, 77, 123, 124, 218, 227, 231, 297
    mystic's disregard of, 2
imaginary twin, 198–200
imaginative conjecture, 24, 75, 78, 93, 119, 269, 331
immune system model, 57, 216
"incarnation", 49, 67, 107–108, 127, 162, 209, 228, 233, 316
    concept of, 52–54
indeterminacy, 89, 262
induction, by gesture and voice, 184–185
ineffability, 52, 56, 117, 123, 127–129, 211, 283
infant:
    capacity of to think, 45
    –mother psychotherapy, 178
infantile catastrophe, 130, 206, 207, 294, 324
infantile dependency, 91
infantile neurosis, 38, 41, 81, 130, 181, 212, 222, 275
infantile psychosis, 38, 40
infantile sexuality, 38
infinite:
    internal domain of, 42
    role of, 52–54
infinite container, 139
"infinite man", 37
Infinite Presence, 77
infinite sets, 118, 136, 139, 277
infinity, 89, 112, 138, 232, 318, 325
    and β-elements, 62, 63, 136
    and containment, 157
    domains of, 21
    and dreaming, 68, 263, 265, 267, 275, 277
    and O, 41, 81, 106, 114–116, 118, 130
    and selected fact, 318
    and the unconscious, 47, 52
    zero dimension of, 74
"influencing machine", 61, 303

innate category, 166
Inquiry (Column 5 in the Grid), 88
internal object, 153, 156, 208, 228, 230
    hateful, 103
    importance of, in projective
        identification, 178–179
International Psychoanalytical
        Association, 200
interpersonal communication, 209
    projective identification as, 49–50
interpretation(s), 54, 55, 85, 88–91, 175,
        237, 247, 302
    and binocular vision, 28–97
    Bionian, 27–33, 55
    and Bion's metatheory, 65
    clinical examples, 98–101, 144–145,
        198–199, 287
    and containment, 159, 163, 298–300
    and dreams, 111, 260, 262, 267, 275,
        277, 287
    and evidence, 93
    and feeling of relief, 145–146
    and functions of container, 156, 163
    and the Grid, 88, 247
    and groups, 192, 193
    intuited patterns, 48, 89, 291
    Kleinian, 29–31
    and left/right hemispheres, 84
    mutative, 187
    and O, 58, 96, 117, 127, 221, 231
    part-object, 28
    and projective identification, 173
    and psychoanalytic theory, 86, 225
    and psychosis, 198–201, 204, 205
    and reverie, 83
    role of, 145–146
    and selected fact, 317
    as transformation, 219
    and unconscious phantasies, 302
        effect of, 290
intersubjective communication, 188,
        209
intersubjectivity, 4, 22, 37, 42, 123, 157,
        158, 163, 188, 214
intimacy, phenomenon of, 328
introjection, 85, 177, 180, 183, 269, 295
introjective countertransference, 181
intuition, 2, 73, 77, 79, 124, 132, 156, 186,
        188, 205, 227, 256, 279, 298, 325

analyst's tool, 2, 82, 83, 86, 91, 127,
        225, 226
    faith in, 58
    Bion's contributions to, 15
    concept of, 211
    developing, 247, 248
    and part-object interpretations, 28
intuitionistic mathematics, 16, 230
    Dutch School of, 234
"invariant", question of, 217–218
Isaacs, S., 300

James, W., 40
Joseph, B., 20, 28, 93, 94, 176, 182, 286,
        287
Jowett, B., 305, 306
Joyce, J., 40
Jung, C. G., 24, 105, 128, 129, 132, 210

K (knowledge), 67, 105, 145
Kabbalah of Zohar, 117, 120, 129
Kant, I., 38, 41, 43, 54, 65, 74, 87, 127, 129,
        132–135, 240, 331
Keats, J., 109
Kelly, K., 172
Kernberg, O., 176, 177
Kierkegaard, S., 129
Kipling, R., 140
Klein, M. (passim)
    Bion's analysis with, 19, 20, 40, 119
    Bion's differences with, 25, 41, 42, 96
        on psychoanalytic aims, 38–39
        on theories, 40–42
    Controversial Discussions, 15, 251
    dangerous, omnipotent "combined-
        parent" function, concept of, 108
    death instinct as first cause, 52, 79, 96,
        115, 121, 135, 158, 295, 331
    defence mechanisms, concept of, 174
    drive theory of, 87
    infantile neurosis, theory of, 130
    internal objects, theory of, 224
    intolerance of depression, 309
    Oedipus complex, 100, 192, 225
        archaic aspects of, 192
    ontic science of, 3
    paranoid–schizoid and depressive
        positions, theory of, 47, 90, 121,
        139, 155, 308, 323, 324

Bion's reconceptualization of, 41,
47, 49, 79, 130–131, 293
persecutory anxiety, 158, 172
positivism of, 37, 40, 44, 114, 116
projective identification, concept of,
20, 37, 86, 92, 103, 168–179, 186,
188, 192, 226
psychoanalysis, one-person
conception of, 93
psychoanalytic principles of, 195
splitting, concept of, 86
technique of, Bion's modification and
extension of, 93–95
theories of:
Bion's extension of, 41, 127, 145
context of, 81
transference, theory of, 70
therapeutic importance of the
analyst's emotions, as valuable
analytic instrument, 41
unconscious phantasy, 178, 300
as prime mover, 301
wisdom arising from breast, 95
Klein, S., 14
Kleinian, Bion as, 4, 6, 14, 27, 28–31,
38–42, 90–96
Kleinian analysis, 30, 39, 41, 155, 163
Kleinian technique, Bion's
modifications and extension of,
93–97
Kleinian theory, 28, 73, 115, 116
K link, 53
–K space, 71
Kohut, H., 160, 252
Korbivcher, C., 229, 230, 234
Krause, J., 188
Krebs cycle, as model, 55, 57
Kristeva, J., 182, 184

L (love), 67, 105
L, H, K, 49–51, 237, 251, 254, 296
linkages, 6, 20, 32, 39, 56, 81, 91, 127,
132, 137, 197, 225, 233, 274, 288,
331
emotional categories, 79
evaluations, 49
and passion, 311–314
Lacan, J., 10, 105, 121, 123, 129, 210, 305
Lachman, F. M., 278

language:
"of Achievement", 3, 6, 23, 44, 56, 78,
109–113, 211, 279
primal, of emotions, 15
as emotional communication, 9
"of substitution", 15, 47, 78, 110–113,
211, 279
universal analogue for
communication between
analysts, 15
of unsaying, apophatic, 120
metaphatic and apophatic
mystical, 113
Laplace, P.-S., 53, 107
Lebow, R., 143
left-hemispheric thinking, 23, 86, 92,
101, 225, 237
logical, 23
Lennon, J., 8
Lévi-Strauss, C., 79, 265, 282
libidinal drive, 39, 96, 135
Lies, 147, 150, 255, 273, 296
"lies", and falsehoods, 147–150
life instinct, 40, 41, 42, 79, 97, 115, 206,
331
lines: see Euclidean geometry
listening to patient, 101, 105, 112, 317
Llinàs, R., 170, 181, 183
Lloyd, G. E. R., 84
logic, 15, 25, 104, 281, 309
Aristotelian, 51, 79, 118, 271, 300
asymmetrical, 118
bivalent, 79, 80, 118, 270, 271
symmetrical, 118
London Kleinians, and Bion, 19, 34, 96,
105, 114, 156, 173, 200, 206, 215,
221, 228, 230
López-Corvo, R., xi, xii, 5, 13, 18, 50, 54,
74, 76, 113, 242
Los Angeles Psychoanalytic Society, 32,
245
Luria, I., 105
lying, 28, 51, 148, 149, 150, 273, 313

Maizels, N., 133
"Man of Achievement", 1, 2, 53, 109,
110, 127
manic defence(s), 30, 77, 114, 121, 301
masochism, 179

Mason, A., 185, 294
maternal reverie, 4, 20, 44, 45, 47, 50, 163, 186, 192, 328
mathematical model, 15, 69, 246, 248
    the Grid as, 246, 251
mathematics, 15, 102–105, 118, 127, 167, 211, 224, 232, 233, 325
    intuitionistic, 16, 230
mathematization of psychoanalysis, 239–242
    see also geometry; mathematics
Matte Blanco, I., 74, 79, 80, 106, 118, 262, 268, 270, 271, 277
Maturana, H. R., 215
Maugham, W. S., 128
McCarthy, J., 285, 286, 287
McGinn, B., 53, 113
meaning, assassination of, 325
Meltzer, D. W., xi, 42, 120, 172, 187, 242, 254, 255, 312
"memoirs of the future", 54, 70, 87, 106, 120, 126, 135, 240, 254, 258, 276, 280, 322
memory and desire:
    absence of, 24, 320
    injunction to abandon, 2, 23, 27, 83, 86, 90, 200, 204, 211, 214, 225, 228, 237, 279, 291, 298, 317, 320, 325
    and containment, 165
    and projective identification, 185
    as protocol, 47–50
    and psychosis, 205, 210
    and secondary process(es), 280
mentalization, 60, 80, 91, 122, 136, 263, 271, 272
    of α-elements, 61, 68, 80, 86, 156, 161, 166, 249, 261
    vs.. thinking, 6, 40
messiah aspects of O, 106
messiah idea/thought, 67, 105, 106, 191, 195, 284
metaphor(s), 56, 70, 111, 218, 267, 329, 331
metapsychology:
    concept of, 66
    psychoanalytic, 23, 47
metatheory:
    for psychoanalysis, 213
    Bion's, 16, 25, 32, 65–81, 127, 135–138, 149, 153, 156, 197, 201, 269, 327, 331
Michelangelo, 76
"middle voice", ancient Greek, 3, 143, 183, 266, 307
Milton, J., 1, 325
minus K: see –K
–L, –H, –K, 254, 309, 312–314
mirroring, 160
    selfobject function, 160
Möbius strip, 265
    model, 216, 250, 264
    of dreaming, 264
Modell, A. H., 182, 184
models:
    analogic, 55
    Bion speaking and writing in terms of, 16, 110
Money-Kyrle, R., 181
mother:
    container–, 45, 68, 89, 92, 102, 103, 136, 154, 156, 159, 160, 164, 166, 175, 209, 292, 298
    reverie of: see reverie, maternal
mourning, capacity for, 131
"multiple vertices", 23–25, 292
Murrow, E. R., 285
Muse, 75, 77
mutative interpretation, 187
mutual hypnosis, 185
mystic:
    archetype of, 77
    and Attention and Interpretation, 21
    and binocular vision, 297
    Bion as, 2–3, 22, 91, 102–108, 129
    and concept of incarnation, 52–53
    and dreaming, 283, 284
    and the Establishment, 283–284
    and the group, 132, 192, 193
    and O, 77, 117–118, 123, 137
    psychoanalytic, 2
    "science of psychoanalysis", 24
    spirituality of, 137
    and thinking thoughts, 67
    and transcendent position, 128–129
mysticism, 3, 25, 94, 106, 128, 129, 143
myth(s), 24, 47, 69, 95, 101, 107, 145, 157, 194, 199, 247, 276, 282, 302, 303, 328, 329

domain of, 237
"Garden of Eden", 20, 21, 141, 143, 277
Oedipus, 20, 21, 91, 113, 141, 143, 200, 277
Prometheus, 21, 143
as psychoanalytic tool, 82, 84, 91, 100, 106, 113, 237, 248
as "scientific deductive systems", 47
sense, passion, use of, 82, 84–91, 100, 106, 113, 237, 248
"Tower of Babel", 20, 21, 141, 143, 277
and unconscious phantasies, 83, 84, 91–92, 237, 288

"*Nachträglichkeit*", 214
nameless dread, 119, 269
of trauma, 40
narcissism, 190, 196, 242, 324
essential, 252
and socialism, 268
negation, 51, 236, 238, 246, 250, 253, 255, 268, 300
negative capability, 3, 24, 38, 56, 66, 92, 109, 142, 317, 321
negative container, 21, 151–152, 156
persecutory, 153–154
negative realization, 103, 209, 210
negative therapeutic reactions, 249, 297
negative transference, 32
neuronal synapse model, 23, 57, 78, 215, 216, 217, 236, 257
neurotic patient(s), 24, 177, 198, 200–202, 223, 230, 236, 294, 296, 319, 321, 324
vs. psychotic patient, 203–205
Nietzsche, F., 2, 129
nightmare, 216, 286
night-time vision, as wakeful dreaming, 83–84
"no-breast", 103, 122, 163, 164, 208, 210, 239, 241, 242, 321
Norman, J., 45
no-penis, 242
notation system, 57, 73, 223–224, 253, 309, 311–312
emotional, 312
in the Grid, 245, 249
memory, 88, 261, 263

"no-thing", 71, 72, 119, 228, 240, 241, 253, 319
zero, concept of, 319–326
noumenon(a), 331, 332
and β-element, 59–60, 62, 135–136, 258
and containment, 42
and "curtain of illusion", 231
and dreaming, 278, 293
and Faith, 10, 317, 318
Ideal Form, transformation of, 53
and metatheory, 65, 67
numinousness, 114, 322
and O, 106, 115, 122, 143, 214, 240, 303, 331–332
potential wisdom, 12
and pre-conceptions, 87, 122, 136
realization of, 53
things-in-themselves, 38
and thoughts, 70, 74
and transcendence, 43, 132
and transformations, 77, 139, 142, 214
Novick, J., 172

O (*passim*):
atonement with, 211
"become", 3, 37, 38, 53, 87, 122, 127, 183, 230
Bion's personal relationship to, 119–120
bipolar, 86, 87, 225
chaos, 130
concept/theory of, 15, 32, 58, 68, 96, 106, 114–121, 132, 139, 230
container of, 53
and "*Dasein*", 123
as "deity", 141
discovery of, 114–120
dread of, 44
emotional imprints of, 183
evolutions of, 116, 211, 213, 296
evolving, 3, 37, 39, 45, 60, 79, 96, 116, 136, 161, 254, 261, 270, 276
experience of, 58, 84, 91, 218, 231, 233, 237, 299, 320
Fate, 61, 62
as first cause, 79
ghost of, 59
"god-container" of, 107

O (*continued*):
    impersonal, 122, 131, 138, 233, 265,
        266, 278, 284
        transformation into personal O,
            40, 261
    infinite self of, 102
    infusion with/by, 2
    "intersection" with, 43
    messiah aspects of, 106
    noumena (things-in-themselves), 38
    oneness with, 2, 77, 31
    orphan of, Bion as, 115, 119
    personal, 40, 116, 117, 122, 131, 132,
        138, 261, 265, 266, 270
    raw Circumstance, 115, 278, 297, 300
    Real, 123, 132, 313
    significance of, 231, 327
    symmetry and death instinct, 118–119
    and transcendence, 123
    transformation(s), 2
        cycle of return in, 122–123
        from, 2, 6, 19, 39, 53, 54, 94, 96,
            105, 145, 156, 183, 188, 193, 197,
            230–233, 314
        in, 2, 6, 19, 39, 53, 54, 94, 96, 105,
            118, 119, 156, 183, 188, 193, 197,
            230–233, 314
        of, 60, 116, 240, 276
        bi-polar, 86, 225
        to, 2, 6, 19, 39, 53, 54, 94, 96, 156,
            183, 188, 193, 197, 231, 233, 314
    triangulation of, 41, 79, 95, 165, 270,
        299, 308
    two arms of, 51, 74, 87, 132, 217, 254,
        277, 327
    as ultimate reality, 117–118
    and uncertainty, 135
    union with, 37
    see also Absolute Truth; β-elements;
        godhead; Emotional Truth; Ideal
        Forms; infinity; noumenon(a);
        things-in-themselves;
        Ultimate Reality; unrepressed
        unconscious
object(s):
    absence of, 89, 224, 232, 239, 253
    analytic, 69, 82, 100–101, 110, 113,
        115–120, 126–127, 134, 199, 237,
        247, 248, 270

    bizarre, 206, 323
    internal, 110, 116, 139, 156, 196, 208,
        220, 224, 228, 230, 268, 278, 297
        hateful, 103
        importance of, in projective
            identification, 178–179
        obstructive, 153
        persecutory, 171
    internalized, 158
    obstructive, 21, 103, 152, 153–154, 167,
        207, 229, 241, 322
    persecutory, 303, 316
    subjective, 228
observation(s):
    psychoanalytic, 114
    two forms of, emotional and
        objective, 83
obsessional defences, 301
obstructive object, 21, 103, 152, 153–154,
    167, 207, 229, 241, 322
oedipal situation, 86, 87, 88, 219, 225
oedipal theory, 87, 226
Oedipus, 194, 219
    (Column 4 in the Grid), 88
    complex, 30, 38, 59, 86–89, 95, 100,
        160, 225, 226, 292, 300, 301
        archaic, 192
        archaic part-object, 30
    myth, 20–21, 91, 113, 141–143, 200,
        277
Ogden, T., xi, xii, 7, 13, 14, 17, 24, 92, 146,
    175–178, 184, 187, 279, 280, 286,
    288
omnipotence, 33, 38, 42, 119, 130, 142,
    143, 154, 172, 179, 207, 322
omnipotent phantasy, 37, 103, 170, 175,
    176, 208
ontological science, psychoanalysis as, 3
ontology, 23, 47, 96, 97, 121, 143
O'Shaughnessy, E., 8, 19, 20, 95, 96
Oversoul, 124

paranoid–schizoid position, 324
    and arithmetic models, 73
    and binocular thinking, 165
    Bion's reconceptualization of, 41,
        308–310
    binocular triangulation, 79
    and depressive position:

relationship between, 30, 47, 95, 165
   transformation to, 86, 90, 307
and dreaming, 263, 270, 286, 288, 293,
   296, 301, 302
and the Grid, 226
and group studies, 192, 194
and instinctual drives, 324
and interpretations, 90
and O, 121, 128
pathologization of, 308
as "patience", 41
and persecutory anxiety, 95, 115
and psychosis, 197, 200, 201, 203, 210
and reverie, 324
and selected fact, 58
and thinkers, 66
and transcendent position, 130–132
transcending, 38
and transformations, 139
and persecution, state of, 149
see also P–S ↔ D
part-object interpretations, 28
passion, 2, 69, 150, 200, 247, 312, 317,
   328
   domain of, 237
   and L, H, K, 311–314
   use of, 84–91
   as psychoanalytic tool, 82, 84, 91, 100,
      106, 113, 237, 248
patience, analyst's need for, 48, 85, 93,
   110, 291
Peirce, C. S., 111, 121
penis, 33, 65, 66, 95, 100, 101, 155, 160,
   195, 239
   no-penis, 242
Peradotto, J., 3
persecutory anxiety(ies), 30, 95, 115, 158,
   171, 172
perspectives, shifting, 23, 329, 332
phantasied twin: see imaginary twin
phantasy(ies):
   and reality, 293–294
   symmetrical, 186
   unconscious: see unconscious
      phantasy(ies)
phenomenology, 52, 96, 97
philosophical prescription and
      proscription, technique as, 84–91
Piaget, J., 280, 321

Pindar, 259
Pistener de Cortiñas, L., xii, 258
plane geometry (Euclidean), Bion's use
   of, 240–242
Plato, 4, 10, 38, 41, 43, 52, 54, 55, 65, 73,
   74, 87, 105, 113, 117, 126, 127, 129,
   135, 214, 228, 240, 305, 307, 331
   identification of Bion with Socrates,
      11
pleasure principle:
   dominance of, 63
   and dreaming, 40, 263, 267, 268,
      270–272, 278, 282
   and the Establishment, 284
   and the Grid, 249, 252
   and hallucinosis, 226, 228
   limitations of, 116
   and O, 121
   –pain principle, 295, 296, 300
   and psychosis, 205–206, 255
   and reality principle, 6, 80, 141,
      145–146, 246, 249, 252, 272
   and truth, 294
   –unpleasure principle, 249, 282, 283
Plotinus, 129
Poincaré, H., 85, 127, 167, 211, 251, 317
points: see Euclidean geometry
Porete, M., 129
positive realization, 209
positivism, 2, 37, 41, 96, 97, 114, 116, 200,
   222
   Freudian and Kleinian, 37, 40, 114, 116
   and Bionian uncertainty, 44
   logical, 116, 129, 197
   psychoanalytic, 12
post-catastrophic stage, analysis in, 220
post-traumatic stress disorder(s), 61,
   119, 154
pre-catastrophic stage, analysis in, 220
preconception(s), 47, 72, 83, 86, 89, 95,
   114, 132, 225, 226, 298, 322, 323
   vs. pre-conceptions, 63, 87, 107, 108
pre-conception(s), 320
   of breast, 320
   concept of, 209–210
   and contact-barrier, 50–51, 216
   and the Establishment, 284
   and the Grid, 71–72, 87, 88, 221, 226,
      239, 245, 254

pre-conception(s) (*continued*):
  inherent, 37, 41, 53, 62, 115, 117, 126,
      135, 136, 142, 166, 303, 316, 317
    and acquired, 106, 322
    and O, 37, 50, 51, 60, 74, 87, 106, 108,
        122, 217, 240
  as "memoirs of the future", 120, 135,
      240, 258, 280
  vs. preconception, 63, 87, 107, 108
  and psychoanalytic theory, 58
  release of, 210, 265
  and selected fact, 58, 85
  and thought, 208
  transformation of, 53, 217, 219, 227
  and unbearable emotions, 107
  "unborns", 62, 71
preconscious, transformational forge
    in, 24
pre-lexical communications, 45
  [Kant], 135
primary category, 157, 304
primary identification, 134, 163, 313
primary infantile destructiveness, 21
primary process(es), 51, 79, 80, 145, 248,
        250, 268, 270, 281, 284, 293, 295,
        321, 324
  and secondary processes, 59, 69, 271,
        282–283, 291
    vs. α-function and dreaming, 79–81
    Freud's, Bion's erasure of
        distinction between, 6, 145–146,
        175, 245–246, 249–250, 270, 293,
        295, 297
primary and secondary categories
primitive catastrophe, 153, 207
primitive functions, violence of, 87, 88
Principle of Asymmetry, 80
Principle of Symmetry, 80
probabilism, 262
projection, 153, 158, 169, 170, 177–181,
        236, 323
  -in-reverse, 153–154
  and projective identification, 173–174
  role of identification in, 173–174
  US versions of, 176–178
projective counteridentification, 181
projective identification(s):
  communicative, 20, 22, 41, 49, 57, 67,
        92, 93, 103, 157, 203

  concept of, 30, 37, 86–89, 95, 170–173,
      208, 226
  and containment, 155–166, 298–299
  defensive, 172, 173, 178
  and displacement, 260
  and dreaming, 85
  and group studies, 192
  interpersonal, 49–50, 193
  interpretations based on, 220
  intersubjective, 55, 95, 165, 174
    theory of, 95, 165
  and mystics, 129
  non-defensive, 172
  omnipotent intrapsychic phantasy
      of, 169
  and patient's communications, 152,
      153–157, 203, 236
  and projection, 173–174
  and projective transidentification, 92,
      97, 168–190
  and psychosis, 102, 203, 206–209, 300,
      323
  and transcendence, 131
  and transference/
      countertransference, 70, 71, 101,
      185–186, 223
  and unconscious phantasies, 301
  US versions of, 176–178
  withdrawal of, 38
projective transformation(s), 70, 71, 222,
      223
projective transidentification, 46, 57, 92,
      97, 168–189, 216
Prometheus:
  Bion as, 1, 12, 20–23, 137, 142, 277,
      329, 330
  myth of, 21, 143
prosodic lexical communications, 45
proto-emotions, 45, 156, 157, 166, 192,
      204, 205, 208, 261, 263
proto-language, dreaming as, 266
proto-mental phenomena, 192, 229, 258
P–S ↔ D, 59, 110, 308–310, 316
  and analysand, 91, 100
  and attachment, 155
  and contact-barrier, 51
  and dreaming, 267
  as element of psychoanalysis, 237
  and Klein's analysis of Bion, 119

reversibility of progression and
regression between, 24
see also paranoid–schizoid position
psychic retreat(s), 61, 150, 154, 164, 295,
297
psychoanalysis:
as "dream mender", 301–303
non-linear uncertainty of, 3
psychoanalytic element(s), 237–238
see also α-element(s); β-element(s)
psychoanalytic functions, 235–237
see also α-function
psychoanalytic metapsychology, 23, 47
psychoanalytic mystic, 2
psychoanalytic positivism, 12
psychosis, 19, 20, 40, 60, 103, 107, 130,
242, 322
Bion's studies in, 197–212
infantile, 38, 40
nothingness of, 323
psychotic(s), 18–22, 71, 91, 151, 226–230,
236, 239, 241, 242, 253, 267–269,
295–297, 312, 319–324
and β-elements, untransformed,
60–61
Bion's studies in, 197–213
and dreaming, 267–269, 303
defective, 268
fear of, 85, 86
lack of (negative) containment,
102–103, 154, 163, 175, 297–298
and evasion of truth, 300
and hallucinosis, 229
infantile, 130
catastrophe, 294
lack of thinking/feeling, 103
meaninglessness, feeling of, 323, 324
vs. neurotic patient, 203–205
and pleasure principle, 255
projective transformations, 223
treating, Bion's experience of, 153,
163, 205
work with/study of,15, 51, 85, 91, 151,
153, 192–193
"public-ation", 23, 223

R (reason), 105, 237
Racker, H., 179
Rather, L., xii, 254, 255, 272

"rational conjecture", 23
raw Circumstance (O), 278, 297, 300
reality:
avoidance of, 295
principle, 6, 40, 205, 268, 270–272, 278,
282–284
dominance of, 111, 271
and dreaming, 262, 263, 267, 268,
271, 282–284
and the Grid, 238, 243, 246, 249, 250,
252, 255
and pleasure principle, 80, 145, 263,
268, 271, 294–295, 300
and secondary process, 270
Real, 123, 313
realization:
negative, 103, 209, 210
positive, 209
Register of the Real, 121, 123
regression, 24, 158, 199
relativism, 16, 114, 123, 231
relativity, theory of, 161
religion, Bion's attitude on, 74, 107, 128,
129, 137, 231
religious instinct, human, 31, 106, 129,
137, 211
religious metaphors (models), 56
renal dialysis as model, 45, 157, 298, 157
repetition compulsion, 193, 305
representability, altered, as function of
dream-work, 260
representations, shared, 170, 185
repressed, return of, 158, 300
repression, 78, 80, 157, 158, 176, 203, 209,
249, 261, 263, 269, 271, 298, 300,
301, 312
resistance, 63, 191, 248, 249, 255, 313
analytic, 200
reverie, 2, 6, 22–24, 29, 50, 82, 84, 91, 156,
185, 188, 200, 331
ability to achieve, 3
analytic, 44, 47–48, 54–55, 69, 83, 87,
95, 101, 113, 175, 211, 237, 286,
307, 317
and selected fact, 48, 291, 298, 320
concept of, as analytic tool, 2, 6, 22–24,
29, 41, 82, 84, 91, 185
vs. countertransference, 41, 188, 212
definition, 185

reverie (*continued*):
    maternal, 4, 20, 41, 44, 45, 47, 50, 68,
        93, 155, 156, 175, 279, 296, 321,
        324, 328
        and becoming, 55
        and containment, 163, 186, 192, 209,
            272, 298
        failure of, 209
        transformational state of, 15
"reversible perspective(s)", 6, 23, 24, 62,
    76, 78, 118, 200, 218, 256, 328
    as model of dreaming, 264
Ricoeur, P., 121, 134
rigid motion transformation(s), 71, 104,
    222, 231
        versus projective transformations,
            223–226
Rosenfeld, H., 20, 172, 173, 297

sadism, 179, 202, 203
Salomonsson, B., 46
Sandler, J., 94, 179, 187
Sandler, P., xi, xii, 5, 13, 65, 80, 82, 226,
        227, 254, 257, 273, 288
Sartre, J.-P., 123, 129, 143
Schermer, M., 54
Schermer, V., 193
schizophrenia, 171, 303
    and dreaming, 200–203
Schneider, J., 288
Schore, A., 45, 92, 166, 178, 278
Schreber, D. P., 111, 129
Schwalbe, M. L., 159, 215
science:
    non-linear, intuitionistic, emotional,
        104
    psychoanalysis as, 104
        emotional, 104
        mystical, 104
        ontological, 3
scientific deductive system, 83, 237
secondary process(es), 280–284
    and abandoning memory and desire,
        280
    and asymmetrical thinking, 80
    and binocular thinking, 79
    and the Grid, 51, 69, 236, 243–250, 284
    and primary processes, 59, 69,
        270–271, 281–283, 291

and α-function, 51, 59, 79–81, 145,
    175, 268, 271, 291, 297, 321, 324
    vs. α-function and dreaming,
        79–81
    as binary-oppositional structure,
        146, 271, 282
    Freud's, Bion's erasure of distiction
        between, 6, 145–146, 175, 245–
        246, 249–250, 270, 293, 295, 297
    and psychotic thinking, 295
    unsatisfactory theory of, 283, 293
    and reality principle, 270
    thinking, 51, 246
secondary revision, 214, 275, 287
    as function of dream-work, 260
seething cauldron, unconscious as, 37,
    74, 116, 120, 135, 300, 324
Segal, H., 20, 108, 139, 159
selected fact:
    and act of faith, 318
    and analyst's reverie, 48, 291, 298,
        320
    and binding of O, 247–248
    and coherence of objects, 58
    concept of, 167, 211, 251
    emergence of, 85
    importance of, 24
    locale of, 317–318
    model, bimodal nature of, 5, 59
    and negative capability, 92
    and O, 156
    pre-conception of, 58, 97, 317, 318
    and psychoanalytic models, 56
    and quest for truth, 139
    and "strange attractor", 58, 85
    and wild thoughts, 76–77, 100
self-abnegation, 127
self-organization, 116, 145, 159, 196, 215,
    331
    and transformations, 214
Seligman, S., 178
Sells, M. A., 113
semiology, 323
    preverbal, 184
Senet de Gazzano, M. R., 238
sense:
    domain of, 237, 247
    use of, as psychoanalytic tool, 82,
        84–91, 100, 106, 113, 237, 248

sensory dream images, 40
Seven Pillars of Wisdom, 140
Shakespeare, W., 109, 303
    King Lear, 36
shifting perspectives, 23, 329, 332
"shifting vertices", 6
Simon, B., 326
Slim, Field Marshal, 23
Socrates, 10, 11, 12, 30, 34, 306, 307, 330
Sodré, I., 174
Sophocles, 142
Sor, D., xi, 5, 12, 13, 226, 238
spacelessness, 112
    psychotic, 242
speculative imagination, 75, 83
speculative reasoning, 83
Spillius, E. B., 173, 176, 182, 300, 301
Spinoza, B., 14, 115, 138, 215, 330
spiritualism, 129
splitting, 30, 65, 66, 86–89, 95, 131, 171,
        172, 201–204, 210, 226, 300, 301,
        309, 310
"spontaneous conjecture", 23
Stanislavski, C., 298, 304, 307
Steiner, J., 61, 150, 154, 295, 297
Stern, D., 182, 186
Stitzman, L., 107, 238
"strange attractor" in chaos theory, 58,
        85, 130, 211, 298
subjective object, 228
subjugating third subject, 186, 187
"super"ego, 164, 229, 241, 288
    moralistic, 153, 164, 229, 288
    as a persecutory negative container
        projection-in-reverse, 153–154
    primitive, 154
superego, 121, 153, 167, 171, 179, 180,
        288
    enviously critical, 31
    moralistic, 103, 287
    murderous, hyper-moralistic, 103
    severe, malignant, 21
supervision, xii, 28, 294
    Bion's attitude to, 12, 28
Sutherland, J. D., 20, 41, 194
symbol, 58, 122, 260
symbolic equation(s), 108, 139, 146
Symington, J. D., xi, 5, 13, 14, 22, 24, 120,
        226, 332

Symington, N., xi, 5, 13, 14, 22, 24, 120,
        226, 332
symmetrical logic, 118
symmetrical thinking, 80
symmetry, 74, 81, 112, 262, 275, 277, 278,
        318, 325
    and asymmetry, 79, 80, 271
    infinite, 118
    principle of, 270, 271
sympathetic magic, 178, 184, 187
Systems Ucs., Cs., 49, 161, 216, 217, 260,
        264, 267, 270, 291, 293, 297, 300
    and O, 78–79
    relationship between, Freud's and
        Bion's conceptions of, 47
    Freud's conception of, 47

Ta α, 86, 222–223, 225
Ta β, 86, 222, 225
Tadmor, C., 126, 330, 331
Tagore, R., 26
tangents: see Euclidean geometry
Tausk, V., 61, 303
technique, as philosophical prescription
        and proscription, 84–91
things-in-themselves, 38, 60, 65, 67, 74,
        87, 106, 122, 135, 142, 210, 254,
        258, 265, 277, 293, 303, 331
thinking/thought(s), 125
    analogic, 46
    Aristotelian, 255, 268
    asymmetrical, 80
    autochthonous origins of, 24
    as "becoming", 50
    binocular, 79, 165
    capacity to, attacks on, 45, 54, 69, 115,
        164, 227, 262
    Cartesian (cognitive), 51, 54, 55, 292,
        305
    conception of, Bion's, 47–48
    development, epigenetic course of,
        208
    emotions as template for, 327
    essentially unconscious nature of, 25,
        47–48
    higher-order, 245
    left-hemispheric, 23, 86, 92, 101, 225,
        237
    vs. mentalization, 40

thinking/thought(s) (*continued*):
  meta-, 245
  model for, the Grid as, 246
  origins of, 69–73
  reflective, 246, 271
  secondary-process, 51, 246
  symmetrical, 80
  vs. thoughts/thinking, 54, 207
  wakeful dream, 45, 83
"thoughts without a thinker":
  and α-/β-elements, 62
  and the Grid, 247
  and inherent preconceptions, 117, 143
  and mental indigestion, 216
  and mind, 24, 54, 69, 125
  and O, 66, 101, 125, 136, 278
  projection of, 156, 175
  and theory of transformations, 234
  "thinker of", 18, 76–77, 107, 125, 136,
    234, 299, 332
  and thinking, 54, 292
  "unborns", 73–75
  "wild thoughts", 50, 68, 75–76, 101,
    247
timelessness, 112
topographic and structural models of
  the psyche, 121
"Tower of Babel" myth, 20, 21, 141, 143,
  277
Tp α, 222, 225
Tp β, 70, 222
transcendence (evolution of self), 53,
  122, 127, 128, 131, 328
  dream demonstrating (clinical
    vignette), 123–126
  Kant's theory of, 132–133
transcendental analytic, 87, 132, 331,
  332
transcendentalism, Kant's theory of,
  132–133
transcendent position, 3, 97, 107, 138
  concept of, 121–134
transcendent vs. transcendental, 132
transference:
  to analyst, 10, 21 24
  and countertransference, 49, 94, 101,
    185, 257
  and forms of O, 332

  and interpreting, 200
  manifestations of, 70–71
  negative, 32, 201
  neurosis, 6, 81, 222, 275
  and projective identification, 71, 178,
    185–186, 189, 223
  and schizophrenic personality, 202
  sexualization of, 191
  theory of, 70
  true but lost meaning of, 10
  and unconscious phantasy, 144
transformation(s) (*passim*):
  autistic, 229–230
  of β-elements into α-elements, 40, 67
  concept/theory of, 68, 77–78, 94, 211,
    213–234, 233
  in hallucinosis, 222, 226–229, 231, 258
  models for, 23, 215–216
  in O, 19, 21, 53, 54, 94, 156, 183, 188,
    193, 231, 313
  perspectives of, 218–219
  projective, 70, 222, 223
    vs. rigid motion transformations,
      223–226
  rigid motion, 71, 104, 222, 223, 231
    vs. projective transformations,
      223–226
  theory of, 94, 114, 132, 197, 221, 223,
    230, 234
  types of, 222–226
transformational forge in preconscious,
  24
transformational generative syntax, 45,
  157, 166
transidentification, projective, 168–189
transience, 5, 306
trauma:
  nameless dread of, 40
  post-traumatic stress disorder(s), 61,
    119, 154
"tree of imaginative inference", 90
Trevarthen, C., 45, 266
triangulation of O, 41, 79, 165
"true-self/false-self" dichotomy, 159
true thought, 148, 149
Truth, Emotional (O)/truth (*passim*):
  concept of, 156
  curiosity about, 139–146

drive or instinct, 52, 60, 79, 87, 96, 135–138, 140, 146, 163, 272
emotional, 2, 79, 87, 96, 101, 141, 156, 190, 219, 276, 281, 329
instinct, 139, 290, 293, 295, 296
    and unconscious phantasies, 290–304
instinctual drive, 295–297
principle, 141, 267, 272
quest for, 135–138
vehicular carriers of emotions as, 45
Tucker, K., 121
Tucker, W., 121
Tustin, F., 33, 167, 230, 316
twin, imaginary, 198–200

"*Übermensch*" [higher man/self], 2, 3, 38, 53
Ultimately Impersonal Reality, 2
Ultimate Reality:
    and Absolute Truth, separate status of, 138
    Absolute Truth about:
        and curiosity, 20
        and dreaming, 94, 261, 265, 266
        and emotions, 62, 166
        O, 2, 41, 44, 97, 115, 148, 135, 136, 156, 265, 270
        and psychoanalytic theory and practice, 80
        of raw Circumstance, 295–297, 300
        and transformation, 21, 55, 78, 136, 139, 143–145
        transformation to tolerable truth (K), 40, 143–146, 156
        and the unconscious, 293–297
    location of, 43, 59–60
    and O, 24, 68, 106, 107, 117, 121, 127, 128, 139, 214, 211, 222
"unborns", 73–75
uncertainty:
    and analyst, 110
    anxiety arising from, 276
    acceptance of, 16
    Heisenberg's theory of, 161
    inner cosmic, Bion's, 21, 40
    manic defence against, 114
    and the mystic, 2

non-linear, of psychoanalysis, 3
and O, 32, 41, 44, 58, 76, 96, 135, 197, 211, 230–231, 262
principle, 134, 272, 282
and psychoanalysis, 16–17, 24
and reverie, 298
theory of, 161
tolerance of, 3, 48, 291, 296
and truth principle, 141
unconscious, the:
    analyst's, Faith in creative response of, 2
    ineffable subject of, 54, 126, 127, 187, 266
    as seething cauldron of negativity and destructiveness, 37, 74, 116, 120, 135, 300, 324
    unrepressed, 43, 67, 87, 106, 136, 214, 217, 240, 254
    inherited, 74
unconscious phantasy(ies), 290–304
    concepts of, 300–304
    container and the contained, 157, 161, 297–299
    and dreaming, 276, 277, 280, 282
    effect of interpretation on, 290
    and Faith, 318
    and imaginary twin, 198
    and internal object, 306, 317
    interpretation of, 267
    intersubjective reality, 93
    intrapsychic, 170
    and myth, 83, 84, 91–92, 237, 288
    omnipotent, 92, 178, 185
    patient's, 69
    and projective transidentification, 169–175, 180, 184–188
    and real event, 144–145
    and repetition, 222
    and symbolic equations, 139
    and transference, 10, 144, 178
    and truth instinct, 290–304
unrepressed unconscious, 43, 67, 74, 87, 106, 136, 214, 217, 240, 254

Varchevker, A., 42, 94
Varela, S. J., 215
Vasta, R., 254

Vermote, R., xii
Vernant, J.-P., 143
"void", 63
von Kekulé, A., 125
voyeurism, 179

Wade, N., 274
wakeful dreaming, 83, 91, 92
wakeful thinking, 152, 264, 268
"waking dream thought", 91
Webb, R. E., 113
Weisberg, J., 288
"wild thoughts", 23, 50, 68, 74, 76, 77,
        101, 195, 247, 250, 292, 329, 332
Williams, C., xii, 143

Williams, M. Harris, 119
Winnicott, D. W., xii, 20, 105, 159, 162,
        228, 267, 298, 321
Wisdom, Seven Pillars of, 140
wish-fulfilment, 51, 145, 293
Wordsworth, W., 74
work group, 191, 194, 195, 196, 258

zero ("no-thing"):
    capacity to tolerate, 321
    concept of, Bion's discovery of,
        319–326
    state, analyst's capacity to tolerate,
        320
Zoroastrianism, 129